An Introduction to the Social History of Medicine: Europe since 1500

An Introduction to the Social History of Medicine: Europe since 1500

KEIR WADDINGTON

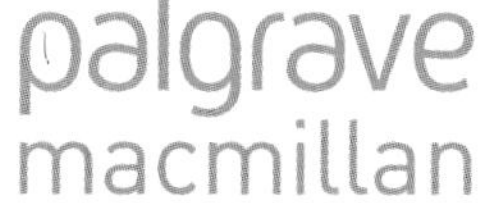

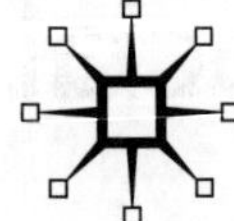

First published 2011 by
PALGRAVE MACMILLAN

Palgrave Macmillan in the UK is an imprint of Macmillan Publishers Limited, registered in England, company number 785998, of Houndmills, Basingstoke, Hampshire RG21 6XS.

Palgrave Macmillan in the US is a division of St Martin's Press LLC, 175 Fifth Avenue, New York, NY 10010.

Palgrave Macmillan is the global academic imprint of the above companies and has companies and representatives throughout the world.

Palgrave® and Macmillan® are registered trademarks in the United States, the United Kingdom, Europe and other countries

ISBN-13: 978–1–403–94692–8 hardback
ISBN-13: 978–1–403–94693–5 paperback

This book is printed on paper suitable for recycling and made from fully managed and sustained forest sources. Logging, pulping and manufacturing processes are expected to conform to the environmental regulations of the country of origin.

A catalogue record for this book is available from the British Library.

A catalog record for this book is available from the Library of Congress.

10 9 8 7 6 5 4 3 2 1
20 19 18 17 16 15 14 13 12 11

Printed in China

Contents

List of illustrations

List of tables

Acknowledgements

It would be hard to thank or identify all those who have contributed in some way or other to writing this book. A debt is owed to all those students I have taught (and learned from) over the years; to all those givers of conference papers I have heard, to colleagues in the Society for the Social History of Medicine, to the staff in libraries and archives who have helped me, and to the numerous colleagues who have been patient enough to discuss the social history of medicine with me. A special debt of gratitude is owed to particular individuals who have provided invaluable support or comments. Roberta Bivins, Bill Bynum, Bill Jones, Colin Jones, Chris Hamlin, Frank Huisman, Pat Hudson, Steve King, Chris Lawrence, Tracey Loughran, Ruth McElroy, Anthony Mandal, Hilary Marland, Kevin Passmore, John Pickstone, Shaun Tougher, Steve Tomlinson, Stephanie Ward, Abigail Woods and Mike Worboys have all offered either encouragement or advice throughout the writing of this book, while Rose Thompson and Anne Hardy have proved unstinting in their support. In the latter stages of writing, Lloyd Bowen, Richard Sugg and Garthine Walker have diligently made useful comments on the early modern sections, while the careful reading of various chapters by Faye Hammill, Kate Gilliver, Martin Willis, Vike Plock and Jonathan Reinarz, and their many useful comments, have been invaluable. A further debt is owed to Martin Daunton, Anne Hardy and the late Roy Porter for setting me on the path that resulted in this book. I would also like to thank Marie-Louise Collard at the Wellcome Library and Jenni Burnell, Felicity Noble and their colleagues at Palgrave for their patience and support.

Keir Waddington

The authors and publishers wish to thank the following for permission to reproduce copyright material:

The Wellcome Library, London, for all images included in this book.

OECD for data showing state expenditure on health from OECD Health Data 2010: Statistics and Indicators, www.oecd.org/health/healthdata

Every effort has been made to trace the copyright holders, but if any have been inadvertently overlooked the publishers would be pleased to make the necessary arrangements at the first opportunity.

Abbreviations

AIDS	Acquired Immune Deficiency Syndrome
BSE	Bovine spongiform encephalopathy
CAT	Computerized axial tomography
ECG	Electrocardiogram
ECT	Electroconvulsive therapy
EMS	Emergency Medical Service
GDP	Gross Domestic Product
HIV	Human Immunodeficiency Virus
IVF	In-vitro fertilization
MOH	Medical Officer of Health
MRC	Medical Research Council
MRI	Magnetic resonance imagining
MRSA	Methicillin-resistant staphylococcus aureus
NHS	National Health Service
RCT	Randomized controlled trial
RSI	Repetitive strain injury
SARS	Severe Acute Respiratory Syndrome
UNESCO	United Nations Education, Scientific and Cultural Organization
UNICEF	United Nations International Children's Emergency Fund
WHO	World Health Organization

Preface

This volume arises out of my research and teaching on the social history of medicine. Although it examines topics familiar to medical historians and common to undergraduate courses, it brings together specialized knowledge with new ways of thinking about the social history of medicine between circa 1500 and the late twentieth century. It explores medicine during a period in which Classical ideas about the body were refined and rejected, in which new models of the body and medicine emerged, new professional structures and hierarchies were established, and new institutions were formed, and in which a biomedical paradigm was established. It was a period that saw both radical and comprehensive transformations in medicine and the delivery of healthcare, and continuities in how disease was understood and treated. In looking at the social history of medicine over five centuries, the volume explores these continuities and discontinuities in medical thought and practice. This approach encourages readers to think about how medicine has been used to fashion and refashion views of the body and disease; how it informed access to healthcare and welfare policies; and how this was related to different political, cultural, intellectual and socioeconomic contexts. The volume focuses not on individuals, institutions or discoveries, but on a comparative examination of key themes in the social history of medicine in Europe.

It is wise to warn the reader that there are obvious problems writing comparative history. There is the danger of superficiality and over-generalization, of ignoring diversity in favour of internationalism or of reading case studies as representative. There are no easy answers to these problems. Unsurprisingly, scholars have seen national or regional studies as richer and more nuanced, or have used cross-national comparative work to examine particular problems or topics; for example, the growth of welfare states. However, there are numerous advantages to using the national state (or colony) as the focus for comparison, especially as the notion of *histoire croisée* suggests that there is no such thing as an isolated entity and that cross-fertilization and entanglements form the fabric of history. The excellent two volume *Western Medical Tradition* (see Further Reading) has already pointed to the convergence of several long-term developments in medicine that produced a particular approach – a Western medical tradition – which was not bound by the nation-state but came to be associated with particular medical organizations, professional structures and scientific values. Approaching medicine in these terms offers the historian a tool to understand the complex processes that shaped medicine, an approach this volume also adopts. Many medical historians have also (selectively) stressed the international dimension of medicine. Epidemics seldom respected borders and improved communications, in terms of transport and publishing, allowed medical practitioners to share medical knowledge across borders. Historians have also warned against creating national histories that ignore wider European influences or trends. As the historian of science Llana Löwy explained in 2007, medical practice may have relied on local medical cultures and been influenced by socioeconomic, cultural and political factors, but modern medicine is transnational in nature.[1] Although during the nineteenth and twentieth centuries there was a growing internationalism in medicine with, for example, responses to epidemics often taking on a global dimension, in the sixteenth, seventeenth and eighteenth centuries medicine and medical ideas equally crossed borders, both within Europe and the wider world. Nor does recognition that every nation is a unique creation of its history inevitably mean that each nation departs from general trends or influences. A comparative approach reveals similarities and differences that can tell historians much about how medicine developed. This is not to ignore national differences. They have been crucial to understanding early modern and modern history. Structural and cultural factors were important, but an analysis on a longer European perspective does provide the opportunity to examine points of contact and discontinuity, not only over time but also between countries.

This volume does not cover every aspect of health and medicine from 1500 to the present or every country. Such a volume would be impossible, or at least impossibly large. Inevitably, therefore there are gaps and omissions. Nor does this volume seek to provide a narrative account. Readers looking for such an approach should turn to the various (and excellent) surveys indicated in the Further Reading at the end of the preface. Instead, the chapters in this volume explore the social history of medicine in Europe since 1500 through an examination of the major themes that have shaped historical inquiry. Rather than describing or chronicling developments, each chapter introduces readers to the key questions that have informed how historians have approached the themes under examination. All locate medicine, medical institutions, practitioners and patients in their socioeconomic, cultural and political contexts, and explore the nature of this change and why it occurred. The aim is to reveal how the adoption of medical practices or ideas was invariably complex; how important linkages existed between ideas, practices, institutions, practitioners, society, culture and politics, and how the social history of medicine does not fit neatly into a history of progress. Although each chapter stands on its own, cross-referencing between chapters allows readers to explore further issues or concepts in detail, while the further reading at the end of each chapter encourages readers to go further in their studies.

Further reading: introductions to the history of medicine

Roy Porter's monumental *The Greatest Benefit to Mankind: A Medical History of Humanity from Antiquity to the Present* (London: HarperCollins, 1997) is perhaps the best starting point for an overview that combines both a chronological account and chapters on individual medical disciplines, while Jacalyn Duffin, *History of Medicine: A Scandalously Short Introduction* (Toronto: University of Toronto Press, 1999) gives a concise and readable overview. On the Western medical tradition and for a thought-provoking survey of medicine, readers should look at Lawrence Conrad et al, *The Western Medical Tradition 800BC to AD1800* (Cambridge: Cambridge University Press, 1995) and W.F. Bynum et al, *The Western Medical Tradition, 1800 to 2000* (Cambridge: Cambridge University Press, 2006). These works can be supplemented by Irvine Loudon (ed.), *Western Medicine: An Illustrated History* (Oxford: Oxford University Press, 1997) and Roy Porter (ed.), *The Cambridge Illustrated History of Medicine* (Cambridge: Cambridge University Press, 1996), or with the two volume *Companion Encyclopaedia of the History of Medicine* (London: Routledge, 1993) edited by Roy Porter and W.F. Bynum which contains chapters on key topics by leading historians. For the Renaissance, Nancy Siraisi, *Medieval and Early Renaissance Medicine* (Chicago, IL: University of Chicago Press, 1990) provides an accessible introduction, while early modern Europe readers should start with Mary Lindemann's excellent *Medicine and Society in Early Modern Europe,* 2010 edn (Cambridge: Cambridge University Press, 2010). More surveys exist of the nineteenth century, with W.F. Bynum's *Science and Practice of Medicine in the Nineteenth Century* (Cambridge: Cambridge University Press, 1994) providing an excellent comparative study of European medicine, while for the twentieth century, Roger Cooter and John Pickstone (eds), *Medicine in the Twentieth Century* (London: Routledge, 2000) provides a thematic introduction. Readers should also consult Christopher Lawrence, *Medicine in the Making of Modern Britain 1700–1920* (London: Routledge, 1994), Anne Hardy, *Health and Medicine in Britain since 1860* (Basingstoke: Palgrave Macmillian, 2001) and Virginia Berridge, *Health and Society in Britain since 1939* (Cambridge: Cambridge University Press, 1999), which cover the nineteenth and twentieth centuries. For those readers interested in approaches to the history of medicine, Frank Huisman and John H. Warner (eds), *Locating Medical History. The Stories and their Meanings* (Baltimore, MD: Johns Hopkins University Press, 2004) is the best starting point, while John Pickstone, *Ways of Knowing* (Manchester: Manchester University Press, 2000) examines the different ways of thinking about the history of science, technology and medicine.

Further reading: introductions to the history of medicine

[illegible]

1

Understanding the social history of medicine: Historiography

The idea that the last five hundred years has seen radical and far-reaching changes in medicine has been widely accepted, but the ways in which historians have understood this process has itself been the subject of considerable change. Before the 1970s, the history of medicine was generally considered to have limited relevance to the wider study of history. However, the growing criticism of Western medicine in the 1960s and 1970s encouraged increasing scrutiny of the idea of medical progress. In response, English-speaking historians pioneered alternative accounts as they explored the social history of medicine. By the early 1990s, social historians of medicine were beginning to feel that their discipline had come of age. Just over a decade later, some historians in the community expressed fear that the discipline had started to grow tired. These claims have proved unfounded. The social history of medicine has continued to take on new approaches and to examine new topics. It has been enriched by historiographical trends in other areas of historical research and by developments in other disciplines. To argue that the social historians of medicine have ignored theory or trends in historical writing is to miss the point of a large body of historical work on medicine, especially as all historical observations are, in some ways, influenced by the approaches that historians adopt, be that empiricism or postmodernism, the questions they ask, and the sources they use. Overlapping discourses and methods from anthropology, literary criticism, psychology, the sociology of science, feminism and postcolonialism, to name but a few, have been incorporated. Even the most empirically minded medical historians have been influenced by these trends. The result has been an enriching of the discipline as new critical readings have emerged.

This chapter examines the broad historiography to explore the major trends in writing and some of the ideas that have influenced the social history of medicine. Later chapters develop these ideas in relation to particular topics. The intention is not to provide a manifesto for the social history of medicine, or to claim the superiority of particular approaches, but to show the ways in which different perspectives have been adopted.

Narratives of medicine

The history of medicine was initially the preserve of medical practitioners, few of whom had any formal historical training. Many focused on how far medicine had come or lauded the contribution of their fellow countrymen. French surgeons in the nineteenth century, for example, celebrated the triumphs of Paris medicine after 1789 and its role in developing a style of medicine associated with the hospital and pathological anatomy [see 'Anatomy']. Later writers were encouraged by the optimism of the 1940s and 1950s in the power of medicine over disease to explore the origins and growth of their profession. In doing so, they examined what they perceived as the triumph of Western medicine over disease. As in other fields, medicine became a story of achievements, often associated with great men, such as René Laennec, Rudolf Virchow or Joseph Lister, and the adoption of technological developments, such as antiseptics or x-rays. For example, early work on the history of psychiatry moved from the alleged brutal treatment regimes of the early modern period through to the rise of the asylum in the nineteenth century and the alleged start of humane and effective treatments [see 'Asylums']. These histories drew heavily on the heroic accounts of nineteenth century reformers to construct a positivist account that stressed progress: periods and treatments were demonized and revolutions were identified with new treatments and institutions. Similar accounts were presented in early histories of hospitals or surgery. This approach asserted the central position of orthodox and male practitioners to focus on the history of medical disciplines to produce an intellectual history that looked back into the past to find the start of modern medical theories or practices. The result was a view that suggested that the French Revolution (1789–99) represented a critical turning point in the history of medicine at the expense of examining earlier time periods. Other medical practitioners, inter- and intra-professional rivalries, and low status specialisms, such as general practice, were marginalized as stress was placed on the growth of hospital and scientific medicine. The emphasis was firmly on describing the changes that had occurred not on explaining why.

As Frank Huisman and John Harley Warner explain in *Locating Medical History* (2004), these traditional histories have often been represented as 'straw figures' to be knocked down as part of a rhetorical strategy to define the new direction the history of medicine took in the 1970s. Early histories of medicine were not unusual in their positivist approach. Other fields of historical inquiry equally adopted a progressive narrative that assumed the present was superior to the past – often referred to as Whig history and associated with modernization theory. However, if early histories of medicine were positivist, in many ways they helped define the discipline.

The social history of medicine

The 1960s and 1970s saw the start of a reversal of these trends. As historians critiqued simplistic ideas of modernization, different views of the history of medicine emerged as professional historians colonized the field. The reasons for this shift were intellectual and institutional, and reflected changing social pressures and growing scepticism of Western medicine. The emergence of a radical sociological critique of medicine, associated with the work of Michel Foucault, Thomas Szasz and Ivan Illich, argued that medicine was a form of repression; a way of defining deviance that exercised a socio-political strategy of power and authority over patients and society. These ideas promoted a re-evaluation of notions of medical progress, the role of medicine in society, and the power of the medical profession. Social pressures, including second-wave feminism, Vietnam War protests, and growing environmental concern further encouraged social historians to turn away from a history of great men, war and high politics. The boom in social history in the 1960s and the growing interest in 'history from below' in the 1970s promoted new ways of analysing the past and an interest in class and marginalized groups. The emergence of a range of historical sub-disciplines, including feminist and gender history, and cross-fertilization from the social sciences, further encouraged historians to reassess the history of medicine. The result was an approach that challenged traditional Whiggish and top-down studies.

What distinguished this new research from earlier studies was a greater consideration of the social and political conditions of medicine. In a series of statements in the 1960s, a generation of British and American medical historians called for an examination of 'the social character of medicine' and for the field to become 'the history of human societies and their efforts to deal with problems of health and disease'.[1] Interest initially focused on eighteenth and nineteenth century Britain and North America to provide the core of scholarship for a new social history of medicine, which gradually came to dominate approaches to medical history. One result was that historians and social scientists came to define the discipline; a move that resulted in disputes between clinicians and historians about the nature and purpose of medical history.

Whereas early medical histories were mainly defined by medical practitioners with a deep interest in medicine, a new generation of historians interested in the social phenomenon of medicine examined the broader social, cultural, economic, political and professional influences on medicine. Rather than being theoretically impoverished as some later critics claimed, early supporters of this new social history of medicine consciously emphasized the importance of context as they sought to integrate medicine and science with wider social history. They stressed the ways in which medicine was a social phenomenon and how medicine affected society. In doing so, they rejected a progressive view of medicine as emanating from a disinterested science and challenged the idea that medical history was the result of great discoveries, technological advances or the achievements of great men free from intellectual, socioeconomic or political influences. A more dynamic view of the history of Western medicine was outlined that revealed that if healthcare has always been a perennial concern, the nature of this care, the doctor-patient relationship, medical institutions, and the role of the state, took many different forms over time and place. As the historian Charles Webster explained in his 1976 address to the British Society for the Social History of Medicine, this new social history of medicine involved 'relegating to a subordinate place any linear account of medical progress in favour of an approach which is primarily concerned with contributing to an understanding of the dynamics of any particular society'.[2]

Many social histories of medicine emerged as new questions were asked, new analytical techniques were applied, new sources were used, and as historians in other disciplines started to work on welfare policy. By exploring the social aspects of medicine, existing fields of interests were re-evaluated and new directions were developed, including the socioeconomic and environmental influences on health. This change in approach is demonstrated by the scholarship on mortality decline encouraged by Thomas McKeown's rejection of the role of medical discoveries and technical developments in reducing mortality [see 'Public health']. As questions were asked about the progressive role of science, historians turned to the ways in which science was used and the authority it conferred on medical practitioners [see 'Science and medicine']. The antipsychiatry movement and the impetus of Michel Foucault's provocative account of the 'great confinement' of the insane stimulated interest in the history of the asylum [see 'Asylums']. Approaches from historical demography, the sociology of science, cultural history, postcolonialism and feminist historiography came to influence research. As a result of the influence of cultural anthropology and Mary Douglas's important work on human culture and symbolism,[3] medical historians started to examine belief systems as demonstrated in scholarship on medicine and religion and in studies of magic and witchcraft [see 'Religion']. Sociological approaches to professionalization came to dominate histories of the medical professions [see 'Professionalization']. Feminist critiques encouraged an examination of the relationships between practitioners and patients and emphasized the sexual politics of sickness [see 'Women and medicine']. If the predominance of studies on English medicine tended to obscure what was happening elsewhere in Europe, growing sensitivity to local and regional histories drew attention to the interactions and the subtle shifts in power and discourses that affected medicine between 1500 and the present.

By the 1990s, the social history of medicine had become more than a blend of social history and medical history, and more than just locating medicine within its social context. Historiographical trends in cultural history may have produced opposition, but they also encouraged new work on disease and the body. Cultural approaches pointed to the ways in which meanings were mediated and contested, and what this meant for how sickness and disease was understood and represented in the past [see 'Disease']. Although some fields of inquiry were influenced by the contemporary questions being asked – for example, about the mixed economy of welfare in the 1990s as evident in work on hospitals and state medicine – social historians of medicine became increasingly sensitive to the dangers of simple presentism. Received views or myths, such as the dominance of Paris in restructuring medicine after 1789, were challenged. Drawing on pre-existing trends in social history, the social historians of medicine put forward longer chronologies and noted continuities that had been overlooked in earlier accounts that had stressed advances [see 'Anatomy']. Research into patterns of disease revealed the extent to which medicine not only reflected socioeconomic realities and political or cultural contexts but also that the history of medicine should not just be limited to histories of medical theories or practices. New collections confidently argued that studying the social history of medicine was now inseparable from general social and institutional transformations. The definition of what constitutes medicine has been extended and deepened beyond the original aim of the early pioneers of the social history of medicine to explore the ways in which medicine affected society and vice versa. Medicine could now represent everything from bedside practices or experiences of illness to laboratory tests and healthcare policy. As Joan Lane made clear in *A Social History of Medicine* (2001), the discipline had become part of a rich social context that could not be separated from political, socioeconomic or cultural changes.

Foucault, discourse and power

One important strand in the social history of medicine has been the idea of power and authority. Here the work of the French philosopher and historian Michel Foucault has exerted a potent and often controversial influence. Although many of the historical nuances of his work have come to be discredited, Foucault opened up the social history of medicine to a range of theoretical approaches and set much of the agenda for the cultural turn in the social history of medicine. His work encouraged medical historians to think about medical knowledge as a form of power and an eclectic adoption of various Foucauldian propositions and critical responses to his work helped define a substantial body of the literature in the field since 1970.

Foucault was one of a number of historians and philosophers who were interested in discourse and the nature of medical power. In the 1960s, the work of Laing, Szasz, Goffman and Illich all reflected growing criticism of the ways in which medical concepts were used to define social, biological and moral pathologies and norms. They argued that the process of defining boundaries between the normal and the pathological was a social construction that drew heavily on medical expertise and ideas. Their views reflected a powerful critique of medicine and growing fears about the influence of an authoritarian medical perspective, which was associated with biomedicine and a collaboration between doctors and the state.

Foucault was particularly concerned with the history of the body and in what ways body politics engaged with structures of power and knowledge to discipline the body within particular spaces, such as the hospital, asylum or prison. In *Historie de la Folie* (1961) – translated into English in 1965 as *Madness and Civilization* – and *The Birth of the Clinic* – published in French in 1963 and translated in 1973 – Foucault historicized the shifts in Western responses to madness and the appearance of the clinical gaze in the late eighteenth and early nineteenth centuries. In both accounts, he rejected ideas of liberal humanism. Foucault was interested in the distinction between the normal and the pathological and emphasized how psychiatry and medicine were part of a discourse of power and discipline that he associated with the process of institutionalization. For Foucault, language and discourses were crucial to understanding history; that radical ruptures in understanding – or epistemes – could occur over a relatively short time. In adopting this approach, Foucault offered insights into the intellectual construction first of insanity and then of hospital medicine or what he labelled 'the birth of the clinic'. Foucault denied that change was part of a history of progress. Instead, he concentrated on French experiences and what he believed was a radical rupture in ideas around the French Revolution. He rejected Whiggish accounts in favour of a view that emphasized the development of rationalism, the rise of absolutism and the growth of medical authority, or how power was corporealized. This approach can also be seen in his three volume *History of Sexuality* (1976; 1984). Here Foucault challenged conventional judgement of sexual liberation by showing the ways in which changing ideas about sexuality from the emergence of sexology in the nineteenth century to the psychoanalytical ideas of Sigmund Freud served to create new controlling systems.

Although all of Foucault's work examined the expanding and tightening boundaries of power, in several essays in the 1970s he explicitly addressed the wider notion of medicalization – the process by which conditions and problems were defined and treated as medical conditions and came under the authority of health professions – and developed the concepts of biopolitics and biopower. For Foucault, starting in the eighteenth century the maintenance of health turned medicine into a force for social control as human existence, behaviour and the body were brought into an increasingly dense network of medical authority. Foucault's concept of governmentality linked the state and medicine together in creating a set of practices or discourses that operated on bodies. Medical practitioners became experts in the service of these discourses.

Foucault's work represented a challenge to all historians, questioning hidden assumptions about the character of modern medicine and the state. For some, it offered a powerful new approach. *The Birth of the Clinic* explicitly demonstrated the ways in which scientific, social and political factors were entangled. It stimulated interest in the history of hospitals and the clinical gaze as reflected in Mary Fissell's *Patients, Power and the Poor in Eighteenth-Century Bristol* (1991) [see 'Hospitals']. *Madness and Civilization* inspired a revisionist history of psychiatry as evident in Andrew Scull's *Museums of Madness* (1979) or Roy Porter's *Mind*

Forg'd Manacles (1987) as historians tried to historicize Foucault and tackle the nature of the great confinement he proposed [see 'Asylums']. More generally, Foucault encouraged interest in biopolitics. This was linked to the coercive aspects of twentieth century states and ideas of social control, most visible in work on eugenics and racial hygiene [see 'Healthcare and the state'].

Foucault's ideas equally generated hostility, and not just from empirically minded historians. Foucault seemed to embody a poststructuralist approach that over-privileged language and texts. If Foucault never pretended to be an historian, he was attacked for his use of historical narrative and for his work's fundamental empirical flaws. He was criticized for misunderstanding the relationship between the ambition to improve and the desire to control; for confusing intellectual ideas, institutional reform and social reform; for concentrating on a few leading men, and for making generalizations based on his reading of French experiences. Foucault was equally criticized for predominantly focusing on language and not on the ways in which power was mediated through gender, age or class, or by other social, economic or institutional constraints. However, Foucault proved hard to ignore. The impact of ideas of social control on social history in the 1970s and 1980s, and the influence postmodernism had in challenging grand narratives and in questioning modernity, created a receptive climate. Notwithstanding the hostility generated in some quarters by new trends in cultural history and the growing interest in language and texts, historians could no longer ignore the discourses that surrounded medicine or the importance of power. Ideas about the birth of the clinic, medicalization, and the growing authority of the medical profession and the state encouraged new and important trends in the discipline. Soft versions of Foucault were employed to rethink the role of the state, asylums, hospitals, race, gender and sexuality. Medicine was no longer seen as a disinterested science, but became a form of power.

Medicalization quickly became a key concept in the social history of medicine and offered historians a means to explore the ways in which behaviours came to be defined medically or pathologically and the fundamental links between the body and political power. If medicalization was never adequately defined and was shown to seldom be an explicit or conscious process, for the historian Paul Weindling it reflected 'the extension of rational, scientific values in medicine to a wider range of social activities' at the end of the nineteenth century, as can be seen in medical attitudes to homosexuality or criminality.[4] Work on the late nineteenth century social purity movement, degeneration, colonial medicine or on pronatalism in the interwar period, for example, illustrated the growing power of doctors and the state to define the normal and the pathological [see 'Healthcare and the state']. Frequently accounts presented medicalization as a harmful process. In part, this was because this approach owed much to the influence of contemporary critiques of medicine and unease about the power of biomedicine, and reflected the historical interest in eugenics or the Nazi extermination campaigns. This created a distorted view of how modern welfare states governed medicine, the body and the individual.

Studies in the 1980s and 1990s increasingly came to present a more intricate picture of medicalization that did not fall into the trap of exaggerating the biomedical power of the medical profession or the state. Scholars started to reveal how the relationship between doctors and the state was more intricate than a simple model of medicalization would suggest; that doctors often resisted state control and that patients had agency [see 'Healthcare and the state']. Attention continued to concentrate on the nineteenth and twentieth centuries to explore the subtle shifts in power and discourse that occurred. Work on hospitals and asylums, for example, indicated how they were prized by doctors more for the professional opportunities they offered than as a way of segregating the deviant [see 'Hospitals']. However, the general idea that medical practitioners were gradually co-opted into a therapeutic state where they played important roles in administering health continued to inform studies, while research on the growth of a biomedical outlook on the management of populations continued to broadly conform to Foucault's notions.

Medicine and markets

Interest in discourses, power and authority was not the only trend in the social history of medicine. As social historians embraced work by medical sociologists and medical anthropologists, ideas about patients' rights, and feminist and gender history, they offered insights into the ways in which the sick negotiated treatment and consulted a range of practitioners. Whereas earlier historical writing had tended to place the physician at the centre of medicine, a view reinforced by ideas of professionalization, new studies pointed to the variety of sources of medical care that reflected contemporary interest in ideas of agency and patient choices. For the sociologist Nicholas Jewson, the influence of patronage provided a means of explaining the relationships between physicians and their patients which put the patient in charge.[5] If Jewson's approach owed much to a Marxist model and highlighted the connections between medical knowledge and social relations, an understanding of medicine as a market offered historians new, more flexible ways of thinking about power and agency. Influenced by the free market ideology of the Thatcher era of British politics (1979–90), and economists' interest in what was happening in competitive markets, the concept of the medical marketplace stressed the economic dimension of medical encounters and the importance of consumption, an approach that drew on a rich vein of historical research on the birth of consumer society. It offered a model of market relations as a way of unpicking the interactions between the supply and demand for medical services.

First used by Harold Cook in *The Decline of the Old Medical Regime in Stuart London* (1986), the marketplace model encouraged historians to rethink the role of other healers, such as quacks or astrological healers, and about patients as active agents. It proved useful for understanding not only the relatively unregulated English context but also as a tool for examining wider structures in European medicine. Studies of early modern Europe revealed the ways in which medical assistance was sought from a variety of practitioners to explore questions of status and authority [see 'Professionalization']. Other tools came to be used to extend analysis. Whereas Laurence Brockliss and Colin Jones in *The Medical World of Early Modern France* (1997) focused on power relations between the orthodox medical community and the medical penumbra, David Gentilcore in *Healers and Healing in Early Modern Italy* (1998) emphasized medical pluralism, both in terms of the types of healers and the sources of healing used. Work by Dutch historians revealed the importance of more immaterial exchanges: how social and symbolic values also needed to be considered alongside economic exchanges.

In thinking about the medical marketplace, new studies of early modern medicine revealed how the boundaries between practitioners were frequently blurred and ill-defined. Although the rhetoric of physicians and their efforts to secure a monopoly continued to dominate studies, eighteenth and nineteenth century practitioners – regular, alternative and quack – became entrepreneurs as historians explored the influence of social and commercial factors on medical knowledge and care, an approach epitomized in Roy Porter's seminal *Health for Sale: Quackery in England, 1650–1850* (1989). In exploring the medical marketplace, the nature and treatment of disease, far from being dominated by doctors, were shown to be negotiated, a move that saw ideas of medicalization reworked. Historians became more sensitive to the intellectual and social diversity among practitioners and patients. The result, as the historian Andrew Wear explained, was that 'a much richer medical world has been uncovered'.[6]

Patients' perspectives

If the social history of medicine encouraged a radical reinterpretation of health, as Roy Porter explained in 1985 even those sceptical of medicine's past and 'sensitive to the self-serving features of professionalization' nevertheless 'implicitly endorsed the view that the history of healing is par excellence the history of doctors'.[7] The early pioneer of the social history of medicine George Rosen had urged in the *Bulletin of the History of Medicine* for a change in approach in 1967 by emphasizing the need to study people, but this call to consider the experiences of the patient was slow to take hold. In the 1970s, the sociologist Nicholas Jewson offered one way forward by highlighting the importance of patronage and agency in shaping medical encounters. However, it was not until the 1980s that historians started to explore the choices patients made. Influenced by medical sociology and medical anthropology, by the intimate connections that existed with social history, by ideas about patients' rights, and by gender history and the medical marketplace model, historians began to assert the need for a more patient-centred approach.

Roy Porter called for a change in perspective: he wanted to rewrite the history of medicine from the patient's perspective. Writing during a period when a social turn had come to dominate medical history, Porter argued that by concentrating on medical practitioners, historians had distorted history, especially as 'a great deal of healing in the past' involved 'professional practitioners only marginally'.[8] Porter did not put forward a coherent theory or embrace a 'history from below' methodology. Influenced by contemporary debates on patient rights, he asserted the importance of agency to privilege the patient in his version of medical history from below. Porter argued that through an imaginative use of sources it was possible to produce a history of the sick and the choices they made to show that patients were not subservient to doctors. If Porter over-privileged elite or middle-class patients, his article and subsequent monographs with Dorothy Porter on medicine in seventeenth and eighteenth century Britain revealed the strength and continuity of lay healing cultures, and asserted the need to examine the complex choices the sick made.

Porter's call for a new perspective in medical history helped set a new research agenda as evident in Guenter Risse's *Hospital Life in Enlightenment Scotland* (1986) and Lucinda Beier's *Sufferers and Healers: The Experience of Illness in Seventeenth-Century England* (1987) as historians examined the patient's experience. However, Porter was not the only one to argue for a history of patients. Alternative approaches were suggested. Jewson's emphasis on the disappearance of the patient's voice with the rise of hospital medicine was embodied in Fissell's *Patients, Power and the Poor in Eighteenth-Century Bristol* (1991). The influence of the social sciences, specifically socio-cultural anthropology, on the social history of medicine further broadened understanding of experiences of sickness, the systems of beliefs, images and symbols involved, and the decisions patients made in response to illness. Tuberculosis and mental illness provided attractive subjects for exploring patients' conceptions and experiences of disease.

Notwithstanding Porter's championing of medical history 'from below', patient-centred accounts were slow to emerge. Studies were often empirically driven and were mainly about understanding the doctor-patient relationship or evaluating claims that hospitals were 'gateways to death' [see 'Hospitals']. Although a radical rewriting of the history of medicine did not emerge, the idea that patients were relatively passive was increasingly rejected. Patients were shown to have bargaining power in the medical marketplace, but historians also noted that this power and their experiences of sickness and treatment were shaped by a range of factors from class, gender and race to social, political, economic, familial and psychological factors. The idea that medical history should take into consideration patients' experiences was accepted but notwithstanding this, the patient's voice remained muted in many studies.

Constructing medicine and disease

Influenced by new trends in cultural history, studies in the 1980s started to explore not just the biological, physical or psychological nature of disease but also the ways in which disease was constructed and the power relations created around the body and medical practices. In this work, the body and disease were not just taken for granted, but were invented. Just as anthropologists demonstrated that beliefs about health and disease were widely variable, social historians of medicine came to recognize that experiences and understanding of diseases changed over time. This encouraged them to seek other means of explaining disease.

More culturally minded scholars turned to the sociology of knowledge and social constructivism for answers. Often its critics have misunderstood the approach but for some historians 'social constructivism' offered a way of understanding disease from a social, cultural and patient perspective. Social constructivism suggested that social and cultural forces influenced even the most complex theoretical claims. Medicine appeared to offer a promising field for analysing the ways in which theories about disease were social constructs. Susan Sontag in her groundbreaking *Illness as Metaphor* (1979) had already pointed to the metaphorical possibilities of disease, focusing first on tuberculosis and cancer and later on AIDS. If her work encouraged interest in disease as metaphor – for example, for sin in the case of venereal disease – social constructivism pointed to the value of more cultural approaches. Social constructionists wanted to show that 'ideas necessarily carry or mediate values, that making and using medical knowledge cannot be so neatly separated, and that understanding the social meanings of natural knowledge is preferable to making moral judgements about the propriety of practitioners'.[9] This view made language and texts central to understanding the ways in which disease ideas were relative to the social and cultural position of those who produced them, and how these ideas were informed by race, gender, class, age, nationality, etc. The historian Ludmilla Jordanova argued that by ignoring this social and cultural dimension historians risked applying contemporary concerns to the past. She believed that a social constructionist approach allowed historians to move beyond an analysis that was limited 'to the social reception or historical context of an idea or set of practices'.[10] David Harley went on to suggest that the approach should stand at the centre of medical history because health and healing were 'rhetorical constructs created in particular social locations'.[11]

Social constructivism proved controversial, however. Critics caricatured the approach as ignoring the material dimension of life, of asserting medicalization, and for claiming that disease was not real, that only practices exist. For them it appeared to represent the worst excesses of postmodernism. For those working on epidemiological, demographic or economic reconstructions of health and disease this was going too far. They vehemently rejected social constructivism, preferring instead a biological or epidemiological history of infection.

The American historian Charles Rosenberg in part resolved the tensions between these approaches. Instead of constructing disease, Rosenberg proposed in the *Milbank Quarterly* (1989) that it should be framed.[12] He believed this offered a more flexible and less charged metaphor. Rosenberg argued that seeing the meaning and impact of illness as varying according to the cultural context was also dependent on the underlying biological reality of the disease. Rosenberg's idea of framing suggested that disease entities were social players. He encouraged the use of complex narratives in which doctors, patients and their diseases all became historical agents.

As the novelty of social constructivism declined, the approach it suggested reminded historians that medical knowledge and practices were constrained by the culture in which they were produced. Encouraged by the collection Rosenberg and Janet Golden edited, entitled *Framing Disease: Studies in Cultural History* (1992), historians recognized that disease had a biological reality but that social, cultural and economic perspectives allowed an account of not just medical knowledge but an integration of the ways in which health, sickness and healing were culturally defined. In adopting this approach, interest initially focused on such diseases as plague, cholera, tuberculosis and syphilis, but gradually historians started to move beyond a style of descriptive histories of disease to adopt some form of social constructionism. Historians became more sensitive to the ways in which medical knowledge and practices were influenced, for example, by local cultures, religious ideas, gender, race or class.

This growing sensitivity encouraged social historians of medicine to become increasingly aware of the pitfalls of applying modern interpretations to past practices, a methodology often referred to as retrospective diagnosis. As Harley explained, it was not just 'a question of the same phenomena being given different clothing' but of looking at the rhetoric and cultural understanding of health and disease as expressed by patients and practitioners.[13] For example, historians working on the relationships between women and medicine highlighted the extent to which medicine was laden with cultural assumptions about women's reproductive roles [see 'Women and medicine']. Medical knowledge and ideas about, and experiences of, disease were contextualized. Work on the sixteenth century, for example, revealed how ideas about the body and disease were shaped by the social, intellectual and religious upheavals associated with the Reformation and Counter-Reformation [see 'Religion']. Medical knowledge and practice came to be seen as integral to socio-cultural history as culturally specific beliefs and social structures were shown to create local realities that defined health and illness. Few scholars would now doubt that diagnoses are socially constructed. One result of this trend is that historians have increasingly sought to understand the ways in which people thought about and understood disease, and to explore the various factors that shaped this thinking. The result has been to show that empirical views of disease that concentrate on classification or observation are no longer satisfactory.

Dominant narratives/discourses

Although historians have abandoned progressive narratives of the rise of modern medicine and a focus on great men or medical innovations, even the most sophisticated have been unable to ignore the new narratives that have come to replace Whiggish views. If historians have rejected triumphalism, it has proved harder to escape from the impression that medical knowledge and practices have progressed, particularly when looking at the nineteenth or twentieth century. Ideas associated with the problematic category of modernity, secularization and the rise of science, professionalization, the medical marketplace, the institutionalization of medicine, medicalization, the triumph of biomedicine, and the growing role of the state, have created their own narratives, even if traditional chronologies have been disrupted and challenged.

If medical historians have become sensitive to ideas of continuity and change, and the contested nature of medical ideas and practices, there remains a belief that certain periods, decades or countries saw important changes – or paradigm shifts – in the nature or structure of medicine. For example, the period 1780 to 1830 has been represented as a watershed associated with the rise of the modern hospital, pathological anatomy and professional regulation, and moves connected to Paris medicine, while the period 1880 to 1970 has been linked to increasing medical authority and the rise of biomedicine. In this later period, first Germany and then the United States became paradigmatic of these shifts.

For some scholars, cultural approaches have offered an alternative to these narratives. Others have turned to micro or regional histories to construct different narratives. If this might seem like a return to reasserting the importance of context, a further way forward is to develop comparative studies to enrich historical understanding of medicine in the past and to open up new research questions. By exploring the social history of medicine in a comparative context, it becomes possible to move beyond the findings of national or local studies to examine the broader narratives – for example, professionalization or institutionalization – to reveal in what ways practices differed or converged.

The end of the social history of medicine

Writing in the *Historical Journal* in 1993, Ludmilla Jordanova wondered if the history of medicine had come of age. Jordanova preferred to see the discipline in its childhood because its archival potential had barely been tapped, there remained huge gaps in the topics or areas covered, and because historiographical debate was limited. If the social history of medicine was not without its controversies, for Jordanova it was 'not yet fully confident in tackling areas of major historical debate'.[14] Other historians quickly joined the debate. Of these, Roger Cooter provided a pessimistic reading that in a more laconic moment he equated to writing his own academic obituary. He lamented that the social history of medicine was 'never much of a discipline to begin with' with few canonical texts and fewer orthodoxies. In a series of pessimistic assessments of the discipline, he believed that many of the key questions that had initially animated debate remained unresolved. Drawing on academic debates more familiar to historians in the 1980s and 1990s, Cooter argued that the cultural turn had effectively 'derailed' the discipline.[15]

If some historians have been swayed by the idea that the cultural turn has robbed their work of meaning, pessimistic claims about the social history of medicine ignore the ongoing vibrancy of the field. To attack the discipline by returning to a controversy largely exhausted in other fields of historical writing, and by recycling the criticisms of the literary critic Hayden White that academic history is a literary genre, succumbs to the same trap that critics believe social historians of medicine have fallen into. Few medical historians would disagree with the claim that the social history of medicine has enriched our understanding of the medical past. Although not all social historians of medicine are self-conscious theorists, this does not mean that medical history has itself become sterile or self-serving. Nor that it has ignored theory or wider historiographical debates. Social historians of medicine have continued to be informed by ideas from the social sciences, literary criticism and other disciplines. This is more than an eclectic borrowing of half-understood theories. For example, the idea of hybridity and entanglement from postcolonial and literary theory has enriched studies of colonial medicine [see 'Medicine and empire'], while actor-network theory has influenced studies of, for example, healthcare in the twentieth century. At the same time, the initial focus on the eighteenth and nineteenth centuries has broadened as Renaissance and early modern scholars have turned their attention to the problems of health and disease, the medical marketplace, medical beliefs, and public health.

This is not to suggest that the social history of medicine has become a coherent field. There are numerous overlapping topics and concerns. As David Harley explains, 'intellectual historians are interested in the development of medical ideas, economic historians in the income of practitioners and the distribution of services, social historians in the creation and consolidation of professions and institutions, historical demographers in the incidence of birth and death, and cultural historians in the representation of race, gender, or the body'. The result is a series of overlapping sub-disciplines. If this might encourage a sense that the social history of medicine lacks a coherent set of distinctive questions, methods or approaches, it has in Harley's words created a 'stimulating complexity' and considerable critical analysis.[16]

This complexity is revealed in how social historians of medicine have pointed to the intricate connections that existed in the past between diseases, ideas, practices, individuals, practitioners and institutions on the one hand, and environment, gender, race, society, culture and politics on the other. Social historians of medicine have revealed how the relationship between medical theory and practice was not straightforward, and how new ideas or institutions were not always translated into new practices. Ideas of power – for practitioners, patients or the state – have become important themes, while the medical marketplace and ideas of pluralism have emphasized the range of healers and healing. More sensitive readings of class, gender and race have informed studies from nursing to colonial medicine. Issues of continuity and discontinuity have offered alternative ways of looking at medicine and questioning ideas of modernity. To return to Wear's claim, the result has been a growing sense of a much richer, complex medical world. It is this world that the following chapters address.

Further reading

Notwithstanding claims that the social history of medicine has stood apart from other areas of historical writing to understand the discipline it is important to have an overview of the broad historiography. Numerous texts tackle how historical writing has developed. A good starting point is Stefan Berger, Heiko Feldner and Kevin Passmore (eds), *Writing History: Theory and Practice* (London: Hodder Arnold, 2003). Rather than focusing upon abstract theory, the volume explains key concepts and the ways in which they have informed historical work. Unlike other areas of history, there are few competing assessments of the historiography of the social history of medicine. The edited volume by Frank Huisman and John Harley Warner (eds), *Locating Medical History. The Stories and their Meanings* (Baltimore, MD: Johns Hopkins University Press, 2004) offers a mixture of biographical assessments and overviews of the discipline, although it presupposes some degree of knowledge of the discipline. A shorter introduction is presented by Gert Brieger, 'The Historiography of Medicine', in W.F. Bynum and Roy Porter (eds), *Companion Encyclopaedia of the History of Medicine*, vol. 1 (London: Routledge, 1997), pp. 24–44, while Dorothy Porter, 'The Mission of the Social History of Medicine', *Social History of Medicine* 8 (1995), pp. 345–59, explores how the discipline developed in Britain. Foucault's work has produced a larger body of literature. For his ideas on health and medicine, a good starting point is Colin Jones and Roy Porter (eds), *Reassessing Foucault: Power, Medicine and the Body* (London: Routledge, 1994). On ideas of medicalization, Robert Nye, 'The Evolution of the Concept of Medicalization in the Late Twentieth Century', *Journal of History of the Behavioral Sciences* 39 (2003), pp. 115–29, offers a compelling introduction, while Patrick Wallis and Mark Jenner (eds), *Medicine and the Market in England and its Colonies, c.1450–c.1850* (Basingstoke: Palgrave Macmillan, 2007) survey the medical marketplace. On the patient's perspective, Roy Porter, 'The Patient's View: Doing Medical History from Below', *Theory and Society* 14 (1985), pp. 167–74, remains the obvious starting point, with Flurin Condrau, 'The Patient's View Meets the Clinical Gaze', *Social History of Medicine* 20 (2007), pp. 525–40, providing an assessment of the impact of these ideas. Ludmilla Jordanova's article, 'The Social Construction of Medical Knowledge', *Social History of Medicine* 8 (1995), pp. 361–81, remains the standard text on social constructivism and how it applies to the social history of medicine. Roger Cooter offers numerous pessimistic readings of the future of the discipline: among the best is 'After Death/After-"life": The Social History of Medicine in Post-Modernity', *Social History of Medicine* 20 (2007), pp. 441–64. For one response to this argument, see Rhodri Hayward, '"Much Exaggerated": The End of the History of Medicine', *Journal of Contemporary History* 40 (2005), pp. 167–78.

2
Disease, illness and society

The ubiquity of disease has been a familiar theme in early modern and modern thought, with diaries and letters pointing to more or less daily symptoms and long lists of complaints. New diseases like whooping cough and cholera appeared alongside the more familiar and imprecise forms of fever in the nineteenth century and contemporary literature was immersed in a culture of sickness. Nor did these concerns disappear at the turn of the century. Fears about degeneration were a feature of *fin de siècle* European discussions of race, gender, nation and empire, while studies continued to reveal surprisingly levels of poor health, not only at the start of the twentieth century but also throughout the 1930s. Yet, generalizations have been made about health between 1500 and 1950. If the dominant view reflects an assumption that health in Europe improved as life expectancy rose, historians have become increasingly sensitive to the complexities this generalization conceals: how, for example, maternal mortality rose in the seventeenth century only to fall again in the eighteenth; how there was no clear global decline in mortality between 1888 and 1912, and how stark regional contrasts existed. Historians have equally become attuned to how the patterns, experiences and even the nature of disease were shaped by environmental, political and cultural factors, and by the material circumstances of everyday life. Hence, rather than a simple model of mortality decline, historians have become aware of the intricate patterns of mortality and morbidity (or the state of being diseased), and how these states have been perceived and explained in the past. Two broad approaches have emerged: one evaluates the socioeconomic, demographic and cultural consequences of disease; the other how people understood disease.

Although disease and sickness were widely portrayed, for the historian they are not always amenable to study. Health, disease, sickness and illness are not straightforward concepts. Ideas of ill health were not always connected to particular diseases in a biological sense, and much is unknown about how contemporaries experienced or perceived ill health in the past. The acutely ill seldom left records, while illiteracy and debility prevented certain groups from writing about their suffering. To get round this problem some historians have employed present-day medical understanding to the diseases described in historical texts. This retrodiagnosis has rightly been criticized for privileging modern definitions and categories of disease to distort our understanding of the past. What we would now refer to as symptoms were often seen as diseases in themselves, while how diseases were understood, as we shall see below, altered according to the historical context. Most historians have hence come to rely on mortality statistics to give an indication of levels of health.

However, there are problems with using mortality figures. In most European countries, records of births and deaths were not kept consistently until the nineteenth century. Diagnosis was frequently unreliable and misdiagnosis was common: for example, in plague epidemics, deaths routinely ascribed to plague were often due to other causes, while during the 1918–19 influenza pandemic, pneumonic complications were often recorded as the cause of death. Diagnostic categories have also changed, as have doctors' ability to recognize particular diseases according to contemporary medical knowledge or the diagnostic technology available to them. Cause of death was equally open to negotiation, often to avoid stigma. For example, during the Florentine plague of 1630–33 doctors recorded something different to spare respectable families the dishonour of a mass burial. States also minimized levels of disease, especially epidemic outbreaks, to protect trade or prevent panic.

The assumption that a fall in the death rate means that populations were becoming healthier is problematic. By their very nature, mortality statistics disguise chronic ill health or disability and tell us little about day-to-day experiences or the levels of sickness over an individual's lifetime. Even in the harshest epidemic, individual experiences varied greatly and not all sicknesses posed a significant risk of death. With improvements in the ability to identify and treat disease, and with public health programmes that sought to reduce opportunities for infection, the chances of dying from infectious diseases fell in the nineteenth century, but this did not mean that populations inevitably became healthier.

Historians have consequently come to recognize that the epidemiological past is hard to know. Health and disease are complex issues; made more so by the fact that most sufferers/patients/doctors frequently moved between the biological and the social when talking and writing about illness. Experiences of sickness depended on a range of factors that included season, geography, class, age, gender, occupation and ethnicity, and were influenced by other factors, such as trade, climate, war, famine or colonization. Sickness levels responded to short-term factors, such as a harsh winter, and to long-term trends, such as rising living standards, but the connection was not always straightforward: for example, harvest failure and a rise in the price of bread did not always mean more disease. Sickness equally involved not just grave ailments, but also minor complaints, which were seldom recorded. There are therefore dangers to generalizing as health and ill health were influenced by socioeconomic, political and geopolitical factors in complex ways.

Nor is there a simple relationship between disease in its biological sense and its social dimension. One way round this problem has been to turn to other sources, such as diaries, letters, almanacs, and literature, and to think in terms of how disease was socially constructed or framed [see 'Historiography']. For social constructivists, the social and cultural context informed how disease was understood and represented, offering an approach that allowed for diseases to change their meanings over time and for those meanings to be contested. Although medical historians have vigorously debated the usefulness of a social constructivist approach, sickness in the past was laden with multiple meanings and prompted a wide range of reactions that expressed cultural, religious, political or socioeconomic values. Names changed, as did diagnostic categories, and this was shaped by patients' account of sickness, by social and cultural perceptions, and by medical knowledge and professional concerns. Disease and sickness are not then stable historical concepts.

In this section, we have seen how morbidity and mortality are not simple questions of statistics and how a range of factors influenced disease, sickness and ill health. Diseases are complex biological, socioeconomic, political and cultural entities that were subject to a range of meanings. In the following sections, we will explore these ideas to examine the impact of epidemics and everyday illness, and how sickness was explained.

Epidemics: 1600–1900

Early modern Europe was beset by pestilence. If the long-term consequences were not as dramatic as might be supposed, epidemics had a short-term impact that could devastate communities and generate fear. Epidemics were frequent and unpredictable. Although most ran their course in a few months, until the 1720s scarcely a year went by in many communities without an outbreak of pestilence. Epidemics might kill hundreds at a local level but spare nearby towns, but occasionally they swept across nations, killing thousands. These epidemics were more than just natural phenomena. They were also socioeconomic, cultural and political events that are central to understanding mortality in Europe and community responses to disease until the nineteenth century [see 'Public health'].

It was not therefore the everyday diseases that afflicted early modern populations that dominated contemporary accounts or captured historians' imaginations, but epidemics. There are clear reasons for this. Epidemics generated a considerable body of evidence for historians to work with from bills of mortality to first-person accounts. As dramatic events, they cast light on attitudes to disease and reveal tensions in communities. Of these epidemics, plague had the most resonance. Oral and literary recollections along with printed treaties kept memories about plague alive between visitations. They helped impose order on the horrifying nature of the disease and set out (sometimes contradictory) programmes of action. Historians have used these accounts to reconstruct the socio-demographic and cultural impact of plague on early modern Europe.

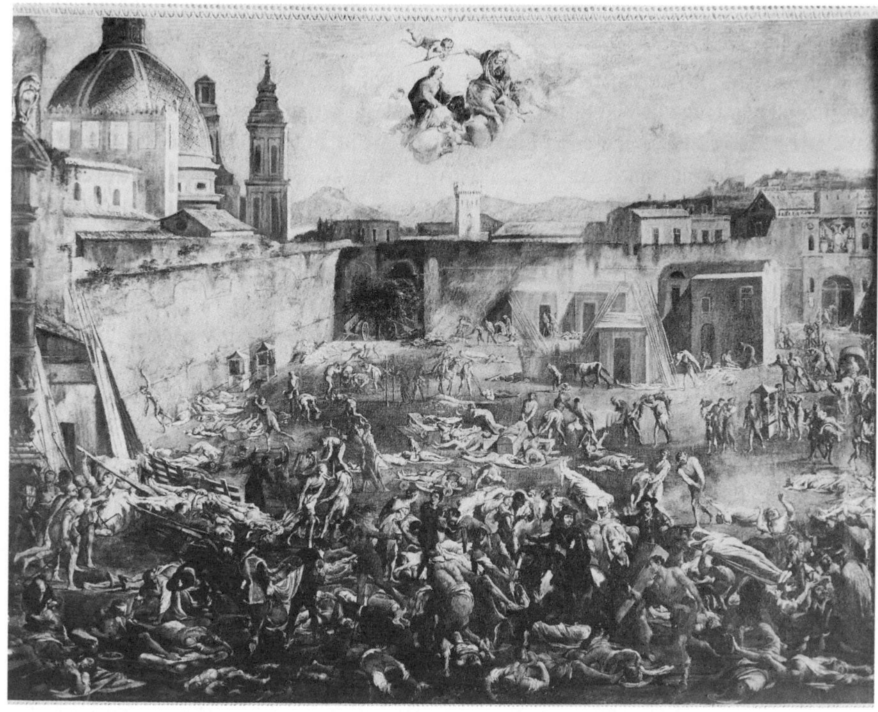

Figure 2.1 The Pizza Mercatellow in Naples during the plague of 1656. The painting illustrates how the plague was viewed as a devastating event.
Source: Wellcome Library, London.

The mid fourteenth century had witnessed a devastating pandemic, the Black Death, which killed between a third and two-thirds of Europe's population. Plague remained endemic, but in the sixteenth century a new, virulent strain emerged that coincided with the appearance of other new diseases, notably typhus and smallpox, and increasing urbanization, which put plague-infected rats in close proximity to humans. By the seventeenth century, plague ravaged northern Italy, southern and eastern Spain, France, Holland and England. Some countries fared better than others did: In England and Italy, epidemics were often separated by decades, but in France, plague was ever-present on a regional or local basis between 1500 and 1770.

Notwithstanding these regional patterns, plague represented the most terrifying disease affecting Europe. Symptoms varied and were difficult to determine, even for experienced physicians, but contemporary accounts describe a rapid and dramatic assault on the body that killed quickly and horribly, often in a manner that was the antithesis of contemporary ideas of a 'good death'. Although the number killed or suffering from plague is often hard to calculate,

60 to 90 per cent of those stricken died. In France, it is estimated that between 1600 and 1670 alone plague was responsible for between two and two and a half million deaths, ensuring that most people living through the period probably lost a relative, friend or neighbour to the disease. Death rates were as high as 40 per cent nationally, and even higher at a local level. In Santander in northern Spain, for example, at least 75 per cent of the town's inhabitants died from plague in 1596–97, while Lyon lost half of its seventy thousand population to plague in the 1628–30 epidemic. The rich fared better than the poor if only because they could, as one slogan advised, 'flee soon, go far, come back late'. Among those left behind, mortality varied: for example, those occupations, such as bakers or butchers, which attracted rats, suffered noticeably higher mortality. Individuals were expected to balance their obligations of kinship and service against their duty of self-preservation, but the concentration of the plague in poor areas often pitted rich against poor, while explanations were advanced that blamed ethnic groups, such as Jews, or immigrants and travellers, for spreading the disease. Plague was therefore far more than a biological entity. When plague arrived, the whole tenor of urban life changed. Trade suffered: shops and churches closed and work often stopped.

Visitations of plague declined unevenly in Western Europe from the mid seventeenth century onwards. Although plague disappeared from England following the London epidemic of 1665–66, most of Italy was free from plague a decade earlier. Elsewhere plague lingered. In France the last great plague epidemic occurred in 1720, in Russia in the 1770s, and in the Balkans in the 1840s. Why plague declined is unclear. Climate change, better nutrition, improved personal hygiene and housing conditions, and growing immunity have all been suggested as explanations. One popular theory attributes the disappearance of plague to the displacement of the black rat (*Rattus rattus*), which lived in houses, by the hardier brown sewer rat (*Rattus norvegicus*). Proponents of this theory argue that as brown rats did not live in close proximity to humans, infected fleas could not easily infect them. There are problems with all these explanations. For example, there is little evidence to support improved nutrition in the seventeenth century. Environmental improvements, such as better housing, were slow to take hold. Nor does the chronology of the spread of the brown rat match the disappearance of the plague: accounts suggest that brown rats were not found in Paris or Spain until after the plague had declined. Recent studies have therefore pointed to the importance of public health measures in limiting the spread of plague [see 'Public health'].

The disappearance of the plague in Western Europe does not tell the entire story. Images of plague and its effects continued to live on in literature, particularly French literature, as seen famously in Albert Camus's *La Peste* (1947). Although a number of plague cases were recorded in Europe in the twentieth century – it was reported as Malady No. 9 in Paris in 1920–21 to prevent a panic – the epidemiological focus shifted east. Between 1894 and 1929, over 24,000 cases of bubonic plague occurred in Hong Kong. India was harder hit. At least twelve million died in the two decades after the 1896 outbreak in Bombay where deaths from plague in the city alone reached 172,511 by 1910. The massive fatalities had a corresponding socioeconomic impact that suggests parallels with early modern experiences. By the 1930s, plague had retreated to a few small pockets of infection, but cases were still reported in the twenty first century, most recently in Libya in 2009.

A focus on plague obscures the other epidemics that regularly affected early modern Europe. Although records are patchy, the sixteenth and seventeenth centuries witnessed the emergence of new epidemic diseases, such as the 'English sweats', the French pox (*morbus gallicus*), typhus and typhoid, as well as epidemic outbreaks of established diseases such as malaria, influenza and dysentery. If levels of leprosy declined dramatically in the sixteenth century, smallpox assumed an increased demographic importance, accounting for 15–20 per cent of deaths in some nations. Between the sixteenth and eighteenth centuries, levels of tuberculosis rose at a dramatic rate, while syphilis appeared in a particularly malignant form in the sixteenth century. Others diseases, such as diarrhoea and measles, were endemic and periodically reached epidemic proportions. Epidemics of fever were common: at least sixteen influenza pandemics and epidemics occurred in Europe between 1700 and 1900. Just like plague, these epidemics could have wide-ranging and devastating effects, not only on mortality but also on social, political and economic life. Epidemics could see the population of individual towns fall dramatically, and decline was often slow to reverse. Existing social inequalities were heightened during epidemics, which in some cases led to riots or attacks on social or ethnic groups. Trade and the economy were equally damaged. This often had a more disruptive effect than deaths from epidemics.

As disease is influenced by socioeconomic, political or cultural events, the social dislocation produced by famine, economic decline or war – for example, during the late fifteenth and early sixteenth centuries – saw levels of infectious disease rise. A move into towns and the growth of trade created a growing pool of susceptible victims and increased opportunities for infection. With little expansion in urban infrastructures, and with chronic overcrowding in inner districts, many towns struggled to adapt. Under these conditions, urban living (at least until the twentieth century) went hand-in-hand with infectious disease. At the same time, the intensification of trading networks combined with greater migration and movement between towns allowed diseases to spread more rapidly between towns and nations. Colonial expansion and troop movements equally played their part [see 'Medicine and empire']. This was not a one-way process as shown by the movement of malaria and yellow fever between the Americas and Europe, and by the suspected arrival of pox (probably syphilis) to Europe from the New World.

By the mid nineteenth century, epidemic and endemic infectious diseases were of major political and medical importance. Efforts to improve urban conditions were offset by changing living and working patterns, and by improved

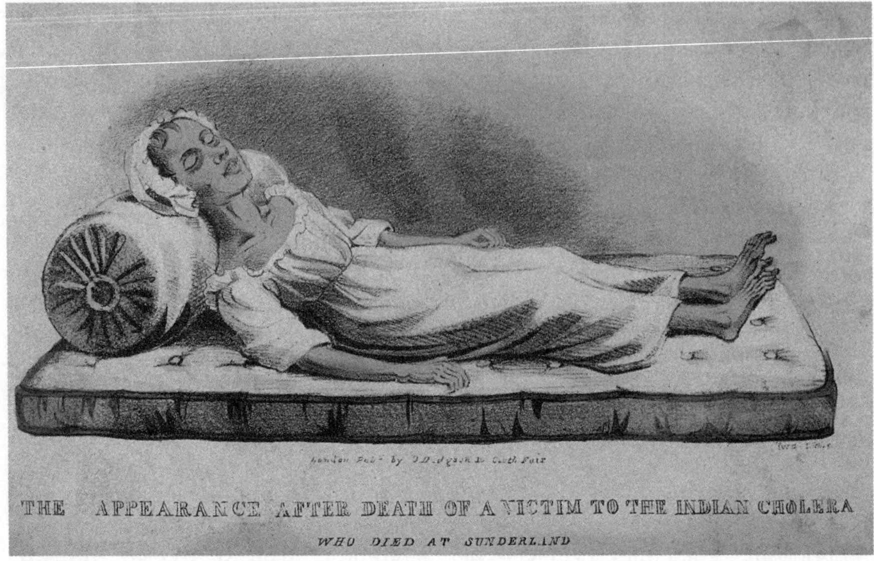

Figure 2.2 A Sunderland cholera victim, 1832. The picture illustrates the characteristic blue tinge of cholera victims.
Source: Wellcome Library, London.

transport routes, which created new avenues for epidemics to spread in Europe and the wider world. Of all the epidemic diseases that threatened nineteenth century Europe, cholera was the most visible and frightening. Although the term 'cholera' was not new – it had been used earlier to describe non-specific gastroenteritis – Asiatic cholera was a severe and often fatal diarrhoeal disease that was unknown in Europe before the 1820s. It spread from India along trade routes in several pandemic waves, the first in the 1820s and 1830s, the second from 1841 to 1851, the third from 1863 to 1875, with the fourth wave from 1881 to 1896. Hitting densely populated areas hardest, to some cholera seemed like the return of the plague. Cholera appeared relentless, killing quickly, with the death of 40–60 per cent of those afflicted. With no effective treatments, cholera had a psychological impact and inspired desperate attempts to protect against the disease at an individual and national level [see 'Public health'].

The growing global risks posed by epidemics in the nineteenth and twentieth century is exemplified by the 1918–19 influenza pandemic, which killed over forty million worldwide. The strain responsible was particularly rapid in its attack and was unusual in that young adults were predominantly vulnerable. Although outbreaks of influenza were not uncommon during the First World War (1914–18), by November 1918 it had spread worldwide and states struggled to respond. By April 1919 the pandemic had passed. Conditions in 1918–19 were favourable to the spread of influenza: demobilization and the privations of war all contributed, while post-war dislocation meant that some European powers were unable to cope. If the long-term demographic impact of the pandemic was small, the psychological and physical impact of the pandemic was considerable, with the consequences of subsequent pandemics being constructed in relation to the 1918–19 pandemic.

It was only in the early twentieth century that the risks from serious infectious disease declined considerably in Northern and Western Europe. As we will see in a later section, the decline of epidemics altered the pattern of disease, allowing chronic and degenerative diseases to assume a greater importance as a cause of ill health and death. However, although the implementation of public health measures and the development of new drugs, for example new vaccines, in the nineteenth century provided a means of limiting disease, epidemics did not disappear in Europe. In the 1950s, an epidemic of polio was feared and the period also saw new strains of influenza emerge, with the 1957 Asian flu killing over two million worldwide. By the late twentieth century, new diseases and drug-resistant strains created the possibility of new epidemics and pandemics.

Everyday illnesses

War, famine and epidemics often brought death on a large scale, but a concentration on these dramatic events conceals the geography of disease and the impact of other diseases that contributed to high levels of ill health. With the poor eating a limited diet until the nineteenth century, many were prone to infection and to a range of nutritional diseases, such as rickets. As shown in Chapter 12, towns exerted a considerable toll on health, and measles, smallpox, scarlet fever and other infectious diseases were endemic in early modern towns. Although the countryside had a lower mortality, it should not be seen as a rural idyll. Malaria, for example, was common in the countryside. More broadly, diarrhoeal diseases, influenza, pneumonia and other respiratory diseases remained important causes of death until the twentieth century. Venereal disease was widespread in the seventeenth and eighteenth centuries, as was measles, while tuberculosis was a feared cause of disability and death until the 1960s.

For most, experiences of ill health were mundane if no less debilitating. Chronic or long-term illness imposed a considerable strain on families, but if sickness was an important cause of poverty, ill health was commonplace for many. Accounts illustrate how the majority of the population in early modern and modern Europe suffered from colds, headaches, ill-defined fevers, indigestion, and a host of other non-threatening illnesses, such as rotten teeth or eye diseases. Evidence on nineteenth century motherhood and working-class communities highlights high levels of chronic illness – with respiratory diseases and muscle and joint problems commonplace – that brought pain and discomfort but were suffered as they were not considered life threatening. Each season brought its own afflictions: diarrhoea in summer or respiratory diseases in winter. Constipation, gastric disorders and diarrhoea were widespread. The same was true of intestinal worms, ulcers and sores, as well as various skin diseases that could become infected. Minor and chronic illnesses were a daily problem for many and contemporary diaries and letters are full of accounts of illness. The diary of Ralph Josselin, a seventeenth century vicar in Essex, vividly revealed a life where colds, eye and skin disorders, and other endless discomforts plagued individuals. Nearly three hundred years later, Pember Reeves's studies for the British Fabian Women's Group exposed how low levels of health were the norm within working-class London communities, with lung diseases and obstetric disorders commonplace.

Countless others suffered from a range of physical disabilities. Rickets produced its characteristic bowlegs; smallpox scared faces, caused blindness and impotence; syphilis led to ulceration and in severe cases the collapse of nasal bones. Tuberculosis of the joints or bones resulted in chronic inflammation, accompanied by decay and ulceration. Urban living created numerous opportunities for accidents that could result in disability, although the modern concept of the disabled did not emerge until the twentieth century. Work was equally hazardous and the regulation of factories remained minimal until the mid nineteenth century. Hours were long and conditions in many workshops contributed to respiratory diseases. The hazards of mining were all too obvious, but even shop work had its associated health problems as many shop assistants worked in small unventilated premises. Apart from the general debilitating effects of work, particular diseases characterized certain occupations. The production of hats, along with mirrors and makeup, involved the use of mercury, which was poisonous. Only gradually was a medical connection established between particular diseases and certain trades.

Given the high levels of sickness – mundane, chronic or otherwise – that persisted into the mid twentieth century, individuals actively tried to avoid disease and protect their families or communities. Sufferers were not just victims of disease. Although medical advice was sought from a range of sources, sufferers in the past responded to ill health through self-medication. Efforts extended beyond taking herbal or over-the-counter medicines. They included wearing warm clothing, avoiding environments associated with disease, staying out of cold or wet weather, eating healthily, exercising or following a particular regimen or health fad. As shown below, these efforts to avoid disease reflected medical and popular understanding of disease and its causes.

Mortality and morbidity transition: 1870–2000

A decline occurred in mortality and in infant mortality in Western and Northern Europe from the last decades of the nineteenth century to the middle of the twentieth century. For example, in France, the death rate fell from 22.9 per thousand of the population in 1880 to 17.2 per thousand in 1920, while in Italy the shift seemed even more dramatic, with the death rate falling from 30.9 per thousand in 1880 to 19 per thousand in 1920.[1] If the 1918–19 influenza pandemic acted as a temporary setback, the European average life expectancy rose from 50 in 1870 to 64 in 1940. A less favourable picture existed for Eastern Europe where mortality remained higher, but even here death rates fell. Although contemporaries in Western Europe pointed to the spectre of degeneration, mortality decline represented both a quantitative shift and a qualitative change in life expectancy at birth. Although historians agree that sustained mortality decline was in evidence by 1900 – even if different countries and regions experienced different patterns – the theories why this occurred have proved controversial.

Debate on why this decline occurred has been shaped by two broad views: whether or not a reduction in mortality was primarily a by-product of improved standards of living, as reflected in better nutrition, or whether it was the result of public health programmes. The first view builds on ideas of progress associated with industrialization and democratization, and is epitomized by the writings of the medical historian and leading proponent of social medicine Thomas McKeown. Drawing his evidence from mortality patterns in England, he argued that medicine had little effect on mortality before 1950. Instead, he attributed mortality decline to rising living standards. Although many historians agree with McKeown that specific therapeutic treatments had a minimal role in the timing of mortality decline, his overall thesis has not stood up to scrutiny. Associating mortality decline with modernization and rising living standards is problematic, especially as industrialization disrupted social and economic patterns and often contributed to mortality. Whereas some historians have advanced the idea that certain diseases declined in virulence – smallpox is often cited as an example – the main assault on the McKeown thesis has come from scholars who have emphasized improvements in preventive medicine – what the demographic historian Simon Szreter has defined as social intervention – personal hygiene practices, or the introduction of social welfare initiatives. Although, as Chapter 12 demonstrates, not all public health initiatives were successful, after 1870 a change in understanding about how infectious diseases were spread combined with improved access to healthcare, helped promote personal hygiene and preventive strategies, which had a positive effect in reducing mortality from the major infectious diseases.

With a decline in incidents of epidemic disease, other chronic and degenerative diseases – cancer, heart disease, diabetes – emerged to take their place in Europe if not in Africa, Asia and South America where epidemic diseases continued to exert a considerable toll. In Europe, new diseases generated medical and popular concern; for example, morphine addiction and alcoholism emerged as new diseases and became sensational topics, while cancer attracted increasing attention throughout the 1920s and 1930s. Fear was expressed about the effects of social diseases, such as tuberculosis and venereal disease, on the strength of the nation. However, if chronic and degenerative diseases became important causes of mortality and morbidity, the extent to which they had previously been under-diagnosed complicates any assessment. Regional patterns also pose problems. Malaria remained a major killer in Italy where it accounted for up to 100,000 deaths a year in the early twentieth century, while Germany experienced an increase in mortality rates in most age groups in the mid 1930s. Large variations existed between affluent and poor districts, something contemporary commentators did not fail to miss.

By the second half of the twentieth century, many people in the West appeared healthier than they had ever been before. If class differentials in health were just as marked in the 1970s as they had been during the 1930s, there were impressive improvements as demonstrated by rising levels of life expectancy at birth (see Table 2.1).

Rising living standards, better housing, therapeutic advances, and public health campaigns have all been identified as laying behind improvements in health. National systems of welfare were introduced which enhanced access to medical services [see 'Healthcare and the state']. Penicillin and other antimicrobial drugs reduced mortality from many bacterial infections, while new medical technologies, such as kidney dialysis, prolonged life. Major childhood infectious diseases were virtually eradicated in Western and Northern Europe following the implementation of large-scale immunization programmes. Successful national campaigns against tuberculosis saw levels of the disease continue to decline throughout the 1960s and international programmes to eradicate smallpox were successful in 1979, although less progress was made with malaria which continued to kill between one and three million a year in the 1990s.

It would be unwise to overstate these gains. Although mortality from infectious diseases fell along with perinatal and maternal mortality, levels of cancer, heart disease, diabetes and the diseases of ageing all rose. Increased affluence brought with it the capacity to consume more alcohol, cigarettes and processed foods, all of which increased the risk of disease. Cardiovascular disease emerged as a major cause of death after 1945 associated initially with smoking and then with obesity and lifestyle. Depression, degenerative disorders, such as Alzheimer's, diabetes and eating disorders, became important concerns in the late twentieth century along with allergies and asthma. However, cancers generated most alarm. Although overall death rates from cancer did not increase between the 1930s and 1980s, cancer became a feared killer associated with a painful and lingering death. Often the management of cancers and other conditions, such as eating disorders, involved long-term care, which increased pressure on welfare services [see 'Healthcare and the state'].

If life expectancy rose and levels of chronic disease fell, sickness rates and incidences of non-fatal illnesses appeared to rise across Europe after 1945. Rising levels of sickness are, for some historians, evidence of a medicalization of society and the greater attention directed at the early signs of illness as the range of behaviours and conditions that necessitated medical intervention expanded. The earlier detection of disease through improved methods of surveillance, such as mass miniature radiography in the 1950s for tuberculosis, screening such as

Table 2.1 Life expectancy at birth, 1970–2000

Year	*UK*	*France*	*Germany*	*Italy*	*Spain*	*European Region (average)*
1970	72	73	–	72	72	–
1980	73	75	–	74	74	72
1990	76	78	76	77	76	73
2000	78	79	78	80	80	74

Source: WHO European Health for All Database (HFA-DB). Courtesy of WHO.

the introduction of pap smears in 1943 for cervical cancer, and better diagnostic methods contributed to this apparent rise in sickness. Illness and injuries that would previously have resulted in death became more amenable to medical or self-management, reducing mortality if not morbidity or disability. However, rising levels of sickness could also reflect changing attitudes to illness (see below) and a growing culture of alarm. Allergies are a good example of this. Changes in lifestyle, working behaviour, and the growth of pensions and insurance schemes contributed to rising life expectancy, but with people living longer they became more likely to experience health problems, especially in later life. Although death rates had declined in the twentieth century, this did not necessarily mean that medicine had conquered disease or that an overall improvement in health had occurred.

Emerging illnesses: twentieth century

Just as the changing experiences of mortality and morbidity in the twentieth century should be questioned, so too should the idea that medicine in the same period was successful in combating disease. In the second half of the twentieth century, there was a resurgence of old infections and the emergence of new diseases. The appearance of supposedly new diseases is not unique to the twentieth century: a new strain of syphilis was believed to have been introduced from the New World in the sixteenth century, while cholera arrived in Europe from India in the 1820s. However, with the twentieth century came new problems. Although some, for example radiation-related diseases, were by their very nature limited, the emergence of drug-resistant and new diseases in the second half of the twentieth century became a global problem, encouraging predications of new pandemics. Such fears were evident following outbreaks of Severe Acute Respiratory Syndrome (SARS) in China in 2002–03, bird flu (H5N1) in 2005, and swine flu (H1NI) in 2009, with the latter quickly reaching pandemic status.

Although some of the problems encountered were far from unique – population movements have always aided the spread of disease – after 1945 the demographic, technological and socioeconomic changes associated with the twentieth century created new work patterns and environments that brought with them new epidemiological threats and health issues. New occupations produced new risks, such as asbestosis, while changing patterns of work involved new chronic health conditions, for example repetitive strain injury (RSI). Other complaints were made visible by new medical technologies or drugs. Although an equation between poverty and disease was a familiar one [see 'Public health'], changes to the global economy, rising inflation and industrial uncertainty after 1970, along with political and social dislocation, war and ethnic conflict, rising immigration and climate change, all had a detrimental effect on biological and social systems. From the mid 1980s, renewed attention was directed at widening health inequalities as levels of infectious disease rose among socially deprived groups: for example, epidemic diphtheria reappeared following the collapse of the Soviet Union (1985–91). Cases of tuberculosis among immigrants, refugees and the homeless equally rose, reversing the global pattern of decline.

However, the re-emergence of infectious disease was not just a problem of the underclass or nations that experienced political or social restructuring. In Britain, growing anxiety about vaccination, in particular following alarm about the MMR – measles, mumps and rubella – vaccine in 1998, led to lower levels of compliance and a rise in measles and mumps in young children eligible for the vaccine. Food-related diseases, as vividly demonstrated in the late 1980s in Britain by the salmonella scare surrounding eggs or by the alarm generated by bovine spongiform encephalopathy (BSE), raised difficult questions about food safety. Alarm over the escalation of untreatable infections, made visible by the appearance of Methicillin-resistant staphylococcus aureus (MRSA) or the superbug eroded faith in medicine's ability to eradicate infections.

Acquired Immune Deficiency Syndrome (AIDS) was the most visible and far-reaching of these emerging diseases. Although AIDS was probably circulating in the 1970s, it was identified in the United States in 1981, appearing at a time when Western countries felt confident that they had surmounted the major infectious diseases. AIDS, spread through sexual intercourse and through blood, was quickly associated with the homosexual community, recipients of blood transfusions, and intravenous drug users, although it was homosexuality that dominated representations of AIDS. By 1983, French researchers had identified the Human Immunodeficiency Virus (HIV) responsible, and by the 1990s, HIV/AIDS had become pandemic, promoting something near panic in many industrialized countries. The West responded with a massive research programme, expensive drug therapies, and a range of public health responses – including a large number of poster campaigns – which raised questions about the balance between civil liberties and community interest.

If the development of drug therapies in the twenty first century saw AIDS reconfigured as a chronic disease, a different picture existed in Africa, Southeast

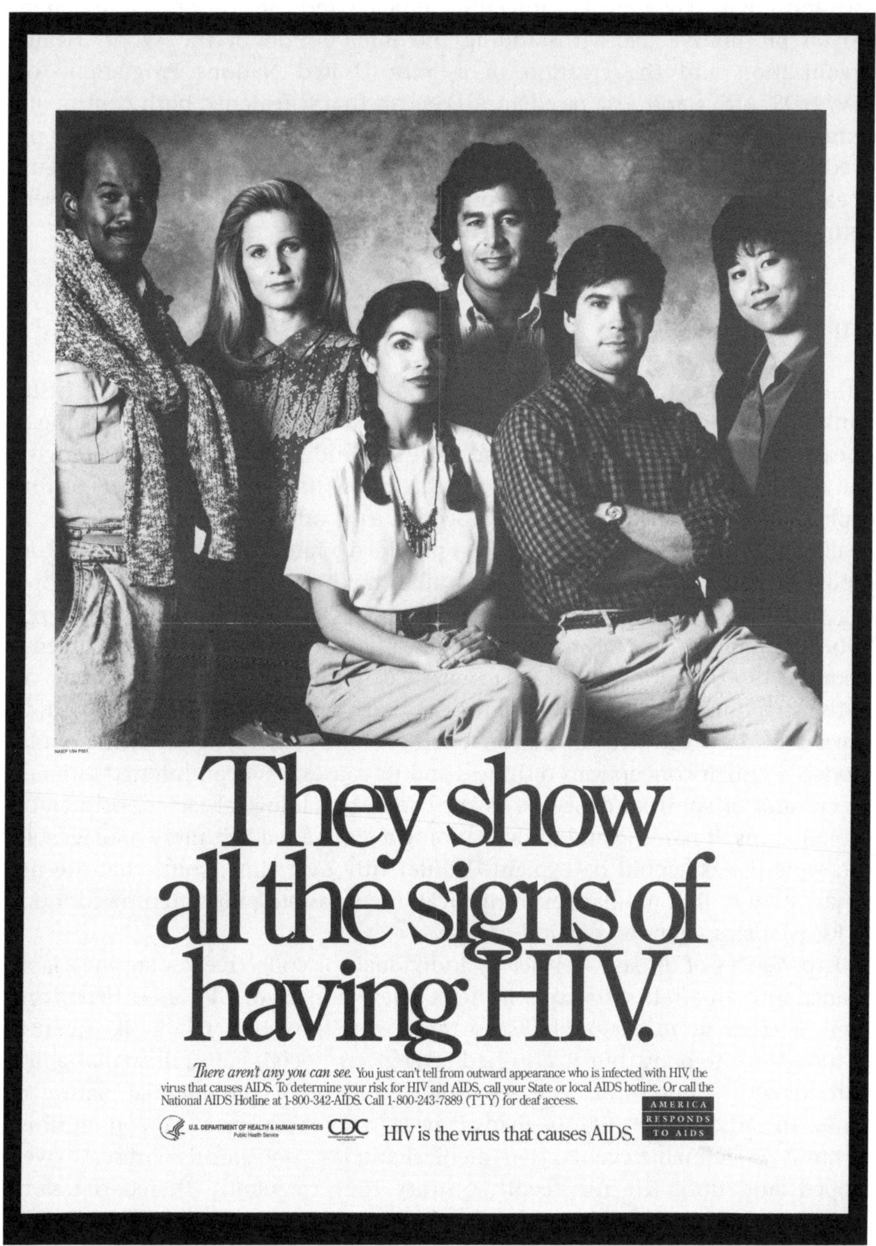

Figure 2.3 Poster produced as part of the United States AIDS campaign warning about the invisible signs of HIV, 1994.

Source: Wellcome Library, London.

Asia and Russia. Here rates of infection spiralled and the cost of drug therapies proved prohibitive. Notwithstanding the intervention of the World Health Organization and the creation of a Joint United Nations Programme on HIV/AIDS, Africa and Asia faced an AIDS crisis that threatened both continents' demographic and economic stability. By 2009, the fact that 33 million people lived with HIV/AIDS worldwide is a vivid example of the effects of emerging diseases. When thinking about the broad trend of mortality decline in the twentieth century, it is important to consider these experiences.

Explaining illness

Although it is hard to escape from our own medicalized views of disease, historians have become more sensitive to how medical and popular understanding of disease was shaped by historical and cultural conditions. Work by sociologists and cultural anthropologists has highlighted how the need for sufferers to find explanations for illness is deeply embedded as it offered some control over ill health. Although early modern doctors provided a range of shifting explanatory models for illness, the sick and their families not only domesticated this knowledge, but also put forward their own explanations that reflected an avid interest in health and disease. Nor was this just an early modern phenomenon. Evidence from the 1960s demonstrates how for many common ailments the 'average man in the street' used a range of explanations that shared boundaries with medical views and drew on ideas of personal responsibility and longstanding popular models. Popular conceptions of illness and its causes were conditioned as much by cultural or spiritual concerns as they were by biological factors or medical explanations. If naming and understanding a disease made it more manageable, the same disease could be explained differently over time; shifts that are not always easy to link to changes in medical understanding but often owed much to ideas of class, gender, religion or race.

Experiences of disease – either by individuals or collectively – are invariably shaped into a narrative to explain them. These narratives allowed sufferers and their doctors to understand disease and why they had fallen ill. Sickness occurred in the body, but it also had a religious, social, cultural, spatial and a chronological dimension. The seemingly random or providential nature of illness in early modern Europe made it necessary for sufferers and communities to pin it on definable events. Here medical and lay conceptions of disease overlapped, and until the nineteenth century they frequently shared the same language to explain the onset of sickness. Disease was invariably represented as an active force that assaulted the body and it was believed that the most trivial of events could trigger illness. There was a point however. By blaming disease on specific events, it was given meaning.

Galenic or humoral views of the body dominated ideas of disease in early modern Europe even if popular understanding used the vaguer concept of flow-ing fluids. The body was believed to consist of four humors of different qualities – cold, hot, moist and dry. Each individual had their own balance that affected their physical and mental makeup. Disease was the result of an imbalance, either a build-up (*plethora*) or deficiency of humors. This could occur naturally or be affected by other factors – or non-naturals – such as food, drink, sleep, work or weather. A wide range of diseases from the mild to the serious could therefore emanate from the same cause or imbalance. Even minor changes could bring about sickness, making prevention as important as treatment.

In popular and medical thought weather, geography and environment offered durable explanations for disease and explained why certain locations were more prone to disease. Well into the nineteenth century, miasmas or bad air was widely associated with sickness and with epidemics. Places like marshes or wet low-lying areas were closely linked to fevers. Hot and cold winds could bring different types of disease, as did extremes of temperature, with the latter contributing to a literature that stressed the debilitating and dangerous effects of hot climates [see 'Medicine and empire']. Sudden changes in temperature were enough to bring on illness: in women it was believed that a chill might cause sickness or a miscarriage. But the environment had a far wider effect. By the late eighteenth century, urban environments and modern living were felt to cause a range of physical, psychological and moral disorders. With many of the poor living in unsanitary conditions, it should be no surprise that many understood disease in these terms. These ideas found resonance in *fin de siècle* fears about degeneration and the role of the urban environment in creating a sickly, stunted and scrawny poor as a race apart, and were given further form in eugenicist movements of the first half of the twentieth century [see 'Public health'].

Sickness did not come by chance, however. Ideas about the laws of health emphasized how the burden of ill health rested with the individual. Lifestyle was crucial: eating too much, drinking too much, not exercising enough, or wearing the wrong clothes were all considered contributing factors to making an individual sick. In the eighteenth century, a large body of writing emphasized the dangers of luxurious lifestyles and modern living, ideas that were used to explain high urban mortality. However, although personal behaviour was important, Christian and supernatural explanations were used to make sense of illness. As explained in the next chapter, many people in early modern Europe understood that a connection existed between the health of the body and that of the soul. Disease could hence be understood as the result of God's wrath, either to punish human weakness or as a trial of faith, or was the work of the Devil. Nor did these explanations suddenly disappear. Magical and religious explanations and cures persisted in the nineteenth century, especially for those ailments that could not be easily understood.

This idea of blame is an important component in explaining the onset of illness. Blame could be personal – the result of individual actions or neglect. At a prosaic level, individuals blamed disease on not wearing the right clothing or going out in bad weather. For example, in 1808 the poet Samuel Taylor Coleridge attributed his inflammation of the bowels to the wet newspaper he had been reading and the damp street. In the twentieth century, ideas of personal responsibility were enshrined in public health education, which called for individuals to avoid risky behaviours. Yet, blame was also directed at particular groups or even nations. Outbreaks of plague in the sixteenth and seventeenth century, for example, were blamed on the arrival of diseased individuals or beggars. Different groups (ethnic and religious) were branded as disease carriers. Jews, for example, were held responsible in the Renaissance for spreading the plague; Africans were accused of spreading AIDS in the twentieth century. Ideas of blame were incorporated into disease names. Sixteenth century physicians used a variety of labels for the pox – Spanish or French, for example – which associated the disease with their neighbours or enemies. Nor did this sense of blame and responsibility stop at one generation. Popular ideas of heredity in the eighteenth and nineteenth centuries saw the sins of parents visited upon their children to produce hereditary 'taints'.

By the end of the nineteenth century, a new language of disease influenced by the ideas associated with germ theories began to enter popular understanding [see 'Medicine and science']. An awareness of the role of germs was aided by public health campaigns and by the growth of commercial disinfectants and over-the-counter medicine. Although germs offered a new language for understanding disease, other terms were translated from the laboratory as references were made to bacteria and viruses and later to hormones and genes. However, the extent to which these ideas permeated popular explanations for disease should not be exaggerated. Evidence from letters, diaries and oral histories suggests that an understanding of germs was not as important to many individuals as more traditional explanations, which associated the onset of illness with behaviour (including poor diet and not enough fresh air or exercise) or the environment as reflected in twentieth century debates about AIDS.

By appreciating the shifting range of explanations for how diseases and sickness were understood in the past, historians have become sensitive to the range of approaches the sick and their doctors adopted to treat disease. Humoral views, for example, encouraged sufferers to expel excess humors through bleeding and purging. The fact that patients in the nineteenth and twentieth centuries attributed illness to environmental factors, such as damp living conditions, eating the wrong food, etc., further shows how traditional ideas continued to resonate. When it came to understanding disease, medicine did not always have the same answers as the public.

Cultural meanings and metaphors

As the above section has started to illustrate, definitions of the normal and the pathological were determined by medical, social and cultural values. It was only by naming and responding to a disease that it was understood or framed, but this framing was more than just crude biologism. Disease was infused with cultural meanings. Although a social constructivist approach remains controversial, historians have come to accept the idea that disease could be a form of social description that reinforced stereotypes or encouraged victim blaming [see 'Historiography'].

The idea that outward symptoms reflected inner states has proved an enduring one in how contemporaries over the last five hundred years have represented and understood disease. Physical and moral infection were often conflated in the past and certain diseases were stigmatized or associated with degeneracy. The persisting resonance of religious interpretations of disease into the twentieth century associated illness with sin. Plague and other infectious diseases provided an ample repertoire of images for national sin, but more often disease was a metaphor for individual sin. Syphilis was viewed as the embodiment of the wages of sin, while gout or jaundice was associated with drinking too much. Disease might therefore be a symbol of misdeed or certain types of behaviour. In the eighteenth and nineteenth centuries, these ideas about behaviour and disease were reconfigured but not rejected. For example, diabetes was attributed to a sedentary life and overindulgence, epilepsy to habitual masturbation and alcoholism. Disease labels were applied to behaviour, such as masturbation, and to social or racial groups, which were perceived to be deviant or a threat to society. This framing of disease also extended to other types of behaviour. For example, if in the eighteenth century the tight lacing of corsets was believed to condemn women's intestines to disorder, the fashions that followed saw medical practitioners point to growing levels of chest complaints in women. Disease has therefore been readily associated in the past with particular character types, groups, activities and even dress, not only in the popular imagination but also in medicine as medical practitioners drew on a range of moral and social explanations. Nor did these associations disappear in the twentieth century. Sexual and racial theories continued to be used throughout the twentieth century, as evident in how HIV/AIDS was represented, but also in how sickle cell anaemia was racialized.

Disease was also used as a language of social description and was employed in discussions about the state of society or particular issues. Venereal disease was used satirically in anticlerical rhetoric in the sixteenth century, while eighteenth century fears about the spread of atheism were reflected in a language that compared it to plague. Ideas of a sick society featured in the philosophical writings of Thomas Carlyle and Friedrich Nietzsche and in the language of eugenics. If in Weimar Germany (1919–33) ideas of health and sickness were widely used when discussing the defeat of 1918, Camus in *La Peste* (1947) used the plague-torn Algerian city of Oran as a metaphoric treatment of the French resistance to Nazi occupation. Defining nations, economies or particular groups as sick and in need of cure provided a way of arguing for or against specific policies. Connections between social and biological disorders have therefore been an integral part of political, cultural and social representations of disease over the last five hundred years, giving particular diseases meanings beyond their biological manifestations.

Attitudes to health

At least until the late nineteenth century, anxiety about health was present in many contemporary memoirs and diaries. Although health was often seen as something unobtainable, disease was recognized as an ever-present reality. It was to be endured, but this did not mean that sufferers in the past were indifferent or stoic. Health was actively pursued. For the poor, the seriousness of being deprived of work encouraged them to ignore disease or cope with ill health in the best way possible. If, as Chapter 5 demonstrates, this meant that many resorted to any means available that promised a cure or relief, it also saw the chronic sick and disabled adapting their life and work around their infirmities in an attempt to maintain independence or from necessity. Others, particularly the middling orders, became obsessed with health – their own, their neighbour's, and society's. Concerned observers at the start of the eighteenth century feared that hypochondria had become widespread. Newspaper reports on outbreaks of plague in eighteenth century France saw many work themselves into a frenzy, and a growing popular and medical literature convinced some that they were susceptible to disease. Throughout the nineteenth century, a morbid interest was expressed in all things health related, even when the subject matter was condemned as prurient.

Numerous popular and medical manuals, as well as newspapers and periodicals, fuelled this concern about health and offered practical advice on how to attain and maintain health. A humoral understanding of disease causation asserted the importance of regimen, which outlined rules for the conduct of everyday life and the maintenance of the bodily constitution. Much of this advice was active, often drawing on traditional folk practices and Christian belief, and stressed moderation in all things. Temperance in diet and alcohol consumption was recommended, along with rest, exercise and morality. By the 1860s, such advice also included sexual continence and by the end of the century extended to beauty tips in girls' magazines. Proprietors of patent medicines actively exploited such concerns [see 'Self-help']. However, although individuals received health advice from all sides and had a personal responsibility to maintain their health, good health was often considered an unexpected bonus.

Only by the end of the nineteenth century did health begin to be considered a normal state. Notions of health, fitness and beauty became associated with modernism and a state of physical, mental and social wellbeing. Emphasis was placed on promoting health as a national and moral duty as anxiety was expressed about the health of city dwellers – fears that fed into a series of movements concerned with national renewal and into a range of commercial interests from Kelloggs to the exploitation of bodybuilding. Many drew on fears of degeneration and eugenicist ideas associated with physical and moral improvement and a holistic understanding that also found expression in public health campaigns [see 'Public health']. These ideas were not just expressed in Nazi Germany (1933–45) or Fascist Italy (1922–43) but across Europe. For example, in Greece commentators noted the educative and moral benefits of athletic exercises following the first Olympic Games in 1896. Food reform movements, such as vegetarianism, dietary fads, physical education and sport were promoted. Fashions were revised to encourage healthy bodies and there was a boom in self-help and baby-care manuals. Daily exercise became vital to keeping the body in good working order, and in France and Britain numerous organizations to promote hiking, youth hostelling and other outdoor pursuits were established to encourage the development of young healthy bodies. This emphasis on exercise was gendered. If men and boys were to take part in team games, athletics and gymnastics, women were targeted in campaigns to promote the values of a hygienic home to combat the spread of disease. Hygiene, nutrition, domestic upkeep and work were all represented as crucial to healthy individuals and nations.

As mortality in Western Europe declined in the second half of the twentieth century, expectations of health increased and the promotion of health became an important social and political goal of post-industrial welfare societies. Although a new generation came to take health and access to healthcare for granted, anxieties about ill health intensified. For some commentators this preoccupation pointed to a growing culture of alarm, fuelled by the media and the rise of the 'worried well'. For others, it was an indication of the medicalization of society. Perceptions of what constituted health and ill health changed, as did the understanding of risk and disease. Renewed emphasis was placed on individual responsibility for maintaining a healthy lifestyle, a message that sat uneasily with rising affluence and an increase in lifestyle diseases such as obesity. By the twenty first century, media coverage of diets, exercise and healthy lifestyles and the leisure and pharmaceutical industries were encouraging Europeans to eat well, take vitamins and be healthy. However, as the above section has shown, these concerns about health and lifestyle need to be seen as part of a much longer European concern with health and disease.

Illness and gender

Whereas wealth, occupation and location shaped illness so too did gender, and poor health has been seen as a feature of many women's lives in the past. If for the most part women suffered from the same range of everyday complaints as men, as discussed in chapter four, pregnancy and childbirth accounted for a wide range of minor and serious medical conditions in women until the mid twentieth century. Many of the resulting ailments were accommodated as part of women's daily lives as economic, cultural and political constraints prevented them from giving in to sickness or gaining access to medical care. The growing use of birth control from the 1870s helped cut the birth rate, but in the 1930s many British women found that the drudgery of housekeeping, childbirth and inadequate medical care ensured that maintaining health was a struggle.

There was more to the relationship between health and gender than experiences of sickness based around pregnancy and childbirth. The idea that women were generally more often ill than men was repeatedly asserted from the seventeenth century onwards. As Chapter 4 explains, doctors were certain that women were driven by their reproductive cycle, and associated their biology with weakness, debility and sickness to create a stereotype of the delicate female that many historians have found appealing. Menstruating girls and women were perceived as ill and vulnerable. Puberty was considered a perilous time – it was felt that as emerging women, girls were susceptible to numerous diseases, a view reinforced in contemporary literature and magazines. The idea that different illnesses had different manifestations in men and women was accepted in the seventeenth and early eighteenth centuries along with the idea that women, because of their leaky and moist natures, were more susceptible to certain diseases (such as smallpox) than men. In the nineteenth century, certain diseases were labelled female maladies like chlorosis (also known as 'green sickness' and associated with anaemia), while women were believed to be prone to others, such as tuberculosis. This perceived pathological weakness assisted in the social and cultural construction of gender roles, while women were blamed for high levels of ill health. Whereas women were seen as spreading certain diseases, particularly venereal disease, at a more general level they were held responsible for maintaining the health of the family.

Yet disease need not always be debilitating. The sociologist Talcott Parsons first proposed the idea of the sick role in *The Social System* (1951). He argued that the occupant of the sick role was exempt from responsibility for their incapacity and normal social obligations relative to the nature and severity of the illness. Although Parsons put forward an abstract model, the idea of the sick role has been used by historians and literary critics, particularly in relation to ideas of gender, illness and empowerment, to understand how sickness could be used by individuals. Given that women until the mid twentieth century were constantly told of their predisposition to sickness, some women made use of their illness or perceived disability. By thinking in these terms, hysteria can be characterized as a subconscious way of expressing discontent or anger; anorexia as an expression of powerlessness. Some women appeared to have mimicked sickness to escape their duties, but the sick role could also give individuals power and the ability to control and regulate visitors. It gave privacy and a degree of authority as shown in the English social theorist Harriet Martineau's work, *Life in the sick-room, or, essays by an invalid* (1844). In adopting a sick role, women were placed under a medical diagnosis that allowed them to dominate the household and freed them from the obligations of family life or the sexual advances of their husbands. Illness was one way of escaping restraints. Gender then was important in shaping both the experiences of disease and the understanding of sickness, but as the above discussion of the sick role indicates, disease need not always be disabling.

Conclusions

Many contemporaries from the sixteenth to the early twentieth century, along with the worried well in the twenty first century, would agree with the English poet Keats that 'Everybody is ill'. By thinking in these terms it is possible to see how there was more to disease in the past than epidemics or changing patterns of mortality. Disease, sickness and illness are not straightforward concepts that are easily quantifiable. Mortality rates and epidemics can only tell historians part of the story as outside of epidemic years many continued to face everyday ailments, as well as the dangers of infectious diseases, accidents, and diseases associated with work or living conditions. Illness was often subjective and even everyday illnesses were liable to a range of meanings. Disease was not therefore just a biological entity: it served a number of functions from labelling behaviours or groups as deviant through to giving some individuals a form of power or in other cases an identity.

Further reading

There are few overviews of health, sickness and mortality, but *Disease and the Modern World: 1500 to the Present Day* (London: Polity Press, 2004) by Mark Harrison places disease in an international perspective. Kenneth Kiple (ed.), *The Cambridge World History of Human Disease* (Cambridge: Cambridge University Press, 1993) offers clear histories of individual diseases, while the *Encyclopaedia of Plague and Pestilence from Ancient Times to the Present* (New York: Facts on File Inc, 2001) edited by George Kohn describes the major epidemics. Readers interested in social constructionism should start with Ludmilla Jordanova, 'The Social Construction of Medical Knowledge', *Social History of Medicine* 8 (1995), pp. 361–81. Susan Sontag, *Illness as Metaphor and AIDS and its Metaphors* (London: Penguin Classics, 2009) and Sander Gilman in *Disease and Representation: Images of Illness from Madness to AIDS* (Ithaca, NY: Cornell University Press, 1988) which explore ideas of representation in different ways, with Margaret Healy, *Fictions of Disease in Early-modern England: Bodies, Plagues and Politics* (Basingstoke: Palgrave Macmillan, 2001) concentrating on plagues. For an understanding of disease in early modern Europe, see the chapter on sickness and health in Mary Lindemann's excellent *Medicine and Society in Early Modern Europe,* 2010 edn (Cambridge: Cambridge University Press, 2010) and Mary Dobson, *Contours of Death and Disease in Early Modern England* (Cambridge: Cambridge University Press, 2003). The best studies of plague include Paul Slack, *The Impact of the Plague in Tudor and Stuart England* (Oxford: Clarendon Press, 1990), Ann Carmichael, *Plague and the Poor in Renaissance Florence* (Cambridge: Cambridge University Press, 1986), and John Alexander, *Bubonic Plague in Early Modern Russia* (Oxford: Oxford University Press, 2003). On explanations for mortality decline readers should start with Simon Szreter's groundbreaking 'The Importance of Social Intervention in Britain's Mortality Decline, c.1850–1914: A Reinterpretation of the Role of Public Health', *Social History of Medicine* 1 (1988), pp. 1–37, or Alex Mercer, *Disease, Mortality and Population in Transition* (London and New York: Continuum, 1990) and James Riley, *Rising Life Expectancy: A Global History* (Cambridge: Cambridge University Press, 2001). Among the best studies which deal with a range of epidemic and endemic diseases (and the responses to them) are Terence Ranger and Paul Slack (eds), *Epidemics and Ideas: Essays on the Historical Perception of Pestilence* (Cambridge: Cambridge University Press, 1995), Anne Hardy, *The Epidemic Streets: Infectious Diseases and the Rise of Preventive Medicine, 1856–1900* (Oxford: Clarendon Press, 1993), and Peter Baldwin, *Contagion and the State in Europe, 1830–1930* (Cambridge: Cambridge University Press, 2005). Whereas Roy Porter's 'The Patient's View: Doing Medical History from Below', *Theory and Society* 14 (1985), pp. 175–98, shows the value of looking at the patient's perspective – this approach is adopted in Lucinda Beier, *Sufferers and Healers: The Experience of Illness in Seventeenth-Century England* (London: Routledge, 1987) and Roy Porter and Dorothy Porter, *In Sickness and in Health: The British Experience 1650–1850* (London: Fourth Estate, 1988). On the day-to-day experiences of sickness, James Riley, *Sick, not Dead: The Health of British Workingmen during the Mortality Decline* (Baltimore, MD: Johns Hopkins University Press, 1997) offers a good starting point. On work and health, see Paul Weindling (ed.), *The Social History of Occupational Health* (London: Routledge, 1985) or Roger Cooter and Bill Luckin (eds), *Accidents in History: Injuries, Fatalities and Social Relations* (Amsterdam: Rodopi, 1997). There is a diverse literature on popular views of sickness, with Athena Vrettos, *Somatic Fictions: Imagining Illness in Victorian Culture* (Stanford, CA: Stanford University Press, 1995) and Janis McLarren Caldwell, *Literature and Medicine in Nineteenth-Century Britain* (Cambridge: Cambridge University Press, 2004) approaching illness through literary representations. Degeneration and eugenics have an extensive literature and those interested should look at the Further Reading for Chapter 12. Individual diseases have their own histories. For the impact of the 'pox', see Jon Arrizabalaga, John Henderson and Roger French, *The Great Pox: The French Disease in Renaissance Europe* (New Haven and London: Yale University Press, 1997) and on venereal disease more generally Linda Merians (ed.), *The Secret Malady: Venereal Disease in Eighteenth-Century Britain and France* (Lexington, KT: University Press of Kentucky, 1996) and Roger Davidson and Lesley Hall (eds), *Sex, Sin and Suffering: Venereal Disease and European Society Since 1870* (London: Routledge, 2001). On cholera, Christopher Hamlin's *Cholera: The Bibliography* (Oxford: Oxford University Press, 2009) draws together the experiences from various countries, while Richard Evans' influential *Death in Hamburg: Society and Politics in the Cholera Years, 1830–1910* (London: Penguin, 1991) provides a more detailed examination. On the 1918–19 influenza pandemic, see Howard Phillips and David Killingray (eds), *The Spanish Influenza Pandemic of 1918* (London: Routledge, 2003), while for tuberculosis David Barnes, *The Making of a Social Disease: Tuberculosis in Nineteenth-Century France* (Berkeley and London: University of California Press, 1995) and Linda Bryder, *Below the Magic Mountain: A Social History of Tuberculosis in Twentieth-Century Britain* (Oxford: Clarendon Press, 1988) offer excellent social histories. There is a growing historical literature on AIDS, with Mirko Grmek, Russell Maulitz and Jacalyn Duffin, *History of AIDS: Emergence and Origin of a Modern Pandemic* (Princeton, NJ: Princeton University Press, 1992) and Virginia Berridge and Philip Strong (eds), *AIDS and Contemporary History* (Cambridge: Cambridge University Press, 2002) offering good starting points along with Peter Baldwin's comparative *Disease and Democracy: The Industrialized World Faces Aids* (Berkeley and London: University of California Press, 2005). For books related to miasmas and environmental explanations of disease, see the Further Reading for Chapter 12, while for colonialism and disease see the Further Reading for Chapter 14.

3
Medicine and religion

Christianity was a healing religion and the Christian requirement to aid the sick and the afflicted was embedded in European culture. If in early modern Europe sickness and suffering were intimately bound up with Christian beliefs, medical historians have often been more interested in professionalization or in the transformation of hospitals from pious to clinical institutions than in the relationship between religion and medicine. When Christian beliefs or the medical work of religious orders has been examined, their relationship with medicine has often been represented in essentialist terms of conflict or harmony or secularization. Such an approach has emphasized how the Enlightenment (eighteenth century) ushered in a new faith in reason that resulted in an inevitable conflict between religion and science with the ultimate triumph of secular medicine. This rather traditional reading has been supplanted. New scholarship on the sixteenth and seventeenth centuries has revealed the connections between theology, politics, science and medicine and the ongoing significance of Christian beliefs to attitudes to disease and in shaping medical knowledge and healthcare. Insights into the medical marketplace have shown how witchcraft, religious healing and superstition were all part of the early modern medical landscape [see 'Self-help']. The idea that secularization was an inevitable consequence of modernization is equally problematic, concealing as it does how religious and supernatural beliefs were part of how the world was understood. Rather than arguing the merits of sharp contrasts between an 'Age of Faith' and an 'Age of Reason', this chapter argues that if the contribution of religion to medicine shifted between the Reformation and the twentieth century, it should not be undervalued.

Theology and medicine in early modern Europe

Christianity was so embedded in early modern European culture that it formed an everyday part of how life, the body and health were understood. Until the sixteenth century, there was little obvious conflict between Christianity and medicine, or between magic and religion. Religious and medical practices rested on similar assumptions that supernatural forces influenced nature. Christian beliefs explained why disease occurred and how it was healed. These beliefs shaped interpretations of sickness, which medical attendants were to be

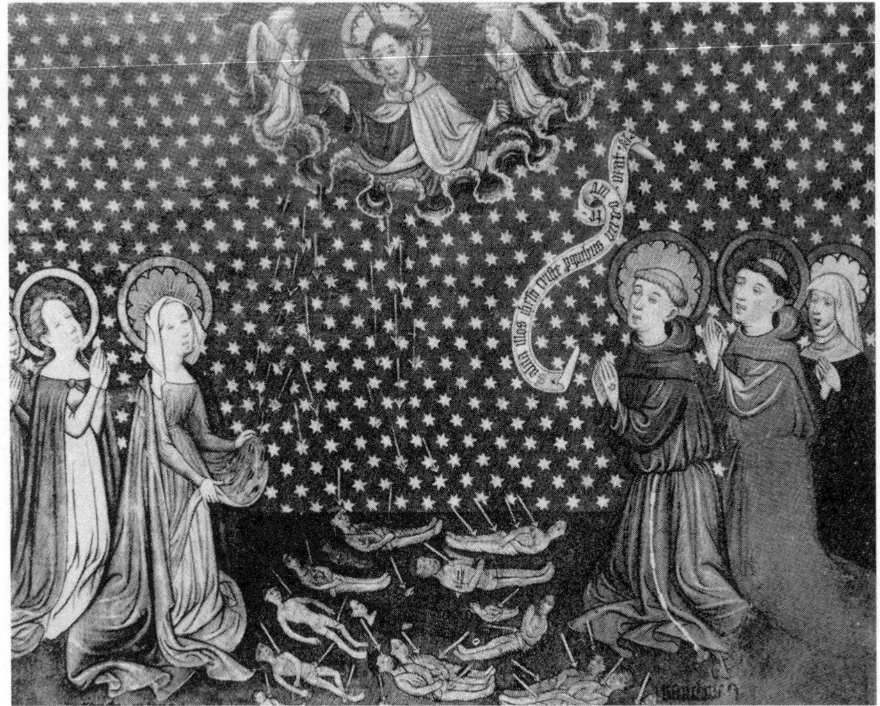

Figure 3.1 Altarpiece in which Christ throws down arrows (of plague) and saints intercede, commissioned for the Carmelites of Göttingen, 1424.
Source: Wellcome Library, London.

consulted and what behaviour should be adopted in the sickroom. Within this Christian framework, health and illness were viewed as God-sent as a gift, test or warning as seen in the altarpiece commissioned for the Carmelites of Gottingen. Clerics were keen to show sickness had a spiritual function and profound connections were made between the health of the body and that of the soul. If not all diseases were the result of individual sin, diseases, such as leprosy or plague, were shown as punishments for individual transgression or as a sign of moral failure, either on the part of the individual or in the case of plague as a warning to the nation to repent. Illness with its connotations of bodily corruption became a metaphor for sin [see 'Disease'].

Although disease was sent by God, this did not prevent people from seeking, and being advised to seek a cure. Church leaders drew on the image of Christ the Physician and medical metaphors in their teachings. Clerics stressed that people had a duty to care for their bodies because it was the temporal home of the soul. They explained how medicine was divinely ordained for this purpose. The clergy hence emphasized the importance of prayer and penitence to healing and encouraged the godly to consult learned and pious medical practitioners. Doctors were expected to recognize that they were the servants of divine will, but in return, Christian teaching provided medicine with legitimacy. If the connections between the soul's and body's health were 'medicalized', physicians stressed the close affinity between saving souls and healing bodies.

God was therefore the source of the disease, medicine and the outcome of treatment as the miraculous and the mundane, the theological and the material existed on the same continuum. Many sufferers moved easily between prayer and medical cures. For example, when plague arrived in Milan in the 1570s penitential processions and public prayers were held alongside efforts by the health magistracy to limit infection. Tensions might exist between spiritual and administrative responses to disease, but the laity readily mixed different types of care available from a range of healers with domestic medicine and religious healing. This covered a multitude of practices from invoking saints to magic, along with prayers, pilgrimages and supplications to treat or prevent disease. Certain saints were associated with particular disorders and were credited with healing powers; for example, women in childbirth called on St Anne, while those afflicted with plague could invoke St Sebastian or St Antony.

Just as God could send disease, so too did demons and witches. The idea that benevolent and malevolent forces shaped peoples' lives was widely accepted in early modern Europe. Rather than acting supernaturally – only God could do this – it was believed that witches and demons manipulated the occult powers of nature to cause sickness. The view that contemporaries turned to demonic explanations when no other causes could be determined has been replaced by an analysis that highlights how demonology, popular belief and medicine often overlapped. Physicians were expected to know the difference between the natural and the demonic, and the sick had to consider the possibility that individual ailments might be the result of witchcraft or demonic intervention. Since demons acted through natural causes, when magic or demonic possession were identified physicians either used natural cures or advised patients to visit the priest for sacramental remedies.

Reformation and post-Reformation medicine

The Reformation has traditionally been perceived to mark a break with these ideas and the beginning of the secularization of medicine. Seen as a sixteenth century movement for reform of the doctrines and practices of the Catholic Church, the starting point of the Reformation is often given as 1517 when the German theologian Martin Luther launched his protest against the corruption of the papacy. The Reformation signalled a reorientation of attitudes towards belief and worship and broad cultural changes that altered the relationship between the human and the divine, undermining popular religion and threatening social stability. In the 1990s, historians began to argue that there was no single process of reform but a series of Reformations. In Switzerland, for example, Calvin moulded reformist opinion into a more explicitly doctrinal and revolutionary theology and Calvinism became the driving force of the Reformation in western Germany, France, the Netherlands and Scotland, where it was linked to political struggle. In England, the Reformation was a more halting and insular process. In Southern Europe, the Catholic Church underwent its own reformation or Counter-Reformation. Modernizing changes were made: the papacy retreated from claiming the special healing powers of the clergy but reaffirmed traditional beliefs and practices.

The Reformation was not just a religious phenomenon that culminated in the emergence of Protestantism. It affected all aspects of sixteenth and seventeenth century European life: it gave expression to socioeconomic grievances and saw cultural chaos, persecution, migration, wars and widespread change, including an erosion of the role of the Church in healing, particularly in Northern Europe where Protestant views were strongest, along with bitter disputes between rival medical systems. Protestants' condemnation of the miraculous powers of the clergy and a range of superstitious practices has been represented as a crucial cultural development that transformed the relationship between religion and healing; a transformation associated with increasing secularization, the decline of magic and rise of science.

However, whereas the Reformation disrupted existing patterns of popular belief and religious observance, and saw new medical and scientific explanations put forward, the outcomes of the Reformation were complex and ambiguous. Reform was not sweeping or, as the Counter-Reformation demonstrates, characteristic of one side of the religious divide. New patterns of belief took time to establish and Christian doctrine remained the dominant way of understanding the world in the sixteenth and seventeenth centuries. As scholars came to accept that early modern science was eclectic and that the Reformation did not usher in a neat rejection of earlier ideas, they pointed to the constructive influence of theological ideas on science. Charles Webster in the *Great Instauration* (1975) provided not only the classic work on the seventeenth century political and scientific revolution but also revealed how theological ideas continued to inform how medical knowledge was generated and received. Here the work of the Swiss-born Paracelsus – Theophrastus von Hohenheim – is significant, not only in terms of his influence on medicine, but also for understanding how theology remained integral to medical debates in the sixteenth and seventeenth centuries.

Paracelsus was not a medical outsider. The son of a physician, from whom he received his early training in medicine and alchemy, Paracelsus studied for a time in Italy before travelling throughout Europe collecting information on folk medicine and visiting the centres of traditional (or Classical) Galenic medicine at Paris, Montpellier and Salerno. He spent time in Salzburg and Strasbourg as a physician and held a faculty appointment at Basle. Here Paracelsus so outraged his colleagues by burning revered medical texts and by admitting Barber-Surgeons to his lectures that he was forced to flee in 1528. Thereafter, he wandered through Central Europe as an itinerant practitioner vigorously extolling his views about the universe, man and the nature of disease. His ideas were part of a broad coalition of sixteenth century religious reforms and a major force in encouraging a rejection of Aristotelian-Galenic medicine in favour of a system based on chemical principles. Paracelsus questioned the miraculous powers of saints in his attacks on the evils he associated with ceremonies and idolatry, a view reflected in Calvin's writings. For Paracelsus the common people attributed their diseases to the influence of saints because they had been deceived by clerics and were ignorant of chemical and pathological processes. As part of his skilful blend of medicine and anticlerical and social propaganda, he sought to reveal that the cure for diseases rested not in the manifestations of witchcraft or in the work of saints but in natural and chemical agents. Others followed and took a stand against magical remedies.

The Reformation did not just see new ideas about medicine emerge. It also challenged the learned tradition of medicine that was transmitted through text-based medicine and a philosophical interpretation of Classical views of the body that had dominated medieval medicine. If the idea that the Protestant Church was a liberal supporter of new knowledge does not hold up to scrutiny but was rather small, weak and divided, those doctors influenced by Protestant ideas were suspicious of priests' monopoly of knowledge. Attacks on miraculous healing were useful for physicians. They bolstered their claims to authority and supported their attacks on healers who claimed divine powers and clerics who practised medicine. If nature and the physical universe continued to be understood within a Christian framework, Protestant doctors also started to question older beliefs and began to look at Classical writings in new ways. Paracelsus's religion of medicine, with its emphasis on nature and chemistry, offered a different approach to conceptualizing disease. Paracelsians asserted the value of chemical remedies, or iatrochemistry, and contributed to the decline of Galenic medicine in the late seventeenth century.

These ideas did not spread uniformly across Europe, however. Whereas sanitized versions of Paracelsian medicine were introduced into the medical faculties of some Protestant universities, such as the University of Copenhagen, in Catholic countries its associations with unorthodox (or heterodox) ideas generated opposition. For Catholics there was a clear connection between the new heresy of the reformers and novelties in medicine and philosophy. In Spain, for example, many doctors viewed the new doctrines coming out of the German states, England and Holland with suspicion. The Counter-Reformation affected medicine in Southern and Central Europe in other ways. Portuguese physicians stressed their religiosity and rejected foreign criticism of their conservative Jesuit-influenced medicine. The Inquisition worked to stamp out heresy and was particularly worried about the social influence of heretical physicians. Books by Protestant doctors were included in the *Index Librorum Prohibitorum* (Index of Prohibited Books), circulated in 1559, and traditional medical ideas were defended. Some doctors in Southern and Central Europe used the Inquisition for

their own ends to drive out unlicensed healers or to denounce competing Protestant doctors.

As can be seen from the above, medicine was not suddenly divorced from religion in the sixteenth century. Early modern medical beliefs were eclectic: medical, magical and theological explanations overlapped and the body became a battleground between natural, divine and diabolical interpretations of disease. This ongoing connection between medicine and religion is evident in the work of Luther, Paracelsus, and in the ideas associated with the physician Francis Mercurius van Helmont. For example, Luther argued for a close affinity between theology and medicine. He believed that in the work of physicians and apothecaries it was possible to discern parables of God's spiritual therapy. In doing so, Luther reinforced traditional Christian practices whereby patients should pray to God and confess their sins before consulting a physician since in his view illness was often the result of sin. This medicinal theology attracted a wide following.

It would be easy to assume that the ferment of ideas often associated with what has been labelled the Scientific Revolution of the seventeenth century and its mathematical treatment and empirical approach to natural phenomena encouraged a rejection of the religious and supernatural explanations of diseases. Within this framework, religion and science are often seen in stark conflict. However, in many ways, contemporaries viewed religion and science (or natural philosophy) as separate-but-equal. Science and theology shared the same cultural and intellectual heritage during the seventeenth century and Christianity remained central to the lives of many doctors and natural philosophers. Few were prepared to deny that the natural world was not divinely created or that sin had a pathogenic effect on the body. Preachers did not see their comments on medicine as controversial, while many medical practitioners believed their investigations were part of a wider examination of the nature of the divine. If natural philosophers strove to find physical explanations for how the world and the body worked, the boundaries between what we might label the scientific aspects of their work and the theological ones were often blurred. Theological concepts (Jewish and Christian, Roman and Reformation) had a direct bearing on the philosophies implicit in the sciences that were emerging as a result of increased lay participation in theology and the scientific study of nature. Questions about the inner workings of man familiar to theologians were reflected in mechanical philosophy – a way of explaining all physical properties and processes in terms of the motion of the smallest parts that composed physical bodies. Although mechanical philosophers rejected Aristotelian philosophy, which emphasized the universal, and most of the mystical elements associated with Renaissance naturalism, rather than dismissing theological questions, they appropriated theological ideas and used them to solve problems in new contexts. The competing medical philosophies put forward in the seventeenth century hence often provided an arena for different theological standpoints. However, if physicians and natural philosophers could be allies for the clergy, they could also be dangerous rivals. For example, anatomical investigations ran the risk of being labelled heretical when they questioned the relationship between the somatic and the immortal soul.

Despite efforts by the Catholic and Protestant Churches to eradicate older beliefs and practices, differences emerged between officially prescribed religion and religion as practised. This created a space in which the laity could draw on religious and superstitious explanations of disease within a pluralistic (or diverse) system of medicine. Many continued to associate sin with disease, a view reinforced by municipal proclamations on plague, popular and professional medical texts, and by the Bible, which had become more widely available in the vernacular as a consequence of the Reformation and the growth of printing. Lutheran views of a bond between body and soul, between sin and disease, strengthened popular and medical perceptions of the need to look after the body. Notwithstanding Protestant attacks, miracles and religious healing continued to form an accepted part of experience. They complemented other sources of care and saints' names remained powerful sources of relief or protection. If by the eighteenth century faith in magical healing had begun to wane, at least among the elite, throughout the sixteenth and seventeenth centuries popular magic was part of the religious and healing rituals employed by ordinary men and women [see 'Self-help']. During a period when access to licensed practitioners was limited, especially in rural areas, miracles, prayer, repentance and magic held out a universal possibility of cure.

Just as miracles, saints and prayer could still bring cures, witches and demons continued to be blamed for causing disease. The idea that witchcraft was argued out of existence by scientific and medical explanations has come to be rejected by scholars. At the heart of the Scientific Revolution was a supernaturalist philosophy that maintained a place for occult causation. It was perhaps natural to attribute sickness to malign supernatural influences at a time when sickness was a mysterious and often unpredictable event and when the witch craze saw thousands of suspected witches killed in Europe. Although the connection between witches and healing has often been overstated, an ongoing fear of witchcraft and demons remained throughout the period. This fear is visible in the casebooks of the English astrological physician Richard Napier: over 500 of his patients seen between 1597 and 1634 believed they had been bewitched. Clerics and physicians did manipulate individual cases to serve divergent religious and political agendas, but many accepted harmful magic as one of the risks of everyday life and that magic could also provide protection. If the Church and licensed practitioners sought to control popular belief and attacked popular magical practices, for many contemporaries religion and magic offered important ways of understanding and coping with sickness.

In many ways, the Reformation marked a new synthesis of medical science and faith. Religious reform and medical reform co-existed with medicine affecting religion and vice versa. No matter how varied the religious belief and affiliations of individual medical practitioners, Christian theology offered many an important means through which to understand disease and medicine. This draws attention to the multiple interconnections between medicine and religion in the sixteenth and seventeenth centuries.

Enlightenment challenge: 1700–1800

A persuasive current in the historiography argues that during the Enlightenment, contemporaries moved away from religious ways of thinking about sickness to favour a secularizing, scientific and rationalizing worldview that rejected magic and religious healing and embraced the growing authority of clinical medicine. There is much to recommend this analysis. During the seventeenth century there was a move against popular superstition and in the eighteenth century the growing momentum across Europe (and especially in France and Scotland) of philosophic and scientific materialism created new ways of thinking about the natural world and the body. Literary men, scientists and philosophers increasingly asserted the supremacy of rational enquiry and identified themselves as participants in a European reform campaign based on reason. They cast themselves as proponents of scientific study that would improve life in this world, the application of which was aided by a flourishing capitalist economy and strong nation-states. They rejected what they saw as the superstition, bigotry and fanaticism of the past in favour of what the French philosopher Denis Diderot referred to as the philosophical spirit of observation and exactness.

The growth of scientific secularism and an emphasis on experience and reason did influence medicine. Calls for an empirical scientific basis to medicine merged with growing scepticism about superstition to challenge established medical ideas to forge new approaches to understanding the body and disease that dismiss supernatural explanations of disease. If there remained room for genuine miracles, by the 1720s the role attributed to providentialism was waning in medical debate and doctors were coming to dismiss clergymen who voiced medical opinions as no better than quacks. However, this connection between the Enlightenment and the decline of religious healing is not clear-cut, or a simple question of a growing separation between the treatment of the body and the treatment of the soul. Enlightenment thinking had limits. Ideas of inevitable secularization and a radical departure from traditional spiritual beliefs and the triumph of rationale science should be questioned. Rather than secularization, it might be better to think about a shift from a religious culture to a more self-conscious religious faith. If the eighteenth century did see innovations in medicine and science, doctors did not abandon God or theology in their explanations of disease or in their practices.

Although the co-existence of Enlightenment thought and religion in science might seem paradoxical, for contemporaries the connection between them was natural. In Southern Europe where Catholicism retained a powerful hold, these ideas were strongest. In Catholic Spain, divine explanations of disease and the body remained entrenched. If the ongoing importance of the sacred in Spanish medicine earned the country a reputation for backwardness, in other European countries, both Protestant and Catholic, rather than a rigid division between religion and rationality, the Enlightenment saw a mixing of religious thought and scientific rationalization. Physicians embraced the physical and the sacred. The fashionable English physician, George Cheyne, described a regimen in his popular *Essays of Health* (1724) that attended just as much to the body as to the soul. In France, the physician Jean Astruc was able to combine pragmatic observation with a belief in divine revelation in his textbook for midwives. These were not isolated examples. Debates about disease were often bound up with politics and religion. This can be seen in discussion concerning the proper treatment of fevers or over mental illness and the immateriality of the soul. Many doctors did start to accept the central position of natural causes in their explanations of disease, but they also continued to admit that God had the power to cause or cure sickness, or saw the existence of the divine in the workings of the body. Influenced by ideas associated with mechanical philosophy, doctors asked if the body was as a machine, what moved it? Some found the answer in the soul.

The sick equally continued to call on God, speak of the miraculous intervention of saints, or blamed disease on the supernatural. When the self-taught Bristol accountant William Dyer took medicine, he sought God's guidance. Dyer's attitudes and actions challenge the assumption that eighteenth century medicine was increasingly secularized and professional. Nor was Dyer an isolated case. As the historian Jonathan Barry explains, 'there is evidence to suggest that patients valued doctors of their own religious persuasion, whose healing art might include religious support'.[1] Saints were invoked alongside other forms of treatment. Popular medical texts, such as the *Bibliothéque Bleue* in France, continued to portray illness as sent by God and the value of prayer and supernatural healing was commonly extolled in these texts. Equally, elite attacks on superstition did not mean that ordinary men and women abandoned magic in the face of new Enlightenment ideas. Ongoing belief in magic hence provided not only a rationale for sickness but also a source of treatment. The eighteenth century was therefore characterized by medical pluralism, which included religious and supernatural explanations and cures, rather than the dominance of secular medicine.

This is not to argue against secularization, lay challenges to religious healing, or that the Enlightenment witnessed a growing separation of religion and medicine. Rather that religious beliefs and practices did not suddenly become obsolete or irrelevant to eighteenth century medicine. Because of the very contradictions and complexities of eighteenth century medicine, religion and magic continued to influence how medicine and disease were understood at a professional and popular level, even if their position and the scope of that influence were challenged.

Secularizing medicine: 1800–1900

The nineteenth century has been associated with several contradictory stances on religion: it is either a period of religious boom or growing secularization, of religious self-doubt and conflicts within the Church and between denominations. Although the two centuries following the French Revolution (1789–99) witnessed popular religious revivals, the importance of religion as a factor in social change has been minimized by historians in favour of an account that emphasizes secularization, its links with modernity and the rise of 'objectivity' in science. A conventional account would explain how science – in the form of geology, physics, biology, physiology and psychology – made traditional beliefs increasingly less plausible; how urbanization encouraged individualism; how the erosion of family life made religious institutions less relevant; and how technology gave people greater control over their environment, making the idea of an omnipotent God less credible. Darwinism is often held up as the classic example of this challenge. Ideas of science at a popular, professional and institutional level were being extended, and the clergy were gradually marginalized as science and medicine were professionalized. Medicine was part of this secularizing process, displacing religious and supernatural beliefs with a scientific view of health and disease. Often the basic assumption made about the nineteenth century is that aside from fringe or alternative medicine, medical science overtook the Church in defining illness.

Religious connotations and references to spiritual enlightenment did pose increasing problems for medicine. This antagonism is embodied in French medical hostility to Catholicism. Materialist French physicians challenged the Church's role in the care of the sick: they attacked the healing properties of shrines and suggested that the expectations of the faithful explained supposed miraculous cures. Anticlerical local councils tried to replace religious with secular nurses as part of a process of laicization [see 'Nursing']. It was not just in France that medical practitioners used medicine to challenge religious practices. Nineteenth century doctors developed critiques of supernatural phenomenon and pathologized certain religious experiences. In Germany, for example, doctors attacked the Jewish custom of ritual bathing as unhygienic and associated it with more that thirty different diseases. Medical materialism was employed as an agent of religious reform.

If church attendance declined in the nineteenth century, religion and faith were not static. Catholic and Protestant countries experienced different processes of changing religious belief, with religion and faith meaning different things according to place, education and class, but religion still claimed a significant role in people's lives: it helped shape collective identities and had a central role in the social, political, physical and economic structure of cities. Religious organizations, from missionary societies to charities, mushroomed and were crucial in delivering welfare. People did not necessarily lose interest in religion but during the nineteenth century the role of religion became more restricted. This was true of nineteenth century medicine.

A näive perception of an inevitable conflict between science and religion has perpetuated myths about the extent and nature of secularization. As the case of Spain suggests, secularization was not an absolute process. Here the ruling conservative elite believed that science without religion was blind. Although Spain was an extreme case, even in anticlerical France the Church remained a potent social and political force before the Third Republic (1870–1940) and attempts to laicize public hospitals. Conflict was never a simple question of scientists versus defenders of the Christian faith, but of conflicting views within different scientific or medical communities over the role of religion. A more subtle analysis suggests not outright secularization but a contradictory tension between growing agnosticism, a term itself coined in 1869, changes in religious activity, religious booms, and the ongoing importance of superstition. Secularization occurred but it was not systematic or unproblematic.

Religion and medicine remained compatible for many nineteenth century doctors and clergymen. A medicalization of morality – reflected, for example, in ideas of degeneration – derived meaning from a religious moral framework. Nor were religion and medicine kept in separate compartments. This can be seen in debates over the use of chloroform in childbirth where some doctors joined with clergymen to argue that God's curse on Eve meant they should not limit the pain of delivery. Medical ideas were appropriated by religious denominations to explain supernatural experiences, and many contemporaries did not see religious views as a hindrance to medical science. The question was not whether medicine and religion should be divorced but the nature of religion's role in medicine. Moral and religious references remained a feature of mid-century medical texts. For example, the respected English anatomist and physician, Henry Wentworth Acland, easily mixed moral and religious concerns with medical theories to see cholera as a divine punishment and the result of miasmas. Louis Pasteur remained a staunch Catholic and an anti-materialist. Other Catholic doctors turned to the Church for approval of their methods, particularly in the field of obstetric surgery or in gaining support for smallpox vaccination. Medical schools frequently extolled the virtues of a pious life and stressed the importance of Christianity in the making of a medical gentleman. These examples suggest the numerous interconnections between medicine and religion and the ongoing importance of religion in constructing and framing medical debates, practices and professional values in the nineteenth century.

The permeable boundaries between religion and medicine are illustrated by fringe or alternative medicine. For the contemporary Edinburgh academic Samuel Brown, popular medical reform movements represented a form of 'Physical Puritanism', a label that reflected their links with religious dissent and the connections that existed between the flourishing of religious sects and alternative medical movements in Protestant Europe. For example, at the heart of debates over phrenology was religion, while mesmerism moved from being a secularizing philosophy to being adopted by ministers. It developed into a spiritualist movement that after 1850 acquired links with the supernatural. In

France, this connection between spiritualism and mesmerism was particularly evident. By the end of the nineteenth century growing interest in the occult, prophecy and the miraculous further encouraged the growth of medico-religious movements.

Scientific and medical models did not simply drive out popular or religious beliefs. Popular beliefs and the cult of saints remained widespread, with the Virgin Mary the subject of growing veneration in the nineteenth century. These beliefs were strongest in rural areas where French and British officials bemoaned the entrenched nature of superstitions. Local lore, popular beliefs and rituals allowed the poor to make sense of the world around them at a time of upheaval and uncertainty created by industrialization and popular religious beliefs flourished, particularly during times of epidemic disease. Examples abound of rural inhabitants continuing to blame their illness on witchcraft or demonic possession. One celebrated case was in the Alpine village of Morzine in Savoy in 1857 where over two hundred women and young girls believed that they were afflicted by demonic possession. Magical cures continued to mean something very real for many afflicted with illness. Shrines were potent places of pilgrimage and cure, providing something that secular medicine could not for many desperate men and women who found little relief in other forms of medicine. By the late nineteenth century, annual pilgrimages to Lourdes had become one of the largest mass movements in France.

The medical debate that surrounded Lourdes symbolizes not only the tensions between medicine and religion at the end of the nineteenth century but also how medicine and religion had an uneasy co-existence. At Lourdes, the Catholic Church utilized all the elements of clinical medicine and observation (including post-mortems) to support miraculous cures and to create a new language of therapeutic healing, which was upheld by Catholic physicians. The French neurologist Jean Martin Charcot's widely endorsed claims in 1892 that autosuggestion explained the miraculous cures did little to undermine popular faith in Lourdes. As the medical debates surrounding Lourdes reveal, medicine had not become entirely secularized and professional in the nineteenth century.

Religion and healthcare

Religion has had a central role in the provision of medical services from the medieval to the modern period. It is here, rather than in the relationship between medicine and religion in shaping ideas about disease and cure, that greater continuity can be detected. The fundamental obligation of the godly to aid the sick emphasized the religious dimension of medical assistance. These beliefs inspired the foundation of numerous religious orders and institutions, many of which provided medical care to the sick poor. For example, medieval hospitals were Christian institutions where patrons and benefactors gave money in return for intercessory prayer, confraternity, hospitality and burial.

The Reformation did have important consequences for poor relief and medical care. In many accounts, the connections between economic change and welfare reforms in this period has been emphasized, but as Grell and Cunningham argue in *Health Care and Poor Relief in Protestant Europe* (1997), the Protestant Reformation, religious turmoil and the new ideologies that emerged in Northern Europe also significantly shaped attitudes to poverty and welfare. If this argument does not diminish the importance of socioeconomic change, war or epidemics in disrupting established patterns of welfare and in stimulating reform, it does highlight how Protestant reformers were important in influencing new ideas about poor relief. Protestant attacks on begging, Luther's idea of a 'common chest' to aid the poor, and the emergence of clear distinctions between the deserving and undeserving poor, all influenced the nature of welfare and the institutions established in Northern Europe. For example, in the Hanseatic towns, the development of Reformed or more radical Protestantism shaped the nature of poor relief, while religious upheaval in the seventeenth century hampered the administration of poor relief.

Notwithstanding doctrine there were few differences between the ways in which Protestant and Catholic countries developed welfare agencies in the sixteenth and seventeenth centuries [see 'Healthcare and the state']. At a national and local level, the Catholic and Protestant Churches provided the basis for administrative and pastoral organizations at a time when welfare was highly localized. In Sweden and Finland, poor relief remained parish-based and the Church was responsible for the collection and administration of poor funds. Even in England, where a more centralized system of poor relief was created after 1601, responsibility for collecting the poor rate and the distribution of alms remained at a parish level until the nineteenth century.

The expansion of poor relief did not undervalue the ongoing importance of Christian charity to welfare. Catholic and Protestant confessions used charity in different ways to define their faith, but both saw charity to the sick as an essential Christian duty, albeit one that often served secular ends. The reinvigoration of Catholicism after the Council of Trent (1545–63) renewed charitable impulses, especially in Southern Europe where new, more dynamic charitable organizations were formed. Tensions might erupt over the control of individual institutions, as evident in the administration of the Nîmes Hotel Dieu between the 1630s and 1650s, but this did not mean that religion played any lesser part in the administration of care. In Holland and France, and in many German-speaking territories, the care of the sick continued to be under the management of religious orders. In France, the Daughters of Charity and the Brothers of Charity of St John of God were an essential part of the medical and philanthropic landscape. Here not only were religious orders in charge of how many hospitals were managed, but they also took responsibility for the new *hôpitaux-généraux* established as part of a state policy to control the poor. The Catholic spiritual revival of the seventeenth century saw the creation of new religious orders that were devoted to charitable and nursing activities. Followers of St John of God were especially aggressive in collecting alms and adopted a broad definition of their medical mission. Religious communities of nursing sisters came to dominate the day-to-day management of many charitable institutions that offered and dispensed medical care. They developed a wide range of skills that went beyond their original function of providing care at the bedsides of the sick poor.

The religious monopoly of the hospital and nursing was challenged in the eighteenth century. New principles started to inform the foundation of hospitals that owed much to broader socioeconomic and religious shifts and new conceptions of welfare and mercantilism [see 'Hospitals']. As licensed practitioners struggled to assert their authority, they came into conflict with religious orders over who controlled admissions and diets, and over the function of the hospital as a site for clinical instruction. Disputes were frequent as different conceptions of medical care clashed, as can be seen in French hospitals. However, it was not necessarily the case that religion was a barrier to medical progress: changes in the nature and delivery of healthcare in the eighteenth century were not just the result of changes in the medical marketplace but also were influenced by religious values and ideas. This is evident in the drive to establish hospitals. The voluntary hospital network that evolved in England and Ireland reflected the ethos of the established Church and evangelical zeal. Religious orders also aided medicalization. For example, the Sisters of the Daughters of Charity in France, rather than being anti-medicine, controlled the diet of the sick, dispensed medicines, undertook minor surgery, and provided medical services for many institutions. In Revolutionary (1789–99) and Imperial France (1804–14), nuns were often key players in mediating between the needs of the patient and those of the medical practitioner.

An analysis of hospital appeals in the nineteenth century reveals that charity continued to be regarded as a form of 'fire insurance' for the afterlife. This interpretation of philanthropy sits uneasily with the historiography, which from the 1970s recast charity as a mechanism of social control, middle-class hegemony and identity, and more recently as a form of social capital. Philanthropy did take on secular concerns and involved a range of motives from guilt to gratitude, but it also retained a strong religious dimension. Charity appeared to embody positive values of Christian virtue, conviction, enthusiasm, and individualism, values that contemporary commentators saw as desirable. This was aided by a spirit of evangelicalism with its emphasis on personal service, salvation through individual effort, and conviction. Although hospitals moved away from their religious origins, those running these increasingly secular institutions continued to call on religious feelings and Christian love to motivate the benevolent to fund medical care.

It was not just in how hospitals were funded and represented that religion continued to provide a rationale and focus for welfare provision. Although there was a broad trend towards scientizing and laicizing healthcare, the Church retained a vital role in healthcare. Voluntary and church-based charities expanded alongside the growth of state welfare [see 'Healthcare and the state'] and continued to shape healthcare. Catholic and Protestant traditions of charity underpinned the foundation of general and specialized institutions for the care of the sick, the mentally ill and the disabled, which were aided by a religious revival in the mid nineteenth century. In rural France, religious congregations often served as the main providers of medical services and pharmaceutical supplies. Protestant institutions – such as the Parisian Association for Aiding the Sick and the Practical School for Social Service – were influential in the development of public health policy at a local level. Catholic and Protestant orders were also significant forces in debates about social welfare. In Belgium, Catholic leaders were active in political struggles over the relative merits of mutual aid and other forms of health insurance, while in the Netherlands Christian philanthropy had a crucial part in shaping social policy, at least until the 1889 Labour Law.

Nor should the contribution of religious orders in nursing reform be downplayed in favour of professionalization or laicization [see 'Nursing']. As scholars have looked beyond the role of Florence Nightingale in reforming nursing, they have shown how religion shaped the nature and status of hospital nursing. Throughout the nineteenth century, nursing offered a battleground for different religious denominations seeking to exert their influence – either between themselves, such as in the Netherlands where Protestant pastors took the initiative in developing Protestant nursing as part of their missionary zeal and anti-Catholicism, or with the state, such as in France. Religious orders across Europe afforded single women of all classes the opportunity to undertake a wide range of social and medical services, including nursing. In Britain, evangelical concerns shaped early nursing reform and efforts to improve the moral character of nurses and the bodily and spiritual welfare of the sick poor. A similar process was evident in Germany. Here the Protestant order of Deaconesses at Kaiserwerth provided not only nursing care but also a model for nursing sisterhoods elsewhere in Europe. They stressed the moral and spiritual duty of the nurse and many early nineteenth century nurses were fervent Christians who believed that caring for the sick was a Christian duty. This religious imperative did not come into conflict with their clinical duties.

Although the number of lay nurses increased, there was no wholesale secularization of nursing in the nineteenth century. Sectarian conflicts may have driven some nursing orders out of individual institutions, as can be seen at King's College Hospital, London, but nursing sisterhoods continued to offer important sources of nursing care in the second half of the nineteenth century. In France, nursing orders flooded state institutions under the Second Empire (1852–70), and by the start of the twentieth century some two hundred female religious orders were providing nursing care. Even supporters of the laicization of nursing were forced to admit that they were not enough competent lay nurses to fill the gap. Many of these religious nursing orders, rather than being backward, ran institutions and presided over nursing that by the standards of the day were recognizably modern.

Assumptions that the twentieth century saw the secularization of medical services are not fully justified. Charity was modernized as it evolved new relationships with the state. For example, in Ireland the Catholic Church was crucial to the development of maternity and child welfare services. In France, women helped establish social Catholic organizations and lobbying groups to press for social welfare programmes. In the Netherlands, denominational organizations continued to play a significant role in home nursing until the 1990s when provision was transferred to regional home care organizations. Other examples could be found, especially in a colonial context where Catholic missionary societies retained a prominent role in delivering medical care [see 'Medicine and empire']. Although the field of social services and welfare provided a battleground between the Church and state, it allowed the Church a role in innovating new services. It illustrates how in the twentieth century the role of the Church and religion in healthcare should not be undervalued or dismissed in accounts that stress the rise of the therapeutic state [see 'Healthcare and medicine'].

Conclusions

The idea that over the last two centuries medicine was secularized has been overstated. An emphasis on secularization and de-Christianization has since the late 1980s given way to a wider perspective that is more attuned to the diversity, productivity and symbolism of modern religion. In the twentieth century, religion was under attack as churches failed to adapt and society became more disillusioned, particularly in the aftermath of the First World War (1914–18) and the Catholic Church's support of authoritarian regimes in Spain and Vichy France. However, the rise of fundamentalism around the world in the late twentieth century calls into question earlier observations that we lived in a secular society. In the twentieth century, religion retained a visible role in contemporary debates and in the life of many individuals.

Boundaries between medicine and religion remained permeable in the twentieth century, although for the most part theologians were no longer directly challenging interpretations of the natural and medical world. As Rhodri Hayward's historical research on medicine and spiritualism in Edwardian Britain suggests, scientific models and medical explanations were used to support religious conceptions and explanations of conversion and possession.[2] Religious beliefs equally continued to influence medical research and debates on healthcare. Nowhere was this clearer than in Spain. Under the Francoist regime of the 1940s and 1950s, moves were made to create a Catholic unity of the sciences. If the example of Spain is an extreme one, elsewhere in Europe medicine and religion continued their uneasy co-existence. Italian doctors drew on Christian metaphors in their campaigns against malaria and in the 1940s and 1950s allied with the Catholic Church in constructing definitions of maternity that influenced state welfare provision and attitudes to motherhood. This connection was not limited to Catholic countries. In the 1930s, prodigious cures were discussed in medical journals. As physicians from different religious and secular positions debated the veracity of miracle cures, clergymen supported the idea of the laying on of hands as a means of healing and played significant roles in disseminating lay healing methods. In some regions, such as the borders of Wales, belief in the relationship between magic, witchcraft, health and illness were reported in the interwar period.

It would be all too easy to over-extend these examples. Important differences existed between Northern and Southern Europe, between Protestant and Catholic countries. However, in the late twentieth century, ethical and religious concerns continued to have an impact on medicine and the delivery of medical care. In debates over abortion, stem cell research, euthanasia and care for the terminally ill, to name but a few areas, the religious beliefs of individual doctors, campaigners and broader communities remained important in structuring debate and shaping regulation. Historians of medicine have been uneasy in acknowledging the significance of religion in modern medical debates and in healthcare. Christianity and belief sit uneasily with narratives of secularization and faith in the power of biomedicine. If the English evolutionary biologist Richard Dawkins feared that religion and spiritualism in the early twenty first century were threatening science and medicine, his fears reveal how religion has never been far from medicine, either as a way of explaining disease, as a rationale for healthcare, or as something to oppose.

Further reading

On the significance of religion to attitudes to disease and in shaping medical knowledge and healthcare during the Reformation, see the collection of essays by Roger French and Andrew Wear (eds), *The Medical Revolution of the Seventeenth Century* (Cambridge: Cambridge University Press, 1989) and by Ole Peter Grell and Andrew Cunningham (eds), *Medicine and the Reformation* (London: Routledge, 1993). Charles Webster, *The Great Instauration: Science, Medicine and Reform, 1626–60* (London: Duckworth, 1975) remains an excellent examination of how theological ideas influenced how medical science was generated and received in the seventeenth century. For a more general introduction to the impact of the Reformation and the Counter-Reformation, students should see Diarmaid MacCulloch's exhaustive *Reformation: Europe's House Divided 1490–1700* (London: Penguin, 2005). On the historiography of witchcraft, see Jonathan Barry and Owen Davies (eds), *Advances in Witchcraft Historiography* (Basingstoke: Palgrave Macmillan, 2007). Although many studies have focused on the early modern period, a growing literature has turned to the role of religion in eighteenth century medicine. Here work by Jonathan Barry, 'Piety and the Patient: Medicine and Religion in Eighteenth Century Bristol', in Roy Porter (ed.), *Patients and Practitioners: Lay Perceptions of Medicine in Pre-Industrial Society* (Cambridge: Cambridge University Press, 1985), pp. 145–75, or Caroline Hannaway, 'Medicine and Religion in Pre-Revolutionary France', *Social History of Medicine* 2 (1989), pp. 315–19, are good starting points. If Colin Jones's work 'Sisters of Charity and the Ailing Poor', *Social History of Medicine* 2 (1989), pp. 339–48, and Katrin Schultheiss, *Bodies and Souls: Politics and the Professionalization of Nursing in France, 1880–1922* (Cambridge, MA: Harvard University Press, 2001) highlight how religion was important to nursing reform, historians have often pointed to a process of secularization in the nineteenth century and the collection edited by Steve Bruce (ed.), *Religion and Modernization* (Oxford: Clarendon, 1992) explores this debate. The secularizing influence of medicine is addressed by Matthew Ramsey in *Professional and Popular Medicine in France 1770–1830* (Cambridge: Cambridge University Press, 1988), while Lorraine Daston and Peter Galison, *Objectivity* (New York: Zone, 2007) examines the relationship between objectivity and science. Ruth Harris, 'Possession on the Borders: The "Mal de Morzine" in Nineteenth-Century France', *Journal of Modern History* 69 (1997), pp. 451–71, is a good example of scholarship that shows how religion was important to the understanding of disease, while Paul Weindling, 'The Modernization of Charity in Nineteenth Century France and Germany', in Jonathan Barry and Colin Jones (eds), *Medicine and Charity Before the Welfare State* (London: Routledge, 1991), pp. 190–206, draws attention to the ongoing role of the church in the delivery of medical care. Roger Cooter's edited collection *Studies in the History of Alternative Medicine* (Basingstoke: Palgrave Macmillan, 1988) points to the important connections between religion and alternative medicine.

4
Women, health and medicine

Mainstream histories in the past have tended to ignore women or presented them in sex-stereotyped ways and until the 1970s research on women and medicine was no exception. The impetus given to women's history by second-wave feminism along with the impact of the social sciences on the writing of history encouraged historians to rethink the relationship between women and medicine. Scholarship shifted from positivist accounts that emphasized the contributions of medicine to female health to a model that asserted subordination to a male medical science. Feminist accounts were at the forefront of this approach: they drew attention to the sexual politics of sickness and the exploitative nature of medical intervention. A central feature of feminist theory was to recognize that gender was not fixed but was constructed in relation to specific historical circumstances. As historians started to think about gender and the cultural history of the body in these ways, they explored how masculinity and femininity were separate from biological sex. If not all historians welcomed this move, others felt that by using gender in the same way as other historians used class or race it was possible to examine how medicine was laden with cultural assumptions about women.

Notwithstanding these historiographical tends, numerous studies continue to position themselves in relation to a male medical science and how medical practitioners and the laity interpreted female health and disease in relation to perceived physiological differences and female reproductivity. Part of the reason for this response is the sources historians have used. A reliance on medical texts, many of which emphasized women's inherent weakness and reproductive role, not only ensured that a male voice invariably dominated accounts, but also that environmental, socioeconomic or political forces were pushed to the background as scholars analysed the relationship between medical and social constructions of femininity. This approach has only recently come to be criticized as scholars have begun to recuperate the role of women in medicine, rejecting ideas of a male medical conspiracy and views that women were passive victims of male practitioners to place greater emphasis on how women assisted medicalization.

This chapter builds on the idea that women were not passive objects of a male medical gaze. It explores the extent to which medicine contributed to and expressed social and cultural definitions of women's role in society. By examining medicine and maternity, the chapter traces women's interactions with medicine from conception to childbirth to question the chronology of medicalization. Throughout, the chapter seeks to determine not only the influence of medical ideas but also women's role in constructing medical debates about their bodies.

Defining women

Most historians now accept that the meaning of gender is historically determined. Strongly influenced by Joan Scott's formulation of gender as defined by the meanings given to bodily differences, in approaching gender and the cultural history of the body historians have examined the legal, religious, cultural and philosophical debates that influenced how gender was defined in the past. Given the importance of medicine in expressing these debates, a wide range of historians have used medical texts to understand the ways in which gender and femininity were framed, and how medicine was used to define and justify the subordination of women. In rejecting rigid biological categories of female versus male it became possible to see how socioeconomic, cultural and political forces informed medical definitions of female bodies, and how they were shaped by language, professional concerns and male anxieties.

The common assumption is that early modern medicine, and by extension society, drew on the humoral system to understand the nature of the male and female body [see 'Disease']. In the humoral system, there was essentially one sex – male – with the differences between male and female sexual organs explained not by anatomy but by the physiological mixture of the humors. Whereas men were believed to be the standard of perfection, women's bodies were shown to be lacking in heat. This suggested that they did not have the energy to form external sexual organs and this explained why they were inside the body. Comparison or analogy with the male appeared to reveal how female organs were merely versions of comparable male organs – for example, the clitoris was a female penis. Rather than ideas of what it meant to be female being tied to particular parts of the body – the breasts or genitals, for example – women were defined by the rhythms of menstruation and reproduction. As healthy bodies in the humoral system were in balance, menstruation was regarded as a mechanism to dispel surplus fluids when woman were not pregnant or lactating, although disagreement existed over whether this was to purify or remove excess blood. Disruption or cessation of menstruation could therefore lead to illness, while cultural and religious taboos contributed to a representation of menstruation as a source of corruption. Given that menstruation was vital for maintaining bodily health for women, early modern practitioners monitored the frequency, quantity and quality of women's menstrual cycles and prescribed medicines to regulate its flow. Taboos about male practitioners examining female bodies maintained a distance between practitioner and patient, reinforcing accepted beliefs about the female body and ensuring that many common conditions in women often went unnoticed.

These views had a resonance with social and political trends in sixteenth century Europe. Although texts are never simple mirrors of everyday belief, during a turbulent period when patriarchy was seen to be in crisis, medical theories reinforced social and political ideas that women were ruled by their passions and were physically and intellectually weaker than men. These ideas carried a clear moral and political message; one that emphasized women's reproductive nature and portrayed them as subordinate, suited to a domestic lifestyle. This understanding of the female body helped structure women's experiences and roles in society. As the debate surrounding whether or not England's Queen Elizabeth (1533–1603) menstruated and had a normal female anatomy demonstrates, these ideas could have national and political importance.

However, early modern women were not passive victims of medicine or their bodies. Evidence from commonplace books and diaries suggests that they were just as concerned as doctors were about their bodies. Menstruation was accepted as something to be controlled. If women seldom openly discussed menstruation, letters between elite women reveal how they privately offered reproductive and other forms of medical advice, while medical and popular texts assumed that women had some agency over their bodies and had a role in managing their health. As Laura Gowing explains in *Common Bodies* (2003), women colluded in the strict regulation of the female body, but they also resisted medical advice when this contradicted their own views or experiences.

Established arguments in women's history suggest that the eighteenth century was a period in which men and women's social roles were split. In *Making Sex* (1990), Thomas Laqueur used elite medical texts on reproduction to reveal an associated transformation in how women's bodies were understood. For Laqueur this was based on a physical construction of gender difference: as anatomists rejected ideas that women were imperfect men, new categories of male and female emerged as opposite biological sexes. Laqueur advanced a compelling view that charted the change from a one-sex to a two-sex model to argue that this transformation was not simply the result of new anatomical or physiological knowledge. Key to this transition was the intellectual, political and social context of the Enlightenment. With political theorists increasingly invoking the idea of natural rights, biology was harnessed to justify female subordination as male natural philosophers and anatomists were led by their own views to show how women were physically and morally distinct.

Laqueur's thesis was incorporated into countless studies of gender and sexuality and was reflected in parallel work by Londa Schiebinger who explored how these ideas of gender informed eighteenth century natural history, racial science and anatomical studies (see Further Reading). New ideas surrounding gender and the female body built on debates about women's place in society with anatomical studies focusing on those parts of the body that were most politically significant, as seen in the anatomical illustrations of the French painter Gautier d'Agoty. Women were re-imagined as sexually passive, less intellectually capable, and with larger pelvises, attributes which reflected a new cult of motherhood

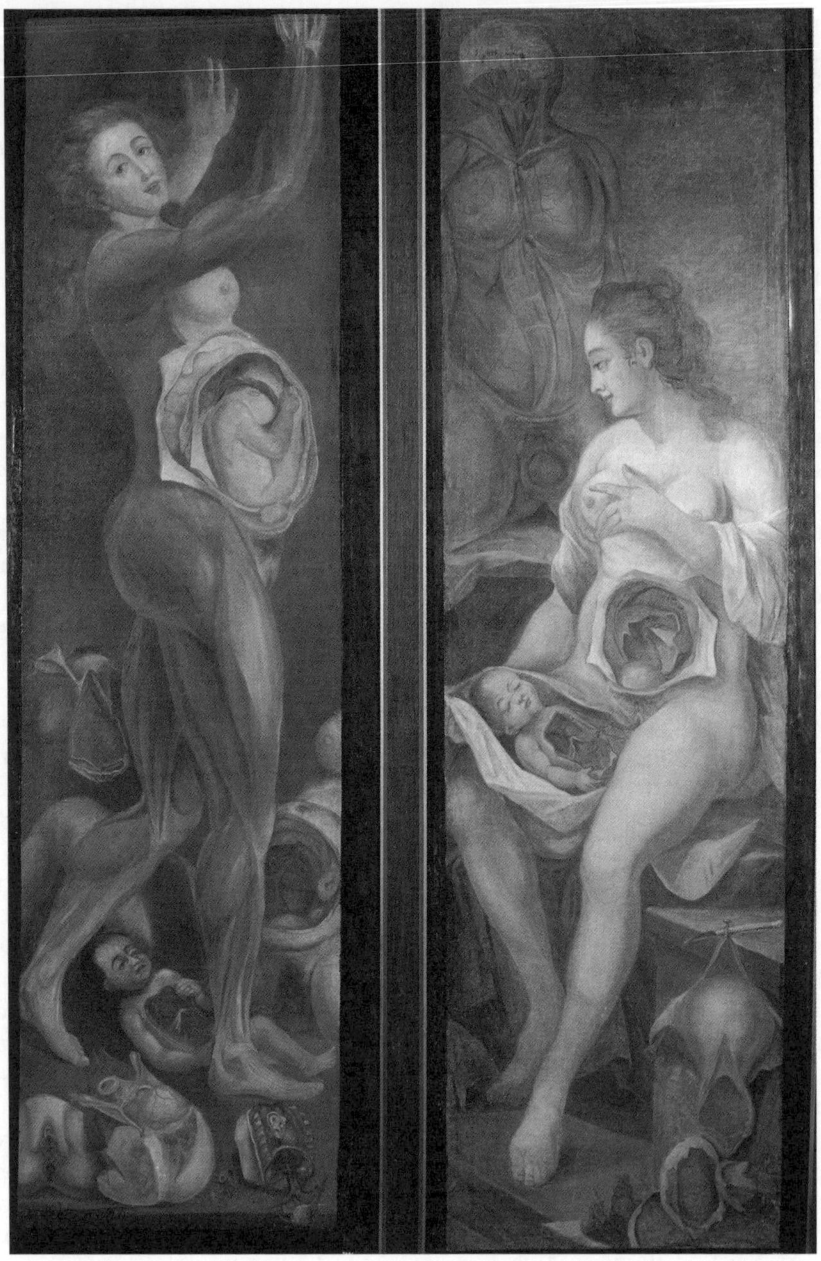

Figure 4.1 Anatomical studies of (left) a dissected pregnant woman and (right) a female dissected woman holding a dissected baby by the anatomical illustrator Jacques Fabien Gautier d'Agoty (1717–1785).

Source: Wellcome Library, London.

influenced by mercantile interests in population growth. The result was a further deterioration in women's social position based around a framework of gender relations in which the boundaries between male and female became clear-cut. As historians examined the ways in which domesticity became a new guide for female behaviour in this period, they drew on an ideology of 'separate spheres' which assigned men and women to distinct public (male) and private (female) spheres based on supposed natural characteristics. Such a framework came to be used as a metaphor for characterizing gender differences and appeared well suited to the values of the aspiring middle classes of Europe.

However, the transition was not as straightforward as Laqueur or Schiebinger suggest. Changes in how women were being defined were happening before 1700. Mary Fissell, for example, argues in *Vernacular Bodies* (2004) how pamphlets, broadsides, medical and other texts questioned the one-sex model, while Laura Gowing in *Domestic Dangers* (1988) used court depositions to argue that ordinary men and women were already stressing sexual difference before the eighteenth century. It is therefore possible to present a more nuanced analysis of early modern medical constructions of gender and argue that the sixteenth and seventeenth centuries witnessed a proliferation of discourses – medical, religious, political, legal, social – that addressed the idea that the sexes were different and that women were inferior. Sixteenth century anatomical investigations were already beginning to discredit earlier notions of the female body based on analogy. Vernacular writing on the female body became less apologetic and more focused on conception and pregnancy, while anatomical studies increasingly drew attention to those sites where they differed from the male to reinforce prevailing social ideas about women's lower status. In the seventeenth century, anatomists pointed to differences in the brain and nervous system to place constraints on women's intellects. Practitioners believed that women possessed unique physiological functions rooted in menstruation, pregnancy and lactation. They observed that diseases appeared to manifest themselves differently in women and considered the impact of their prescriptions on women's bodies, and if necessary altered them accordingly. Nor were eighteenth century ideas of sexual difference monolithic. Ideas about the nature of men and women were often fluid and, depending on the audience, drew on both humoral and contemporary interpretations of gender and the body. The same can be seen in ideas of gender roles as a variety of private experiences point to a looser division of responsibilities rather than a rigid ideology of separate spheres. Representational shifts and gender roles were hence not clear or consistent: men and women were both different and similar.

Despite challenges to Laqueur's thesis, historians are reluctant to abandon how the understanding of sex difference altered in the eighteenth century and how sex and sexual difference became part of a new cultural paradigm. Prevailing ideas about gender difference were more clearly defined by the last decades of the eighteenth century, and new expectations of women were gaining prominence among the middling orders, but changes in the conceptions of gender were not omnipresent or limited to the Enlightenment. A variety of models of gender were available, but many of these were increasingly reinforcing fundamental sexual stereotypes which were upheld by a range of political theorists that built on the idea that certain natural or physiological differences existed between men and women. These ideas emphasized women's delicate natures, as seen in female fashion, their modesty and morality, and sought to restrict middle-class women to the home.

Medical theories were more explicitly harnessed to social and cultural constructions of gender roles in the nineteenth century. In the large number of medical studies in France, Britain and Germany devoted to the subject of feminine nature, a scientific understanding of women's bodies and capabilities were presented that assumed innate physiological qualities. These ideas formed the basis for the development of gynaecology as a medical discipline that emphasized women's unique biological characteristics. Medical texts portrayed women as slaves to their bodies, with their physical frailty explained by the relationship between their ovaries and nervous systems. Ovaries were viewed as the essence of femininity and the key to understanding not only women's bodies but also all women's diseases. Within this framework, puberty and menstruation were shown to be particularly dangerous times: menstruating girls and women, for example, were viewed as essentially unwell, unstable and helpless. This made it all the more important for doctors to be involved in their care. Such medical arguments reinforced a social construction of women as inconsistent, readily exhausted and lacking in self-control, above all vulnerable to emotional upset and consequently suited to the home. Medical theories that women were physically and mentally conditioned by their bodies, and were prone to physical and mental weakness, also allowed woman who stepped outside culturally constructed boundaries of female behaviour to be labelled degenerate or ill, ideas that were used to support claims that they were ill-suited to university education, the professions, or to voting.

Medical ideas of insanity are a good illustration of this gendered perspective. In the sixteenth and seventeenth centuries, many contemporaries felt that women were more predisposed than men to mental illness. Physical infirmities – from gynaecological disorders to difficult births – and the traumatic events of life – for example, the death of a child – were given as reasons. In the eighteenth century, nervous disease became closely associated with effeminacy. Because of their physiology, medical practitioners assumed that women were more vulnerable to insanity than men and experienced madness in a specifically feminine way. Reproductive explanations were extended in the nineteenth century as doctors asserted a connection between the ovaries and the brain and the amount of nervous energy available. The female lifecycle was perceived to be fraught with dangers that could drive women insane. Menstruation was shown to predispose women to madness: too much or too little, too late or too soon, were all dangerous. Puberty was a perilous time, while childbirth ran the risk of puerperal insanity, which ranged from short-term antenatal depression to incurable psychosis. Given the prevailing medical notions that women were prone to the fluctuations caused by their reproductive organs, certain mental conditions became peculiarly female. This was clearest in the case of hysteria and later in the idea of the neurasthenic lady who was highly-strung and too fragile for manual or intellectual labour. That the mad and hysterical woman became a feature of novels, such as Brontë's *Jane Eyre* (1847) and Collins's *The Woman in White* (1860), underscores how these medical views had a strong cultural currency that reflected contemporary anxieties about women's position in society.

There were obvious class differences in these interpretations. Victorian assumptions about women's physical capabilities and lifestyles were based on middle-class perceptions. The bodies of working-class women were problematic, especially when they did not conform to the same characteristics of frailty and physical weakness. The realities of many working-class women's lives sat uneasily with nineteenth century theories of the reproductive body and notions of domesticity. Some doctors explained away this problem by arguing that the organs of working-class women were in better working order than their middle-class counterparts, which they felt were drained by emotion and intellect. Concerns were also voiced about working-class women as sources of contagion, fears that were given force in *fin de siècle* debates about degeneration and anxiety about the spread of venereal disease.

The extent to which women colluded in this construction is open to debate. Some women used definitions of feminine infirmity to their advantage, employing illness to escape their domestic or marital duties [see 'Disease']. Nor were women passive victims of medical authority: women were equally concerned about the reproductive functions of their bodies. They shared with doctors a common concern with menstrual regularity, and sought medical advice for conditions or behaviour they defined as abnormal. Nancy Theriot in her work on nineteenth century British and American medical literature has revealed how doctors 'learned to call "abnormal" what patients described as part of their illness: the inability to manage her household, the tendency to untidiness of person, the propensity to foul language'.[1] Physical or psychological explanations both reflected and constructed female experiences of their bodies and their lives, but they were also redeployed by women. This is evident in how nineteenth century charity workers and the early women's movement used the link between women's bodies and maternalism to their advantage to support roles outside the home. Although the interests of children were frequently placed before the rights of mothers, and even supporters of women's rights expected women to subordinate their demands to male control, ideas of maternity and domesticity shaped the rhetoric female campaigners used in early twentieth century campaigns for social welfare [See 'Healthcare and the state'].

This section has shown how medical ideas about the female body informed debates about women's position in society and how these debates influenced medical theories. Medical ideas about women's inherent weakness and inferiority were reformulated to reflect social, cultural and political views about women's nature and role. Important continuities existed, but assumptions about women's bodies and their position in society centred on reproduction proved hard to dislodge. Research on sex hormones in the 1920s and 1930s, for example, provided scientists with what they saw as the key to sexual difference that firmly associated the female body with reproduction. Although a hormonal understanding of the menstrual cycle reconfigured menstruation as a minor event, a stress on women's reproductive bodies still found expression in the 1940s and 1950s. In post-war Italy, for example, male practitioners contributed to discussions of motherhood that stressed women's maternal nature, combing biology with moral concerns. However, women were not necessarily passive victims of male medical hegemony. Women were not only expected to play a role in managing their health, but they also assisted in the construction of medical theories about the nature of female bodies and the importance of reproduction. If the early women's movement manipulated medical ideas to their advantage, it was only in the 1970s that these long-standing medical constructions were seriously challenged. Feminists and women's groups were at the forefront of critiques of medicine as they expressed anxieties about doctors' control over women and reproduction. Where this encouraged scrutiny of the gendered aspects of the doctor-patient relationship, for many women medical encounters were slow to change. It was only with biomedical research in the 1990s, which pointed to how men and women did not always have the same responses to disease, that constructions of sexual difference held the promise of a more positive therapeutic approach.

Medicine and sexuality

The history of sexuality is closely tied to cultural and medical constructions of the female body. Although feminist scholars have analysed how female sexuality was normalized and scrutinized in the past, the work of the French philosopher Michel Foucault has been important in shaping historical assessments of sexuality. In the *Introduction* (1977) to his history of sexuality, Foucault presented sexuality as the product of discursive practice. He explained how the sexual body became the focus for a range of restrictions during the eighteenth and nineteenth centuries, and how in the last decades of the nineteenth century sexuality was medicalized. If Foucault tended to neglect non-medical discourses – for example, religious or legal debates – and over-privileged the nineteenth century as central to the emergence of modern ideas about sexuality, his work encouraged research into the construction of sexuality and how it was policed.

Much of the research on medicine and sexuality has emphasized the role of medical experts – physicians, psychiatrists, and sexologists – but sexuality can be approached through a number of discourses – legal, religious, moral, medical or cultural – even if these are often hard to separate. Medical and moral discourses, for example, continued to be entwined into the twentieth century. Class also creates problems. If historians know a considerable amount about what Victorian middle-class professionals wrote about sexuality, popular attitudes are less well documented. By looking at different class cultures, different constructions of sexuality emerge. Further questions should be asked about the influence of medicine on popular understanding and practices, and about the extent to which women colluded or resisted constructions of their sexuality. Sexuality is as problematic for historians as it was for contemporaries.

Early modern debates on sexuality were informed by overlapping religious and medical discourses. For the Church, sex was a moral issue, while medical texts repeated Hippocratic and Galenic theories of reproduction in which both the male and female seed was necessary to produce a child. These theories asserted that the production of the female seed was connected to women's experience of pleasure – symbolized by orgasm. If the female seed was believed to have a less powerful role in conception, female sexual pleasure was perceived as necessary for reproduction. At the same time, a humoral view of the body, which saw women as cold and moist and men as hot and dry, suggested that sexual intercourse raised women's temperature. This made women naturally libidinous.

The emergence of new embryological theories in the seventeenth century challenged these views. Anatomical and microscopic studies revealed that rather than sexual pleasure producing the female seed, all female bodies contained eggs. This encouraged a view that conception happened regardless of women's experience of pleasure during intercourse, a view probably more in line with female experiences. These theories of reproduction influenced ways of thinking about sexual difference that emerged during the Enlightenment. Informed by religious, political, philosophical and cultural debates, and by the socioeconomic changes associated with industrialization, ideas about sexuality and sexual difference were put forward that reinforced new social and sexual roles that were being held up as marks of class distinction. The result was that the early modern libidinous woman evolved during the eighteenth century into the ideal of the passive and domesticated women of the nineteenth century.

Few historians would reject the idea that during the eighteenth century medical and cultural representations of female sexuality changed, but the completeness of this transformation is open to debate. Studies of eighteenth century pornography, far from signifying passivity, depict women as seductresses, while accounts by unmarried mothers further indicates that not all women were sexually passive. Popular midwifery manuals made little reference to new anatomical or physiological views, suggesting the more limited impact of new theories of reproduction. For many historians, the eighteenth century was a highpoint in sexual liberation – it was only in the nineteenth century that more repressive discourses emerged.

If the eighteenth century was a period of transition, conventional accounts stress how during the nineteenth century sexuality was medicalized. Yet, for much of the nineteenth century licensed practitioners tended to avoid discussing sex. When they did, it was largely in response to wider social or public health debates, for example, about the nature of prostitution and venereal disease or the role of women in society. Medical views of female sexuality were therefore intimately tied up with the emergence of new role models for middle-class women and ideals of respectability. They were informed by class, religious and moral values, and by the assumption that whereas men had natural sexual urges, which they should control, women had no innate interest in sex – a view that represented a double sexual standard and provided the cornerstone of middle-class ideas about female respectability. Rather than relying on medical evidence, medical practitioners initially employed a pseudo-science based around existing physiological models and cultural prejudices to support the ideal of the passionless woman. Ideas of sexual pleasure for women were rejected and normal female sexuality was defined within reproduction. This made sexuality in women a potential sign of moral failure or madness. These ideas have been closely associated with the work of the British surgeon William Acton. Historians have been keen to emphasize how women whose sexuality did not fit this model were subject to medical treatments as brutally embodied in the 1866–67 scandal that surrounded the British surgeon Isaac Baker-Brown and clitoridectomy.

The above discussion presents only one view of female sexuality. If research on working-class cultures has challenged views of sexual prudery and reticence, neither were ideas about female sexuality static. Although Foucault argued for a medicalization of sexuality during the last decades of the nineteenth century, licensed practitioners continued to be reticent when it came to writing about or discussing sex. Hence, the beginning of a shift in ideas about sexuality in the 1870s was only indirectly related to medicine. Ideas of hygiene, concerns about the regulation of prostitution, and first-wave feminism, voiced fears about the transmission of venereal disease and attacked the double sexual standard. They championed a single sexual morality, reversing earlier constructions to argue that it was women, not men, who were in control of their sexuality. It was not until the early years of the twentieth century that these views gained greater acceptance among a generation more eager to encourage female passion.

This did not mean that medicine was silent. The work of sexologists – for example, Otto Weininger and Richard von Krafft-Ebing in Austria or Havelock Ellis in England – and Sigmund Freud's studies of hysterical women, sought to construct new categories. They emphasized the importance of marriage, motherhood and heterosexuality for women's health. However, whereas Freud insisted that adult sexuality was not biologically predetermined, sexologists responded to *fin de siècle* anxieties about prostitution and venereal disease to reinforce middle-class morality. In presenting a scientific rationale for heterosexual sex, they reaffirmed traditional concepts of motherhood and emphasized male dominance to which women ideally responded. Equally, Freud's views of female sexuality assumed that the penis was the primary sexual organ and pathologized women who failed to conform to stereotypes of motherhood.

In the 1920s and 1930s, debates on birth control, eugenics and pronatalism encouraged a more active discussion of female sexuality. Local and national societies, along with some women's magazines, contributed to a loose sex reform lobby, while social scientists started to question biological determinism. Freudian ideas and sexology focused attention on appropriate expressions of sexuality within marriage. The writings of Marie Stopes in England and Theodor van de Velde in Holland proved enormously popular. Their work reinforced ideas that heterosexual women's sexual drives were natural but like psychological and medical discourses reinforced the centrality of marriage. Only slowly was sex and sexuality separated from reproduction as existing social mores proved hard to dislodge in part because there were high levels of ignorance about sex and reproduction and also because many women appeared to have wanted to adopt a passive sexual role. Censorship, especially in Britain, restricted popular dissemination of sexology. In France, popular marital advice manuals continued to presume that women had no sexual instinct, a view encouraged by the Catholic Church, while in Turkey the state sought to control women's sexual behaviour by requiring them to submit to virginity examinations.

Whereas open discussion of sex was relatively uncommon during the 1920s and 1930s, by the 1950s sexuality was discussed more from the perspective of pleasure than procreation. Anthropologists and sociologists started talking about sex roles as culturally determined and sexology informed couples of attitudes and techniques. The publication of Alfred Kinsey's extensive studies of the sex-life of Americans (1948 and 1953) had a powerful impact and new work in the neurology, psychology and social sciences in the United States started to separate sex from gender. For many, however, the 1960s appeared to mark a sexual revolution. The reasons for change have been associated with the development of the contraceptive Pill, although assessments of changing sexual attitudes should not ignore the role of post-war social reconstruction and socioeconomic changes that led to new social attitudes. For many, the Pill became synonymous with worry-free sexual activity and experimentation, but its use sparked heated discussions about sexuality, contraception and its moral consequences, and made women more dependent on medical practitioners for contraception.

Throughout the early modern and modern period, medicine offered a discursive framework that was frequently co-opted to wider social, cultural, political or economic debates about the role of women in society but it was seldom the dominant discourse when it came to female sexuality. If sexology in the late nineteenth century offered a new scientific language to understand sexual difference, it continued to uphold social norms. Often central to these debates was a connection between reproduction and female sexuality, which was only gradually eroded in the twentieth century. Rather than a clear process of medicalization, views of female sexuality involved complex interactions between medical and social views.

Regulating female sexuality

Although medicine was never the sole authority in defining female sexuality, theories of contagion and medical practitioners were important in policing female sexuality. In exploring how sexuality was controlled, historians have examined how in measures to prevent the spread of venereal disease concerns about deviance, sexuality and gender were combined. Regulation embodied medical and cultural assumptions about female sexuality and gave medical practitioners considerable rights over women's bodies. By looking at nineteenth and twentieth century measures to limit the spread of venereal disease, it becomes possible to explore the myths and contradictions that surrounded female sexuality in the past.

Because signs of venereal disease in women often went unnoticed, it was assumed by nineteenth century doctors that they were the chief carriers of venereal disease. In this discourse, medical pronouncements on the relationship between non-marital sex, prostitution and syphilis – seen for example in the ideas of the French 'hygienist' Parent-Duchâtelet – provided the basis for European governments' efforts to target the bodies of prostitutes. Broadly similar preventive strategies – often called regulationism – were adopted across Europe. Influenced by measures introduced in France during the Napoleonic era (1799–1815), regulation involved the identification and licensing of prostitutes, medical inspection and enforced treatment if a venereal disease was found. This approach was conditioned by a gendered view of female sexuality: it created a separate category of women – the prostitute – and endorsed a sexual standard by which men's sexual behaviour was treated with licence whilst women's was pathologized. In linking prostitution with venereal disease, regulation reinforced a view that sexuality in working-class women was dangerous.

The most notorious attempt to police female sexuality was the British Contagious Diseases Acts (1866–86). Historians have used the Acts to examine a number of contemporary issues relating to medicine, morality and the position of women. The Acts were framed as a public health measure to limit the spread of venereal disease in certain garrison and port towns. They gave a special body of plainclothes policemen the power to identify woman suspected of being a prostitute. Once identified, these women could voluntarily register as a prostitute or present themselves to a magistrate to prove their virtue. Registered women were required to undergo a fortnightly internal examination by a naval or military surgeon. If the woman refused, a magistrate could order her to be examined and sent to a lock (or venereal) hospital if found to have a venereal disease, where she would receive treatment and moral instruction. As in other European countries, moral and medical pathologies were conflated.

The Contagious Diseases Acts prompted a backlash, but the campaign against the Acts had two clear dimensions. For Josephine Butler, who led the campaign, the Acts subjected women to degradation and institutionalized a double sexual standard that targeted women. Examinations were defined as instrumental rape and campaigners argued that the Acts amounted to state sanctioned vice and sexual assault. However, whereas some protested about the attack on liberty and championed women's rights, others sought to prevent and punish what they saw as morally wrong. Often referred to as the social purity movement, they campaigned for further legislation to regulate sexuality. The result was the suspension and then repeal of the Acts and the passing of the 1885 Criminal Law Amendment Act, which raised the age of consent from thirteen to sixteen and provided a mechanism for the further policing of public sexuality.

The British Abolitionist campaign encouraged comparable movements across Europe, and before the outbreak of the First World War the regulation of prostitution and venereal disease control were major topics of public health and welfare debate. As in Britain, discussions were as much social as medical. They involved wide-ranging issues from the policing of the urban environment and sexual behaviour to questions of liberty and medical authority. If Abolitionists initially aimed to challenge existing sexual standards, through their campaigns they created new surveillance strategies and enforced middle-class views of sexual morality. The result was three broad approaches – ongoing regulationism in France and Germany, a voluntary approach in Britain, and 'sanitary statism' in Scandinavia where measures were applied to the sexually active population. In all cases, medical provision was combined with reformative policies that reflected ideas of class and perceptions of women's bodies, appearance and behaviour to target sexually active single women. Eugenic and pronatalist policies further politicized female sexual behaviour, ushering in maternalist policies in the early twentieth century that defined female sexuality through motherhood (see below).

Venereal disease control policies embodied the idea of the sexually dangerous woman. Measures targeted women, particularly young, single and working-class women, who violated social norms. Although the public nature of these debates in the twentieth century provided opportunities to challenge sexual mores, connections between venereal disease, morality and female sexuality persisted after 1945. The overlap of the moral and sanitary aspects of venereal disease control promoted the potent image of the sexually active women as potential reservoirs of infection. By the 1960s and 1970s, anxiety had shifted from prostitution to promiscuity but extramarital sex and female adolescent sexuality continued to be pathologized and targeted in public health campaigns. In regulating female sexuality, medicine provided a powerful agent of middle-class moralism.

Maternity and childbirth

An interest in history from below has encouraged historians to examine the doctor-patient relationship and patients' experiences of medicine. Although much of this research has often failed to consider the gendered dimension of medical encounters, or has focused on accounts of the literate, women often experienced a three-way relationship in their treatment. Relatives and family, who acted as gatekeepers and partly determined what care women received, influenced many women's interactions with healers. If financial resources further limited women's access to medical care, it was through pregnancy and childbirth that women came into regular contact with medicine.

Pregnancy and childbirth were central to women's accounts of sickness. Although maternal mortality was much lower than commonly believed – roughly one per cent of births in early modern Europe resulted in the woman dying – for many women, pregnancy and childbirth brought sickness, injury or even disability. The diaries of the seventeenth century vicar Ralph Josselin highlight how childbirth was not only hazardous, but also how most of the complaints suffered by his wife were related to pregnancy and childbirth. Most women recovered from minor complications or accommodated the resulting ailments into their daily lives as socioeconomic or political constraints prevented them from giving in to sickness. Many suffered in silence unless the problem was too serious to ignore. The growing use of birth control from the 1870s helped cut the birth rate, but mothers in the early twentieth century continued to remember the suffering associated with childbirth.

Given the importance of childbirth to female health, and representations of female bodies as reproductive bodies, historians have tended to concentrate on four main areas of maternity: the scene of the birth, the professional rivalries between male doctors and female midwives, the legal dimension (abortion and infanticide), and medicalization. By widening the scope of inquiry, a richer understanding of the relationship between medicine and maternity becomes possible, one that traces female experiences from conception to birth to show the ways in which class and medical and social constructions of female bodies influenced healthcare.

The development of oral contraceptives – the Pill – in the 1960s has commonly been represented as transforming sexual attitudes and marking the start of a sexual revolution. Medicine had provided a technology that allowed women to take control of their fertility. Such technological determinism ignores the fact that despite the relative ignorance about sexual and contraceptive matters before the late nineteenth century, women in the past had some control over their fertility. Often this had little to do with medicine. In the sixteenth and seventeenth centuries, when the information on contraception available from physicians was constrained by ecclesiastical opposition, oral traditions and popular literature offered fertile sources of knowledge. Abstention, non-coital sexual relations, withdrawal and prolonged lactation were all widely recognized methods of birth control, with barrier methods of contraception dating from the eighteenth century. When these methods of family limitation failed, abortion provided a solution. Court records reveal how women procured abortions by taking oral abortifacients, inserting instruments into their wombs, or by seeking medical assistance under the guise of provoking menstruation.

Although birth rates varied by country and region, and by class – the poor had higher birth rates for longer – there was a general European trend of falling birth rates after 1870. This has been seen as marking a radical shift in the nature of marital relations and as a feature in the development of modern societies. Demographic historians have put forward numerous explanations for this decline. Chief among them is the growing use of contraception. Although medical practitioners often resisted publicizing birth control, or labelled it dangerous, mechanical contraceptives were actively marketed in the nineteenth century as birth control became gradually more respectable. However, birth control had a clear class dimension: in Finland, it was the higher social classes that mostly used mechanical means of birth control, while evidence from Germany and Britain highlights how poorer women continued to rely on traditional methods, such as withdrawal, abstinence or abortion.

New barrier methods of contraception, such as the female cap or the latex condom, were developed in the 1920s and 1930s, and the availability of information on birth control increased considerably, encouraged by a combination of eugenics, liberalism, feminism and socialism, and by Marie Stopes and other campaigners' successful efforts to publicize birth control and improve access. Historians have assumed that together these had a marked impact on practices of family limitation. The use of female methods of contraception, such as the cap, did increase among all groups in the interwar period despite medical resistance, but traditional practices persisted. Notwithstanding the advice from birth control clinics, and medical warnings against the dangers of withdrawal, which included mental illness and sterility, new methods were not always trusted or welcomed. Abortion remained a widespread practice. In countries where pronatalism led to restrictions on the sale of contraceptives, such as Fascist Italy or Republican France, few options were available.

By the 1950s, previous attitudes that contraception was morally dubious had been eroded as post-war anxiety about the dangers of over-population made birth control more acceptable. Although the withdrawal method continued to be popular, pressure was applied to decriminalize abortion, and in Britain, France and Italy changes were made to the law to give women the legal right to choose. The introduction of the Pill in 1960 made birth control more palatable and accessible for many women and saw renewed interest in family planning. Despite the fears that came to surround the side effects of the Pill in the 1970s, by the end of the twentieth century, over 70 million women were using oral contraceptives.

The other side of the equation was medical assistance to help women become pregnant. Promoting fertility was an important early modern and modern concern. Popular midwifery manuals and sex advice literature offered practical advice on how to get pregnant. In the 1920s and 1930s, effort was invested in developing techniques to improve fertility. Research into the role of hormones contributed to a better understanding of ovulation to provide women with new scientific techniques for identifying and managing reproduction. Fertility drugs followed in 1960s and were quickly adopted. More controversial was in-vitro fertilization (IVF). The practice initially provoked outrage in the 1940s, but the British gynaecologist Patrick Steptoe and the physiologist Robert Edwards slowly developed a technique whereby eggs were removed from the ovary using a laparoscope, fertilized, and then returned to the uterus. The process produced the birth of the first 'test tube baby' in 1978 and attracted widespread media coverage. The new technique was controversial: IVF raised difficult moral questions and concerns about the legitimacy of surrogate motherhood. Notwithstanding these concerns and a number of scandals, IVF quickly became popular.

Medical involvement did not cease with conception and restart with birth. If feminist historians have shown how medical concerns were often more about behaviour than cure, uncertainties surrounding pregnancy shaped early modern medical debate. False conceptions were reported regularly as pregnancy was mistaken by women and by doctors for colic or wind, or as a dangerous stagnation of menstrual blood; uncertainties that some women used to secure an abortion. Much of the medical literature therefore emphasized how the detection of pregnancy was not straightforward. If in the seventeenth century considerable discussion focused on the process by which a foetus was formed, in other respects medical ideas repeated religious and supernatural views as evident in the link made between monstrous births and excessive or illicit sexual practices. At a more prosaic level, practical advice was given to early modern women on how to avoid miscarriage and on restorative remedies to aid pregnancy.

Evidence from popular medical and obstetric manuals reveals a growing medicalization of pregnancy in the nineteenth century. If medical check-ups during pregnancy were rare, detailed advice was offered on how to recognize the signs of pregnancy and how pregnant women should behave. Building on traditional notions of regimen, pregnant women were told to engage in moderate exercise, avoid tight clothing and mental excitement, and eat a light diet. Such a regimen reinforced social and biological constructions of femininity. Medical practitioners also advised on the treatment of common complaints, including nausea, indigestion and headaches. Although it was felt that practitioners had relatively little control over these symptoms, it was acknowledged that they could relieve the common complaints that caused many pregnant women discomfort.

However, until the late nineteenth century, most attention was directed at troublesome symptoms or the major complications of pregnancy. Miscarriages and those diseases that led women to miscarry therefore troubled medical practitioners most. In their writings, doctors asserted the importance of pregnant women consulting a doctor if problems occurred. It was therefore not just attendance during childbirth that offered doctors an entrée into the household. The development of laboratory tests to determine pregnancy in the twentieth century and the growth of antenatal clinics not only enabled doctors to detect obstetric abnormalities but also extended their role in defining pregnancy. By the 1920s, attendance at clinics, examinations and tests had become a routine part of pregnancy. A decade later expectant mothers in England could apply for free nutritional supplements from their doctors, and could have regular antenatal check-ups either at the local infant welfare clinic, or by home visits. These trends continued after 1945. The introduction of ultrasound in the 1950s allowed the careful monitoring of foetuses for abnormalities, and after initial concerns became routine. In the last decades of the twentieth century, a range of technological and genetic tests extended monitoring.

Historians have argued that this process of medicalization is evident in childbirth. Traditionally it has been suggested that the growing role of male practitioners in childbirth replaced female control and represented the triumph of medicine over superstition and ignorance. The introduction of the forceps in the eighteenth century is widely cited as the first step in this medicalization, which was followed by growing emphasis on hygiene in the nineteenth century and gradual improvements in obstetric surgery and a rise in the number of hospital births in the twentieth century. Although this neatly linear account has been challenged to suggest how medicalization not only deprived women of agency but also exposed them to greater risk during childbirth, the idea that male involvement in childbirth was limited before the eighteenth century has proved enduring.

Established narratives see women and midwives dominating childbirth in early modern Europe. In the sixteenth and seventeenth centuries, midwives provided assistance privately and through town councils as part of urban public health policies. Many were part of the system of licensing that dominated medical practice and some, such as Louise Bourgeois in Paris, were skilled practitioners. However, midwives did not have a monopoly. Across Europe, controls over midwifery rested with male corporate bodies [see 'Professionalization']. Midwifery and gynaecological texts were often directed at male physicians and surgeons, and in the seventeenth century a stream of books were published by male writers on pregnancy, caesarean section, ectopic pregnancies and difficult deliveries. Anatomical investigations of female bodies and foetuses point to further male involvement. In difficult deliveries, surgeons were called in, but male involvement often went further. For certain obstetric conditions, men were considered experts and male physicians were consulted to clarify problematic cases. Nor should it be assumed that male practitioners did anything different from their female counterparts.

Notwithstanding this male involvement in early modern childbirth, historians have commonly placed the eighteenth century as central to a change in the management of childbirth. This has been associated with increasing male medical intervention through the rise of the man-midwife, the growing use of forceps, and the creation of lying-in charities, which provided institutional care for poor reputable married women during pregnancy and birth. Yet, this process was neither simple nor inevitable. Nor was it purely the result of the impact of new instruments and interventions. A combination of forces – the growing market for medicine, professional concerns, the fashion for male attendance, efforts to promote population growth and reduce infant mortality, and the growth of specialist institutions – encouraged broad shifts in the nature of maternity care. Although the introduction of forceps allowed safer deliveries in difficult cases, the creation of training programmes for female midwives – for example, in Germany – suggests that women were not systematically excluded from practice or childbirth. Equally, the idea that change was driven by male practitioners does not hold up to scrutiny. Adrian Wilson's important work on the social history of childbirth in Britain reveals how women were active in encouraging changes in midwifery. In the *Making of Man-Midwifery* (1995), Wilson showed how the emergence of a new female culture among literate and upper-class women created demand for man-midwives as they sought to distinguish themselves and define their social status.

This is not to underestimate the changes that were occurring. The attendance of a man-midwife became fashionable for those who could afford them and the period saw the growth of lying-in hospitals and maternity charities that aimed to extend care for poor, often married women. Feminist historians have criticized lying-in hospitals as primarily patriarchal institutions that not only undermined female practitioners but also transferred control over birth from mothers to male practitioners. Studies of individual hospitals have questioned these assumptions, showing how they were not the mean and harsh institutions many have supposed. Nor did the growth of maternity hospitals mean the immediate medicalization of childbirth or male domination. They may well have created a bureaucratically controlled environment that conformed to middle-class moral standards, but most of the work in them continued to be undertaken by female staff. Male obstetricians were only generally used for difficult deliveries and their practices do not conform to the image of coercive or violent meddlers.

Nor did the growth of lying-in hospitals and the emergence of the man-midwife see sudden changes as suggested by the painting in Figure 4.2 which depicts what might be seen as a traditional birth scene. Traditional practices and cultures of childbirth continued. If female midwives lost ground with elite clients to the man-midwife, they continued to practise widely among the poor and middling sort. The assistance of female midwives remained the norm until the 1850s, and efforts to improve midwifery were designed to control not displace female midwives. It is also important to remember that women had choices. Experiences varied, but women also welcomed medical intervention. For example, notwithstanding the medical and religious debates that surrounded the use of chloroform in childbirth in the 1840s and 1850s, many women welcomed its use and the subsequent methods introduced to control pain during birth.

The creation of lying-in hospitals, however, did create a new institutional space for childbirth and fashioned the development of obstetrics. Although lying-in hospitals remained peripheral to most women's experiences of maternity in the nineteenth century, the European trend was from home to hospital births, particularly after 1930. This shift saw childbirth become safer as improve-

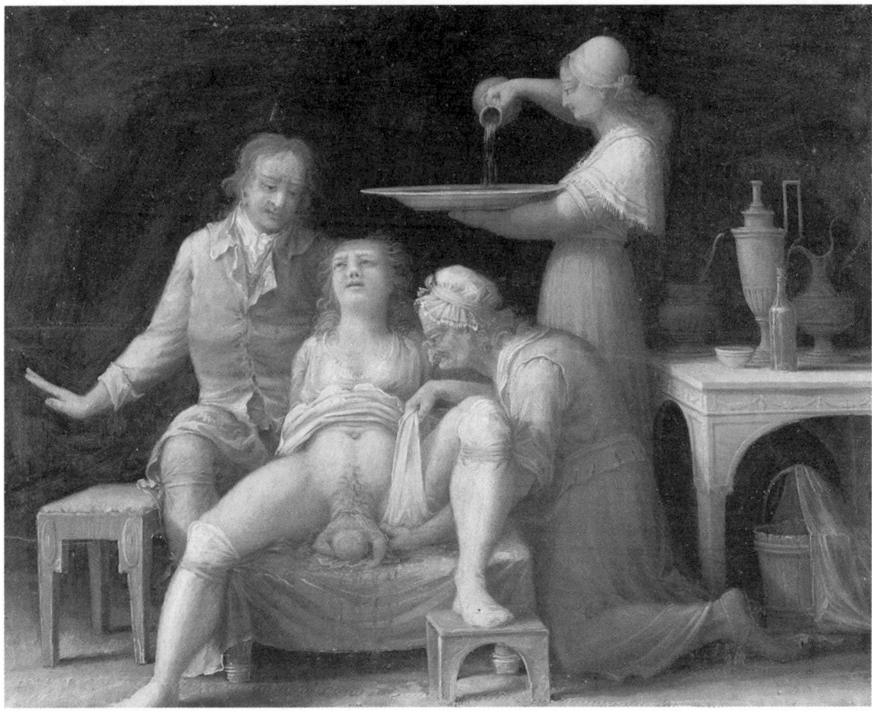

Figure 4.2 A birth scene, 1800.
Source: Wellcome Library, London.

ments to medicine – for example, the introduction of sulphonamides and blood transfusions – combined with improved prenatal care to reduce levels of puerperal fever, toxaemia and haemorrhages. As childbirth was redefined as a medical process and institutionalized, childbearing women became patients. If this was not an uncontested process, pregnant women and medical practitioners changed their habits and expectations regarding the place of birth.

The medicalization and institutionalization of childbirth was assisted by growing voluntary and government intervention in the politics of maternity. Ideas of scientific motherhood and the authority of doctors and other paramedical professionals over maternity were asserted. European states became more actively involved in maternity provision and the need to protect pregnant women [see 'Healthcare and the state']. From the early twentieth century, pronatalist concerns had a strong influence on social welfare, particularly in France under the Third Republic (1870–1940). Policies ranged from controls on women's work and access to contraception to investments in ante- and postnatal care, which in the 1930s were reinforced by the economic climate of the Depression and what might be seen as a broad back to home movement to protect male jobs. If these policies reached a particular intensity in Nazi

Germany (1933–45), elsewhere state provision reflected a desire to reduce infant mortality, protect the future strength of the nation, and preserve the wellbeing of mothers as a connection was made between maternal health and infant survival. Antenatal and maternity services were developed. Midwifery practices were standardized, institutionalized, and brought under the control of male medical hierarchies as evident in interwar Italy under the National Mother and Child Agency. One result was that by the late twentieth century midwives had little professional control over the management of childbirth.

Apart from in Nazi Germany, where considerable ideological emphasis was placed on home deliveries, the idea of a natural birth was replaced by a more interventionist and institutionalized model. Hospital provision of maternity beds rose and among the better-off private nursing homes became popular. Hospitalization for birth was quickly adopted in Scandinavia and other countries followed. New methods of management and pain relief – for example, twilight sleep that sought to remove the memory of pain if not the pain of childbirth itself – were introduced. The use of sulphonamides after 1935 to treat puerperal fever encouraged a steep fall in maternal mortality, and after 1945 the use of drugs and oxygen to induce childbirth and caesarean sections allowed greater medical management. If experiences varied across Europe, depending on socioeconomic and political factors and access to services, by the 1970s hospital births and dependence on qualified midwives, health visitors, general practitioners and obstetricians, and the advice they offered, had become the norm.

It would be easy to assume that this shift to institutionalization represented a state or doctor-driven phenomenon. As the 'women's question' challenged existing social and political institutions in the late nineteenth century, women's reform efforts were most visible in maternal and child welfare. Although feminists have criticized women campaigners for focusing too narrowly on maternity, this assessment underestimates how important these issues were, how they helped prepare the way for social policies and for women's role in them, and how many women benefited. Many women also welcomed these new maternity services. Childbirth was widely regarded as dangerous, a view shared by women and by doctors. Women feared for the health of their babies during pregnancy and after the birth. They sought support from medical practitioners and welcomed the medical management of childbirth, especially as hospital births became associated with safe and pain-managed deliveries. If this did not mean that standards of care or hygiene were always good – they were frequently poor – women used these new maternity services to their advantage. They derived benefits from them, not least in terms of better standards of obstetric care and lower levels of ante- and postnatal complications. Improved knowledge and rising expectations after the 1950s increased pressure from women for these services to be extended.

However, gendered interpretations of welfare often ignore class. Middle-class mothers and female healthcare providers worked with medical practitioners and state officials to promote the medicalization and institutionalization of childbirth, but in so doing they became involved in the development of policies that constrained the lives of other women. For example, before 1914, the French feminist movement successfully used pronatalist and nationalist concerns to pressurize the state to protect mothers. After 1918, these same ideas were used to push women out of the labour force. For poor women access to trained midwives and institutional services was limited. It was constrained by the extent and finance of state welfare provision, by household incomes, and by the geography and nature of voluntary services, which were predominantly urban in nature.

From looking at the experiences of maternity from conception and the management of pregnancy to childbirth, it becomes possible to see a process of medicalization between the sixteenth and twentieth centuries. If male practitioners were often silent on birth control, in the management of pregnancy and childbirth they offered advice and assistance throughout the early modern and modern periods. Rather than a shift from female cultures to male medical intervention, or sudden changes in the eighteenth century, a different process can be detected. It is one that points to gradual changes and growing institutionalization in which women had agency and were often willing partners. Although class was often important, such an account does suggest that our views of maternity provision in the past should not be solely coloured by twentieth century critiques of medicine and maternity.

Further reading

The best place to start when considering gender is Merry Wiesner-Hanks, *Gender in History* (Malden, MA: Blackwell, 2001) and Laura Lee Downs, *Writing Gender History* (London: Hodder Arnold, 2004). Although the bulk of writing on women and medicine concentrates on the modern period, Mary Fissell, 'Introduction: Women, Health and Healing in Early Modern Europe', *Bulletin of the History of Medicine* 82 (2008), pp. 1–17, provides an overview, with Monica Green, 'Gendering the History of Women's Healthcare', *Gender and History* 20 (2008), pp. 487–518, challenging traditional narratives of women and medicine. Thomas Laqueur, *Making Sex: Body and Gender from the Greeks to Freud* (Cambridge, MA: Harvard University Press, 1991) offers a provocative assessment of changes to the understanding of sex and gender, while Mary Fissell, 'Gender and Generation: Representing Reproduction in Early Modern England', *Gender and History* 7 (1995), pp. 433–56, and her *Vernacular Bodies: The Politics of Reproduction in Early Modern England* (Oxford: Oxford University Press, 2004) presents a longer chronology of change, with the collection edited by Londa Schiebinger (ed.), *Feminism and the Body* (Oxford: Oxford University Press, 2000) bringing together classic essays that explore perceptions of the female body. One of the first works to examine how female patients understood their health and illness is Barbara Duden's *The Woman Beneath the Skin: A Doctor's Patients in Eighteenth Century Germany* (Cambridge, MA: Harvard University Press, 1991), with Nancy Theriot, 'Negotiating Illness: Doctors, Patients, and Families in the Nineteenth Century', *Journal of the History of Behavioural Sciences* 37 (2001), pp. 349–68, arguing for female agency in shaping medical views. On the history of sexuality, Robert Nye's *Sexuality* (Oxford: Oxford University Press, 1999) provides a wide-ranging and thoughtful introduction, while Timothy Gilfoyle's 'Prostitutes in History', *American Historical Review* 104 (1999), 117–41, is an excellent historiographical review of prostitution and its regulation. For the literature on birth control, a good starting point remains Angus McLaren, *A History of Contraception* (Oxford: Blackwell, 1990). For the twentieth century, Kate Fisher's *Birth Control, Sex and Marriage in Britain, 1918–1960* (Oxford: Oxford University Press, 2006) is a lively reassessment of the role of birth control, while Lara Marks, *Sexual Chemistry* (New Haven and London: Yale University Press, 2001) outlines the history of the contraceptive pill. There are numerous good studies of maternity and childbirth, and readers should turn to Jacques Gelis, *History of Childbirth: Fertility, Pregnancy and Birth in Early Modern Europ*e (London: Polity, 1991) and Adrian Wilson, *The Making of Man-Midwifery: Childbirth in England, 1660–1770* (Cambridge, MA: Harvard University Press, 1995), while Ann Oakley's *The Captured Womb: History of the Medical Care of Pregnant Women* (Oxford: Blackwell, 1986) provides a feminist reading. For a comparative dimension, see Irvine Loudon's *Death in Childbirth: An International Study of Maternal Care and Maternal Mortality, 1800–1950* (Oxford: Clarendon Press, 1980).

5

Medical self-help and the market for medicine

The sick have never been passive in the face of sickness. In early modern Europe, many people made their own preliminary self-diagnosis or sought one from other family or community members. The sick and their families, especially female members of the household, assessed how serious a condition was, followed by the likely cost of care in terms of money, time or convenience, before turning to all manner of medicines. Medical cultures in early modern Europe were pluralistic and neither patients nor their families were the passive subjects of medical practitioners. They were historical actors who made independent judgements and choices about the treatments they used and the practitioners they consulted. Many turned to domestic or commercial remedies before they chose to consult one of the many types of medical practitioner that existed or would mix the different types of care available to them [see 'Professionalization'].

The concept of the medical marketplace has offered historians a means for mapping these choices. First referred to by Harold Cook in *The Decline of the Old Medical Regime in Stuart London* (1986), and influenced by the free market ideology of the 1980s, the medical marketplace proposed a model of market relationships between patients and healers as a way of understanding the intricate interactions between the supply and demand for medical services. Mainly applied to early modern medicine, the model encouraged historians to think about patients as active agents and practitioners (licensed as well as irregular) as entrepreneurs to examine how social and commercial factors influenced medical knowledge. If a concentration on the medical marketplace has often been at the expense of cultural forces and has marginalized cooperation in favour of competition, the model has proved useful for historians in understanding how the sick sought and negotiated care. The growing complexity of this marketplace in the eighteenth and nineteenth centuries only served to increase the access the sick and their families had to a diverse range of medical care, both within and outside the home. What emerged out of these historiographical trends is a market model of medical encounters in which questions of agency and choice were central to structuring medicine, the choice of practitioner, and the use of popular medicine and self-medication. The result, as Andrew Wear explained in *Medicine in Society* (1992), was a much richer medical world.

This chapter examines ideas of choice. Rather than concentrating on the variety of healers that inhabited the market, it adopts a more patient-centred and domestic perspective to focus on individuals and families. It explores the nature of the medical marketplace by examining medical pluralism from the perspective of popular medicine – defined as the medicine of ordinary people – self-medication and the role of quack and patent remedies, and how an examination of the socioeconomic landscape of medicine can shed light on social issues from religion and lifestyle to political protest. Key concerns explored are the boundaries between popular and learned medicine, how the sick respond to illness by examining the opportunities available to them from popular to over-the-counter medicines, and how this allowed the sick to be their own healers.

Popular medicine and medical self-help

At a time when disease was ever-present, early modern men and women maintained their bodies and even checked on how they smelt to monitor their health [see 'Disease']. When confronted with the inevitable reality of disease, most had a keen interest in healing. With university-educated physicians able to claim few therapeutic successes until the late nineteenth century, and with too few licensed practitioners to meet the needs of most towns, many drew on a wide array of healing measures and turned to medical self-help and more immediate and domestic sources of treatment, or what can loosely be termed popular medicine.

The terms popular medicine, vernacular medicine and folk medicine are often used interchangeably to describe early modern practices of medical self-help. Associated with the feminine and domestic sphere, popular medicine has frequently been dismissed as somehow outside of conventional medicine or based on folk beliefs that were somehow unscientific. As scholars rejected older explanations that equated medicine with a history of progress, popular medicine was shown to embrace a wide spectrum of overlapping systems of medicine, which formed a shared set of mentalities to create individual, collective, local and regional practices. Rigid divisions between learned and popular medicine became suspect as historians became more interested in how academic and other forms of lay and alternative medicine interacted.

People from the sixteenth to the eighteenth century were clear that looking after and preserving their own and their dependants' health was a self-evident duty, a belief reinforced by Christian traditions and by physicians [see 'Religion']. At a domestic level, this was often the responsibility of female household members, who were expected to have some skill in the manufacture of remedies. Historians have tended to emphasize the importance of suspicion or disillusionment with formal medicine in explaining the longevity of medical self-help, but it was more than just an expression of distrust or fatalistic views of disease. It reflected social and cultural ideas about health and responsibility as well as economic realities – it was considerably cheaper than consulting a physician – and limited access to licensed practitioners. Popular medicine was part-and-parcel of wider realities of self-sufficiency and making do with local resources. Rooted in the home and often simple to make, popular medicine represented the most ubiquitous form of medical care in early modern Europe.

However, popular medicine was not monolithic. Structured around oral and printed culture, family and community networks, popular medicine was mapped, as the British historian Roy Porter explained in *Patients and Practitioners* (1985), onto varying socioeconomic circumstances, levels of literacy, class and community perceptions and onto individual and personal circumstances. It was structured by religious beliefs and by gender and geography. This local dimension gave popular medicine shape, meaning and a domain of application, which was shaped by the physical, social and cultural circumstances in which it was made, and in which it was used. Within this framework, it might therefore be better to think of popular medicines and medical pluralism rather than a monolithic popular medicine, at least until the eighteenth century when a proliferation of medical texts and commercially available remedies created more national patterns.

With everyone responsible for maintaining their own health, a certain amount of medical knowledge was indispensable, but if popular medicine in early modern Europe was eclectic, it was not separate from formal medicine. Historians have shown how elite and popular cultures were not unconnected; that there was interaction between the two. The same was true of medicine as evident in Edward Jenner's work on smallpox vaccination, which drew on local knowledge that milkmaids who suffered from cowpox seldom succumbed to smallpox. Although popular medicine was derived from learned medicine, it was not simply a question of learned and popular ideas intersecting. Nor was it a matter of true medical knowledge versus a corrupted lay version. Rather, medical and popular understanding of health and disease shared common ideas about the body and illness.

Licensed practitioners did lay claim to greater knowledge and expertise, but a commonality underpinned encounters between practitioners and the sick. If people frequently used domestic analogies to understand the body, at least until the late eighteenth century, they and learned physicians drew on the humoral system and an understanding that treatment aimed to maintain or restore lost equilibrium [see 'Disease']. The other mainstay of early modern medicine – the idea of sympathy – equally allowed people to cure themselves by transferring their illness to other objects or plants. Within this shared framework, practitioners and the laity drew on similar approaches to particular illnesses, and both accepted that magic had a powerful influence on disease [see 'Religion']. If the power of magic to cause or cure disease lost ground in the seventeenth century, studies of household remedy books reveal how many of the ingredients used in popular medicine between the sixteenth and eighteenth centuries closely resembled those recommended by physicians and sold by apothecaries. Cowslip wine (for measles in children) and rhubarb (for purging), as well as medicines made from animals, such as grasshoppers and swallows for example, were folk remedies and were commonly prescribed by doctors. Comparable roles were assigned to food, regimen and moderation in treating or preventing disease, although most popular remedies tended to emphasize purging and the alleviation of symptoms. Different explanations for using these remedies might have been put forward by licensed practitioners and the laity, but similarities were an important feature of medical practices. Ideas and information was exchanged between the laity and medical practitioners and a common medical culture existed.

Although popular medicine shared common characteristics with the medicine dispensed by licensed practitioners, it also proved highly flexible and was historically and culturally determined. Sufferers and their families developed hybrid and plural forms of medical self-help that was shaped by a wide range of sources, traditions and ideas, and by the availability and affordability of natural and commercial remedies. It was adaptable to local circumstances and beliefs, and was passed on through an oral tradition and family recipe and commonplace books, and later through popular medical texts and almanacs. These texts had a wide readership. They acted as reference books and practical manuals, providing the laity with a high degree of medical knowledge.

Medical self-help covered the management of sickness and the positive pursuit of health. Food, drink and lifestyle (including exercise) were important. Herbs, flowers and roots, minerals and animal matter – ingredients easily grown, gathered and administered – formed the mainstay of therapies in the sixteenth and seventeenth centuries. Certain plants or ingredients had particular properties: for example, rhubarb was used for constipation; goose-grease cured colds; mistletoe aided the treatment of tumours. Objects or charms had healing powers that utilized magical and superstitious beliefs. Amulets worn to heal or avert illness were popular: those containing jewels, bones or coral were worn for the protection of infants and as a cure for kidney disease; fossilized shark teeth (believed to be the tongues of serpents turned to stone) were employed as antidotes to poisons. Such traditional remedies could be combined with the various moral self-help therapies, such as herbalism, vegetarianism or temperance, which came into vogue in the nineteenth century and drew on long-established notions of regimen and the importance of diet and lifestyle in promoting health.

It would be easy to assume that medical self-help was limited to the uneducated, but the idea that the lower orders were the only ones to deal with everyday ailments themselves does not hold up to scrutiny. Popular medicine was everyone's medicine, although the elite appeared to have had a fondness for more exotic remedies containing luxury ingredients like saffron or pearls. Most families were fairly knowledgeable about medical matters, and all income groups took energetic action to protect and manage their health [see 'Disease']. Nor were there rigid distinctions between urban and rural practices. Published texts and almanacs detailing domestic or herbal remedies were widely available. They assumed a basic medical and botanical knowledge, and advised on diagnosis and on treatments that could be prepared at home or by an apothecary. Familiar and medicinal herbs were easily grown and collected, or could be readily purchased from apothecaries, who traded in all but the remotest areas. From 1700 onwards, the use of commercially available ingredients and remedies became more marked as the sick invested in proprietary medicines. By the eighteenth century, the laity were often just as at home using traditional herbal remedies and regulating their lifestyle as they were with proprietary medicines.

Self-management and medication was a common response to trivial conditions but also covered many diseases, accidents and emergencies. Confidence was expressed in the methods adopted because they appeared to work, a happy coincidence aided by natural recovery and the medicinal quality of some of the ingredients. Nevertheless, there were other factors at work. Medical self-help offered the means for the sick, their families and the community to take remedial action on their own initiative and to match treatment to their perceptions of the disease. If for some it was a desperate move, others were motivated by a sense of vanity or a desire to conserve resources. Given that medical practitioners could claim few therapeutic successes until the late nineteenth century, self-medication was not necessarily worse than the other options available. Many regularly took a purge or vomit to remove excess humors and employed a range of remedies, combining different systems of medicine. Families and friends swapped advice, recipes and treatments, which often reflected familial or local networks of information, power and authority. Many households were well stocked with laxatives, purgatives and painkillers (such as the bestselling Dr James's Powder). The widespread availability of opium gave easy access to pain relief, and the growing market for proprietary remedies in the eighteenth century increased opportunities to self-medicate. That William Buchan's *Domestic Medicine*, first published in 1769, informed readers to avoid certain forms of surgery not only reveals how the laity would dress wounds, and even set fractures but that some might attempt more ambitious operations.

Recognizing that most saw self-medication as complementary to care from a practitioner, doctors responded accordingly. They drew on shared ideas and language. Early modern plague texts advised the laity how to prevent or cure the disease. The seventeenth and eighteenth centuries saw an increase in medical manuals, with later texts reflecting an Enlightenment (eighteenth century) belief in the diffusion of useful knowledge and the need to reform popular habits. They had a major impact on medical beliefs and practices at every strata of society. Texts fell into two broad categories: books on regimen intended for an educated audience and more pragmatic advice manuals with their strong emphasis on self-help. In France, numerous compact health dictionaries were published. In Britain, the English Revolution (1640–60) and the lifting of censorship saw a flood of vernacular publishing and the rapid proliferation of domestic medical texts. Publications like Samuel Tissot's *Avis au Peuple sur la Sante* (Advice to the People Regarding their Health, 1761) or Christoph Hufeland's *Die Kunst das menschlichen Lebens zu verlängern* (The Art of Prolonging Life, 1797–98) proved immensely popular. Such texts gave instructions for healthy living that included drug remedies and advice on how to cure a variety of common disorders. In providing this information, they served a somewhat contradictory purpose: they asserted medical authority to protect the public from unlicensed practitioners and brought medical knowledge within everybody's reach. However, they were not the only sources of information. Newspapers reported a wide range of medical and scientific courses, cures and advances. If such texts did not entirely supplant oral traditions, they served to popularize medical knowledge and encourage self-medication.

Peter Burke in his seminal study, *Popular Culture in Early Modern Europe* (1978), argued that by 1800 European elites had abandoned popular culture to the lower orders. Support for magical cures did decline in the eighteenth century, and in the nineteenth century there was growing assault on popular errors that equated popular and folk medicine with superstition and ignorance. Divisions and tensions between the medical beliefs of the learned and the poor, between professional and popular medicine, became more clearly defined, and government intervention in healthcare altered the structure of the medical market.

However, the view that in the eighteenth century elite and medical ideas replaced popular practices is not supported by evidence from nineteenth century diaries or letters. True, informal and formal medicine clashed in the period, but traditional practices that served a function, and beliefs that made sense of everyday ailments, continued to thrive at a time when fevers, childhood diseases, accidents and minor ailments remained widespread. Nor was it just the rural poor who clung to traditional remedies and beliefs. In the lives of many working men and women room remained for medical self-help, especially given the cost of consulting a medical practitioner. Ideas associated with popular medicine were absorbed into the medical fringe. Movements, such as phrenology or mesmerism, not only provided a means to understand the natural world and the mind, but also offered people the opportunity to experiment and make their own medical decisions. Lay responses to health and disease went much further than embracing alternative medicine. They also involved collective strategies. Hospital provision was driven by the laity [see 'Hospitals'], as was public health [see 'Public health'] and poor relief [see 'Healthcare and the state']. These collective strategies represented a different dimension to lay responses to medicine: not only did they transcend the individual and the domestic but they also served to legitimize the authority of the medical profession.

At an individual and local level, middling and poor families throughout the nineteenth century turned to informal methods of treatment, especially for minor or self-limiting ailments. For example, when Adelheid Popp's brother was suffering from an open abscess in the 1870s in Germany, Popp explained that 'Any household medicine, good and bad, was used. My mother went to see an old woman in the city to get an ointment which was supposed to work wonders'.[1] In many rural areas, the labouring poor maintained a framework of local beliefs, superstitions, knowledge and remedies that helped them make sense of the world. But traditional remedies and practices also remained strong in towns. There were continuities, but practices and beliefs, rather than remaining static, were adapted to new circumstances. New ideas from medicine, such as germ theories, were incorporated into popular understanding of disease and ideas of prevention [see 'Disease']. Some customs and remedies were abandoned in the face of new commercial remedies. Others were repackaged, as can be seen in the many forms opium took. Rising disposable incomes and the growth of proprietary medicines as part of a consumer revolution created numerous opportunities for medical self-help (see below) as an unprecedented range of mass-produced over-the-counter medicines flooded the market. Retail chemists grew in number in response to demand, offering an accessible range of remedies for the home. Over-the-counter indigestion remedies and cough mixtures provided symptomatic relief, while disinfectant soaps helped women create germ-free homes. Medical practitioners answered demand for advice and responded to contemporary debates on diet and lifestyle with vigour, publishing numerous advice books. Local and popular medical cultures meshed readily with the medicine provided by doctors.

Sufferers continued to embrace medical self-help for many of the same reasons as their predecessors had – cost, seriousness of condition, ability to control treatment or desperation – while self-help practices formed part of local cultures and traditions of domestic manufacture. Evidence from local newspapers, letters and diaries highlights ongoing distrust of formal medicine. The visibility of disease and epidemics along with sensationalist newspaper reports further frightened patients into trying numerous forms of self-medication. Historians have been keen to emphasize patient agency and choice in structuring medical pluralism, but it should be remembered that socioeconomic and other constraints, including access to licensed practitioners and the scale of ill health, often necessitated some form of self-medication. If it is unwise to overstress antagonism to formal medicine, a powerful nineteenth century ideology of self-help continued to encourage a do-it-yourself approach, as did the cost of licensed practitioners. As George Sturt remembered in *A Small Boy in the Sixties* (1977), people took risks because it cost too much to go to a doctor.

Nor would it be wise to see medical self-help and medical pluralism as somehow vanishing in the twentieth century in the face of the power of biomedicine. The growth of over-the-counter medicines and the ongoing faith that regular doses of drugs or vitamins along with diets and exercise could bring health ensured that many continued to take responsibility and action when it came to maintaining their health. If the expansion of state welfare brought more people into regular contact with doctors, self-drugging continued to be enormous. Individuals and families had their own strategies, which included mixing home-made remedies with over-the-counter medicines. Making medicines from home or bought ingredients remained commonplace in the 1930s, while by 1939 an estimated £22 million was being spent on proprietary medicines in Britain. Wartime surveys in Britain revealed not only that many individuals took a range of medicines from aspirin and headache powders to laxatives and sedatives, but also that many ailments continued to be self-managed as the sick balanced concerns about seriousness with the cost of care, attitudes to consulting practitioners and practitioners' attitudes to particular ailments. It would seem that alternative medical systems and popular medicine were remarkably enduring, aided by the ongoing expansion of newspaper circulation and a vogue for self-help books. Popular and over-the-counter medicines underwent their own rationalizing process to take on new commercial forms or became associated with populist health movements, such as nudism or vegetarianism.

In post-war Europe, the consolidation of state medical services did not see the sick rushing to their doctors or high-tech hospitals for every ailment. Old wives' tales and folk beliefs – feed a cold, starve a fever for example – continued to offer a repository of popular and medical facts. Room remained for self-diagnosis and medication, particularly for non-serious ailments like headaches, nausea, hay fever, and colds (to name but a few). Access to effective over-the-counter medicines, vitamins and other medical-related products from plasters to blood-pressure monitors made self-medication a feature of the high street and provided consumers with numerous opportunities for self-medication. From the 1960s, emerging doubts about medical procedures, about drugs and their side effects, and about individual practitioners, encouraged both growing mistrust of medicine and a desire to regain control over the medical process. For some this meant embracing commercially available alternative medicines, particularly homeopathic remedies; for others, exercise and health fads became the route to health. With the growth of the internet in the first decade of the twenty first century, health advice became freely available and the online sale of medicines flourished. Internet users drew on a similar range of concerns and attitudes to those of early modern individuals when they shopped around for therapies or made informed choices about different systems of medicine or treatments.

Even with the growing contemporary popularity of alternative and traditional herbal remedies, it would be easy to dismiss the role and efficacy of popular medicine. Historians (and indeed modern medical researchers) have become increasingly aware of the dangers of passing judgements on past medical practices, of dismissing domestic remedies as arcane or wrong. As explained above, this presumes a dichotomy with conventional medicine. It ignores how popular and academic medicine overlapped. This was still evident in the nineteenth and twentieth centuries. For example, medical and lay responses to influenza both asserted the need for rest, good nutrition and symptomatic relief. Opium was both a popular remedy effective for a whole range of ailments and was prescribed by doctors. Nor was popular medicine static. Popular understanding was reworked as new ideas were absorbed from medicine. Ideas about germs, for example, were incorporated into popular perceptions of disease and, as Nancy Tomes demonstrates in *The Gospel of Germs* (1998), through the selling of ideas of hygiene came to alter every aspect of everyday life. The idea that popular medicine was somehow backward also obscures the roles it had in making sense of disease, in providing relief, or its socioeconomic or political role. Popular medicine could be an expression of choice or a strategy that reflected the cost of, or access to the care available from medical practitioners. It could embody popular conceptions of health and disease or wider social concerns about naturalism or holism. Rather than dismissing popular medicine, we should see it as integral to individuals' approaches to sickness and health in early modern and modern Europe.

Charlatans, quacks and commercial medicines: 1500–1800

Whereas popular medicine was ubiquitous, the growth of quack and commercial medicines represented the dynamic edge of self-medication and the growing market for medicine. Discussions of the growth of commercial medicines have frequently concentrated on the economic dimension and the birth of a consumer economy in the eighteenth century. Roy Porter's *Health for Sale* (1989) is the most important (and engaging) survey of the topic. For Porter the market was a driving force for modernity and quackery the capitalist mode of production in medicine. Until Porter's study, historians readily dismissed quacks, a view that does injustice to their careers, their patients, and to the medical milieu in which they sold their cures. The increasingly vociferous attacks on quackery by licensed practitioners from the late eighteenth century onwards have created a skewed picture. These campaigns tell us more about the concerns of licensed practitioners than they do about the nature of quackery [see 'Professionalization'], but how to define quackery is problematic. The origin of the term, an abbreviation of quacksalver, is obscure but probably dates from the sixteenth century and was used to describe a range of healers and nostrum pedlars. Licensed practitioners applied the label quack as a term of abuse to attack individual healers, treatments and emerging specialist fields as a means of denouncing competing forms of medical practice. Nor are we making distinctions between licensed and irregular practitioners straightforward. Quacks used the title doctor to acquire status and respectability, and came from a range of backgrounds; licensed surgeons, physicians and apothecaries sold cheap remedies and marketed cures, while many also endorsed patent medicines. One way of understanding quackery therefore is to see the vendors of commercial medicine as medical entrepreneurs who developed the consumer side of medicine.

The expansion of towns and the growth of trade in the sixteenth and seventeenth centuries created new opportunities for the sick to seek out all kinds of medical practitioner and buy remedies. Choice and pluralism were central to the medical marketplace and a variety of (travelling and urban) charlatans across Europe sold simple remedies for common ailments. In rural or under-populated areas, quacks and their remedies formed an essential component of medical care that reflected ideas of choice, medical self-help and economics. These healers mixed care for the body with an understanding of popular culture. They sold

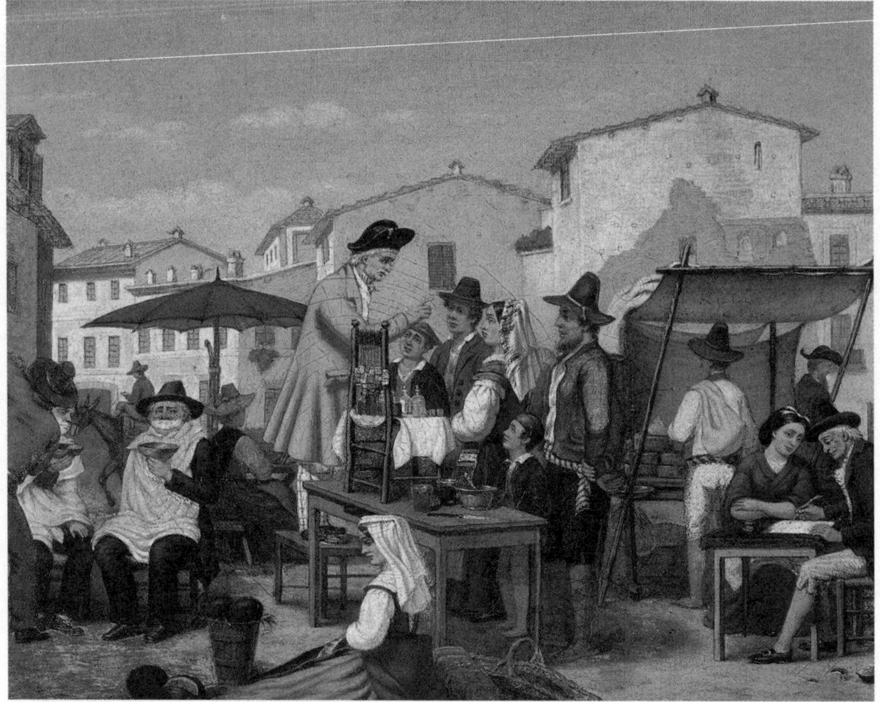

Figure 5.1 A quack and a barber ply their trade in an Italian market square.
Source: Wellcome Library, London.

remedies that were consistent with popular conceptions of disease and took advantage of growing discontent with established medicine. By combining theatre with the sale of medicines, such quacks became popular with crowds everywhere.

There was an increase in the number of remedies available in the seventeenth century as quack and over-the-counter medicines flourished. Some developed into household names – Daffy's Elixir first appeared around 1660 and was advertised into the 1920s – and there were a number of competing brands. Treatments for venereal disease were fertile ground as the powerful stigma attached to sexually transmitted diseases made privacy crucial. If stigmatized diseases (such as syphilis) produced secret remedies, as treatment and health grew increasingly synonymous with taking a drug, commercial remedies flourished as the middling sort started to look outside the home and use commercially available medicines. An expansion in the market for printed material and newspapers along with the growth of postal systems allowed medicines to be sold at a national level, and by third parties, including innkeepers, booksellers and pedlars. It was a phenomenon that coincided with an expansion in the production of cheap consumer goods and non-essential or luxury items. With few legal controls on medical practice, especially in Britain, and with medicine driven by demand and choice, commercial medicine could thrive.

As Roy Porter eloquently argued in *Health for Sale* it was in the eighteenth century that commercial medicine and quackery entered its golden age. If national regulatory systems and economies determined the nature of this market at a national level, the idea that commercial and over-the-counter medicines became a standard feature of an expanding medical marketplace, replacing domestic remedies and challenging licensed practitioners, has become a commonplace in the historiography. Historians have pointed to the growing demands of a medically promiscuous public and a dramatic increase in the number and variety of healers in the eighteenth century. Quackery hence both reflected and fuelled a transition from home remedies to commercial medicines and reinforced the notion that health was a commodity. In meeting demand from the sick and in attracting medical entrepreneurs, commercial medicine served to broaden the opportunities for cure or relief available in an already pluralistic medical marketplace.

There is considerable merit in this analysis. During the eighteenth century, the boundaries between commercial and non-commercial medicines became increasingly blurred and quackery benefited from the growing market for medicine at a time when state and professional controls were weak. This phenomenon has been associated with industrialization and urbanization, particularly in England where Porter argues quackery flourished. Although this argument fails to take fully into account that not all sections of society participated in the eighteenth century consumer boom, it does have an appeal. New methods of standardization and industrial production aided the manufacture of commercial remedies. The rapid increase in population created new mass markets, while the dramatic rise in the number and size of towns made the retailing of goods and services easier. New wholesale and retail outlets emerged to meet demand: for example, the number of druggists grew dramatically. Innovations in commerce, improved communications and levels of literacy, and the growth of the provincial press were all crucial in shaping national markets. Part of the bourgeois public sphere, the growth of the press created what Colin Jones has referred to as a '"Great Chain of Buying" (and selling)' based around the small ad, which made it easier to promote goods and create a demand for brand names.[2] Better postal networks made it more straightforward to sell goods at a national level. Combined these factors encouraged the desirability of consumption that went beyond localism, class, occupation and gender.

This expansion of a consumer society created an ideal environment to promote the business side of medicine, and medicine became a crucial component of this new world of consumerism. The emphasis placed on the maintenance of private and domestic health, and long established habits of medical self-help, offered a rationale and language that helped sell a wide range of medical commodities. As levels of disposable income rose, so too did the amount spent on health, highlighting the strength of demand for medical services. In this growing market, medical diversity and distinctiveness were clear advantages. For many practitioners, the chance to make a medical living and a name for themselves rested with exploiting this market.

With commercial medicines sold at a high price, especially for the poor, other factors are needed to explain the spectacular growth of commercial medicines in the eighteenth century. Drawing on Neil McKendrick's ideas[3] about the eighteenth century consumer revolution in England, the emerging cult of sensibility and social emulation have been presented as key factors as the middle ranks became more self-confident and sought to imitate their betters. Yet, aspiration and emulation are problematic categories to unpick, especially as those buying commercial medicines may have invested them with different meanings. For Roy Porter other factors were responsible from the growing culture of hypochondria – an argument that reflected contemporary concerns – to the value commercial medicines had in providing the sick and their families with reassurance and the ability to exert some control over illness. Porter goes on to argue how as the market for medicine grew, the more sick people came into contact with medical practitioners, which encouraged both a preoccupation with health and a tendency for the sick to try the growing range of medicines advertised in newspapers and available in shops. The other side of the equation was scepticism of formal medicine and distrust of doctors. The therapeutic complexity that characterized the eighteenth century – in which different systems of medicine competed and most practitioners adopted an eclectic approach – provided a space in which quacks staked out their claims.

Eighteenth century quacks ranged from the occasional part-time healer and itinerant pedlars to large-scale capitalists. While most quacks were smaller-scale entrepreneurs, they were by no means poor, provincial or outsiders. Although some lacked medical training, others had a formal medical education and might be physicians or surgeons. A few sold their medicines in enormous quantities and made considerable fortunes. Just like their predecessors, they sold an array of pills, powders, lozenges, tinctures, cordials, plasters, ointments, lotions and oils. Some were patented, giving the producer a monopoly, but most were merely proprietary. There was also a vast array of medical appliances. These included false teeth, spectacles and a profusion of trusses. While some quacks offered specifics, other marketed cure-alls. Producers were free to make any claims they wanted. Cough medicines also purported to cure headaches; nerve tonics to relieve gout. Many commercial medicines professed a blunderbuss quality. Contemporaries were aware that some medicines were little short of miraculous in the cures they promised.

Notwithstanding this diversity, eighteenth century quackery had several common components. It reflected consumer choice and the economics of medical care: quack medicines were cheaper than the cures prescribed by licensed practitioners and were widely available as they made their medicines available nationally through newspaper advertisements, grocers and chemists. They were hence convenient and accessible, and reflected the desire of consumers to self-diagnose, choose their treatments, and self-medicate. Because of this, quack remedies covered the whole range of medical complaints, though desperate or stigmatizing illnesses continued to offer fertile ground for secret remedies and treatment for venereal disease was considered something of a racket in the eighteenth century.

Central to the explosion in commercial medicines in the eighteenth century was how quacks marketed their medicines and made them accessible. They drew on existing advertising schemes employed in other areas of commerce and associated their wares with whatever was convenient and interesting. Quacks used publicity stunts, enthusiastically denounced their competitors, and patented remedies and cure-alls such as Carter's Little Liver Pills or Poor Man's Friend Ointment. Although the methods they adopted mirrored the publicity devices used by licensed practitioners, quacks also exploited new forms of commercialism and the press and took accepted practices to extravagant lengths to get themselves noticed. Advertising provided the cornerstone of success: many were bold and utilized a common vocabulary, often containing a paragraph extolling the virtues of a particular remedy or a testimonial from a purportedly respectable member of society. As skilful psychologists, quacks manipulated desires for reassurance and privacy: they played on latent hypochondriacal tendencies and popular and scientific fads to sell a wide range of medicines to meet every need.

However, quacks were not ignorant fraudsters whose only goal was to exploit the gullible. To accept these claims would be to endorse not only contemporary criticisms of quackery but also a rhetoric of modernization and professionalization. Quacks were not some simple medical 'other' but were closely associated with regular medicine. Indeed, qualified practitioners devised some of the best selling commercial medicines, such as James's Powder, and regularly endorsed their effectiveness. Quackery formed part of a pluralistic medical system and, just like popular medicine, complemented other forms of care. Many remedies were similar to those prescribed by physicians and many followed traditional treatments or repackaged folk or popular medicines. For example, most opium preparations sold by chemists or marketed as patent medicines were only commercial versions of common remedies. What was different was the nature of the marketing and the scale. Nor were commercial medicines limited in their appeal. All social classes used them. Charitable and state institutions for the relief of the poor purchased commercial medicines, which were equally dispensed by physicians and apothecaries. Quacks offered mass market, brand name medicines, making money out of selling medical commodities and devices rather than expertise.

Whereas the above might beg the question 'did such medicine work?' in many ways this is misleading. Attacks by licensed practitioners on quack and over-the-counter remedies were informed by self-interest and questions of integrity and competence are difficult to settle. Investigations in France and Britain revealed striking similarities between commercial medicines and those prescribed by licensed practitioners, but perhaps the main test should be contemporary assessment. Despite opposition from licensed practitioners, in a milieu when regular medicine offered few therapeutic advantages, quack and over-the-counter medicines were regarded as equal to the cures available from licensed practitioners.

If eighteenth century commercial medicine is often discussed in economic terms, studies of the campaigns against irregular practitioners and commercial remedies have done so within a framework of professionalization and medicalization. Competition from quacks did generate considerable anxiety among licensed practitioners. In the sixteenth and seventeenth centuries, attacks focused on fraud and deceit. Alarm about the composition of secret remedies acquired new intensity in the eighteenth century against a background of growing Enlightenment concerns about fraud and the need to verify discoveries. Quacks provided ideal targets. As part of an Enlightenment move against charlatanism, licensed practitioners argued that quacks sold medicines to the sick no matter what their symptoms. This ran counter to prevailing notions in medicine, which emphasized how each case was individual and required a complex course of treatment. Chemical and clinical investigations were undertaken in France and Britain to uncover and damn proprietary medicines, and the public were regularly warned that they were spending their money on potential poisons or useless cures. By the nineteenth century, these concerns played on wider fears of commercial fraud and adulteration.

As competition in medicine increased quacks were denounced for making extravagant claims and were accused of breaking with established medical orthodoxy. Licensed practitioners suggested that quack medicines did not have any virtues. By the mid nineteenth century, critics had partially shifted their stance. Quack and secret remedies were increasingly discredited as worthless or potentially dangerous. Doctors argued that to attack quackery was a public duty to protect the gullible and defenceless from the unscrupulous who exploited ignorance and anxiety over chronic and incurable diseases, but at the root of this opposition were fundamental concerns about intellectual and economic competition. As significant numbers of licensed practitioners invested in training and worked to fashion a professional identity, attacks on quackery intensified. Quackery was seen to represent trade and commercialization from which licensed practitioners became increasingly anxious to distance themselves in their attempts to fashion a professional identity [see 'Professionalization']. Licensed practitioners were alarmed that quackery elevated public opinion over their professional judgement and saw in quackery an affront to the professional standards they aspired to. The accusation against quacks therefore expressed fears of competition and an antagonism between professional medicine and popular medicine; between trade and pretensions to a gentlemanly status for medicine.

The explosion of proprietary medicines in the eighteenth century encouraged licensed practitioners to seek greater legal control to protect themselves and the public. Of course, attempts to regulate medicine were not unique to the late eighteenth or nineteenth centuries. In early modern Europe, official pharmacopoeias set out acceptable remedies and measures to license medical practice existed at a regional and national level [see 'Professionalization']. However, as the market for medicine expanded and licensed practitioners felt themselves under threat, moves to regulate medicine intensified. Fears about quackery and competition provided a rallying point for doctors' demands for regulation, a process seen as fundamental to professionalization. The need to police the remedy trade and medical practice did attract state support. Licensing systems were revised and new measures, such as the 1868 Pharmacy Act in Britain, or moves to regulate patent medicines in Finland in 1928, were introduced to control the sale of certain drugs. As the historian Matthew Ramsey has shown, for European governments the sale of dangerous drugs seemed a more immediate threat than inept practice and was easier to define and prosecute.[4]

Campaigns against quacks and proprietary medicines were often ineffective, however. The realities of commercialization, the nature of property rights, and the growing power of the press, which received considerable revenues from advertising commercial remedies, restricted the field of action. The limits of state control and licensing bodies, which were inconsistent in their behaviour, created barriers to effective regulation. Early modern licensing practices were imperfect and often failed to extend outside metropolitan areas. Eighteenth and nineteenth century licensing was often little better at restricting the sale of quack remedies. In France, the activities of the Société Royale de Médecine in the 1780s and 1790s, the work of the Imperial Commission established in 1810, and the creation of an Académie Royale de Médecine in 1820, all had limited success in regulating secret remedies. Legislation and licensing systems were unable to outlaw secret remedies, or offer a framework that could cope with the rapid growth of the pharmaceutical industry in the nineteenth century. Prosecutions were difficult to set in motion or enforce. Legal loopholes, distance and poor communications, the small number of officials, and the popularity of quack and proprietary medicines, all limited the effectiveness of legislation and ensured that quacks and the sellers of proprietary and patent medicines continued to flourish.

Commercial medicine after 1800

The implication from the historical literature that the rise of modern medicine and the growth of state welfare displaced quack remedies or transformed quacks into alternative practitioners is misleading. This approach downplays the growth of a mass market for over-the-counter medicines and overemphasizes the power of hospital medicine or professionalization. Rather than being squeezed out after 1800, medical entrepreneurs continued to thrive. Some quacks embraced alternative medicines, but more took advantage of the continuing commercial opportunities offered by proprietary medicines. Remedies for virtually every complaint flooded the market. As editorial restrictions were relaxed and illustrations improved, advertising became more ostentatious even if the same marketing strategies that had been developed in the eighteenth century continued to be employed. The market remained highly structured. It ranged from quacks selling their wares at rural fairs through to a wide range of chemists and druggists to commercial manufacturers. Well-established brands continued to thrive and new brands were added as the number of universal cures and specific remedies multiplied. If many overlapped with conventional pharmacy in terms of their composition, they were supplied in a different context.

The forces that had encouraged a dramatic rise in quack remedies in the eighteenth century continued to drive the market for commercial medicines in the nineteenth century. James Woycke in his research on patent medicine in Germany has attributed their continuing appeal to the way in which they blended 'traditional folklore with industrial practices', but market pressures were also at work.[5] The long-term rise in disposable incomes, the growth of the press, improved communications, and a fall in the price of drugs, all aided expansion and fuelled competition. These commercial medicines were priced to sell and were endorsed by celebrities, politicians, practitioners and royalty. When these factors were combined with aggressive advertising, especially in women's magazines, demand was stimulated for mass-produced and marketed over-the-counter medicines. In Germany, over a thousand patent medicines were available by 1871.

However, the nineteenth century medical marketplace became increasingly structured in a way that allowed certain commercial medicines, particularly those developed by the pharmaceutical industry, to become associated with prescription and ethical cures. If some patent or proprietary medicines continued to be branded as dangerous, medical entrepreneurs took on new forms associated with ethical and over-the-counter medicines that utilized modern business methods of industrial production and commercial distribution. Outlets expanded and medicines were readily available from grocers, cooperative stores and chemists, as well as through the flourishing mail-order trade. This demand provided the background for retail chemists, such as Boots the Chemist in Britain, which not only sold proprietary medicines but also their own brands.

By the early twentieth century, brand name medicines were a thriving business. Pressure was applied for ethical pharmacy with standardized ingredients supplied through reputable businesses. Controls were introduced on dangerous, poisonous or addictive substances. New health movements, such as the craze for vitamins, the links made between food and health (seen in Bovril, Oxo and Kellogg's), and the importance of health, fitness and beauty to the nation, broadened the market for medicine and health-related products. In Germany, support for commercial and alternative medicines was fuelled by a perceived crisis in medicine and distrust of licensed practitioners. Although anxieties about orthodox medicine were not as pronounced in other countries, the continued growth of a mass market for commercial medicine was a European phenomenon that drew on new commercial practices and traditional ideas that drugs could restore health. New mass production techniques placed medicine in the vanguard of the commodity culture, while the sugarcoating process for pills made them more palatable. Medical entrepreneurship was refined as it took on new forms; given shape by chemical and pharmaceutical companies, such as Bayer in Germany or Burroughs, Wellcome & Co in Britain. They used notions of scientific modernity and openness to deflect suspicion, investing in research laboratories and providing not only prescription drugs for medical practitioners but also lucrative over-the-counter remedies. This created new divisions in proprietary medicines between ethical and secret remedies. By the 1940s, commercial and over-the-counter medicine represented a multi-million international business and a visible part of individual responses to everyday maladies.

Quacks, commercial medicine and medical knowledge

As historians have reacted to the view that quacks were ignorant and irrational and that the remedies they peddled were dangerous, the medicines supplied by quacks and commercial vendors have been recast to show how they were often similar to regular medicine. Evidence that quacks and licensed practitioners used analogous medicines has contributed to the idea that the boundaries separating the two were not rigid. Hence, rather than seeing distinctions between regular and irregular, it might be better to think about a growing division between commercial and non-commercial medicine. Conventional and quack medicine converged more often than they diverged.

Promoters of commercial medicines associated their products with the mainstream – by the titles given to their medications, through their accompanying medical advice labels and booklets, or through their use of quotations from medical authorities. In terms of composition, numerous contemporary studies revealed how quack and conventional medicines were often little different. In early modern Italy, for example, apothecaries and quacks employed similar ingredients and both subscribed to the Hippocratic-Galenic tradition. Both created and sold substances for self-medication. Until the late nineteenth century, the only difference between licensed practitioners and quacks was often little more than how they interacted with their clients.

Quacks and the makers of patent medicines played on the latest fads and co-opted the language of orthodox medicine, assimilating innovations from medicine. It was a move that lay behind the growing mass market for painkillers following the introduction of ether and chloroform into medicine in the 1840s; that saw disinfectant soap or carbolic vaporizers come onto the market in the late nineteenth century as the public were exposed to germ theories. All ostensibly drew on scientific information. If the growth of modern pharmacology and the introduction of synthetic drugs in the 1880s widened the gap between proprietary and prescription medicines, the makers of commercial medicines were quick to absorb the same values and findings. They too invested in laboratories and research as evident in the transformation of Beecham's or Boots, which set up the largest surface culture plant in the world to produce penicillin. The relationship worked both ways, with pharmaceutical companies investing in proprietary medicines and vitamins, which were an important source of income.

Quackery and commercial medicines contributed to the functioning of orthodox medicine in a number of ways. Through their experimentation with a variety of techniques, quack ideas and medicines could enter the mainstream. The use of electricity as a therapeutic agent moved from the margins to the mainstream in the mid nineteenth century as practitioners redefined the social and philosophical rationale behind electrotherapeutics. Aspirin was introduced as a proprietary medicine by Bayer in 1899 and quickly became the 'Drug of the Century'. More importantly, as Roy Porter argues in *Health for Sale,* quacks showed how unpleasant life could be without doctors and contributed to the medicalization of society. For example, the hero of Jerome K Jerome's *Three Men in a Boat* (1889) was so alarmed by a circular for a patent liver pill that he consulted a doctor.

Commercial medicines hence served vital and contradictory functions. Their growth encouraged a change in popular medical habits to favour over-the-counter remedies. Opposition to them shaped medical reform, but also how licensed practitioners perceived and organized themselves. They allowed patients to circumvent medical advice and contributed to a medicalization of society. Above all, they developed the commercial side of medicine and provided numerous opportunities for the sick to self-medicate in a changing medical marketplace in which choice and agency remained vital and not all medical encounters were with licensed practitioners but covered a range of popular, proprietary, commercial and domestic remedies.

Further reading

On the concept of the medical marketplace, readers should start with Frank Huisman, 'Shaping the Medical Market: On the Construction of Quackery and Folk Medicine in the Dutch Historiography', *Medical History* 43 (1999), pp. 359–75, or Patrick Wallis and Mark Jenner (eds), *Medicine and the Market in England and its Colonies, c.1450–c.1850* (London: Palgrave Macmillan, 2007). Mary Lindemann's book *Medicine and Society in Early Modern Europe,* 2010 edn (Cambridge: Cambridge University Press, 2010) provides an excellent overview of medical self-help in early modern Europe. The collection *Patients and Practitioners: Lay Perceptions of Medicine in Pre-Industrial Society* (Cambridge: Cambridge University Press, 1985) edited by Roy Porter offers a solid introduction to the nature of popular medicine in pre-industrial England, while Lucinda Beier's *Sufferers and Healers: The Experience of Illness in Seventeenth-Century England* (London: Routledge, 1987) is a more detailed examination of the middling orders. For France and Italy, students should consult Colin Jones and Laurence Brockliss, *The Medical World of Early Modern France* (Oxford: Clarendon Press, 1997) and David Gentilcore, *Healers and Healing in Early Modern Italy* (Manchester: Manchester University Press, 1998). The best study of eighteenth century quackery remains Roy Porter's *Quacks: Fakers and Charlatans in Medicine* (Stroud: Tempus,

2003) an illustrated edition of his groundbreaking 1989 work *Health for Sale*. Although far less has been written on patent medicines in the nineteenth or twentieth centuries, James Woycke, 'Patient Medicines in Imperial Germany', *Canadian Bulletin of the History of Medicine* 9 (1992), pp. 41–56, and Carsten Timmerman, 'Rationalization "Folk Medicine" in Interwar Germany: Faith, Business and Science at "Dr Madaus & Co."', *Social History of Medicine* 14 (2001), pp. 459–82, show how patent medicines remained important. For those interested in medical pluralism, Waltraud Ernst (ed.), *Plural Medicine, Tradition and Modernity, 1800–2000* (London: Routledge, 2002) covers a variety of contexts. For students interested in alternative medicine, W.F. Bynum and Roy Porter (eds), *Medical Fringe and Medical Orthodoxy, 1750–1850* (London: Croom Helm, 1987) and Roger Cooter (ed.), *Studies in the History of Alternative Medicine* (Basingstoke: Palgrave Macmillan, 1988) still provide excellent essay collections, while Roberta Bivins, *Alternative Medicine: A History* (Oxford: Oxford University Press, 2007) is a thoughtful study of how alternative medicine has adapted, survived and prospered.

6
Anatomy and medicine

Gunther von Hagens's controversial travelling exhibition, 'Body Worlds', put dissected cadavers on display (as art?) and provoked predictable reactions, mostly of disgust. Von Hagens was keen to show that the human body anatomized was an amazing object that had to be understood. In doing so, he shared a common vision with Renaissance anatomists. If historians cannot be accused of viewing the body in the same way, they have equally been fascinated by anatomy, its relationship to shaping views of the body and disease, and how, much like anatomists in the past, anatomy reflected broader social, religious and cultural concerns. Most historians agree that important changes occurred to anatomy in the sixteenth and seventeenth centuries as inquiry focused on first recovering and then questioning Classical texts; that this movement encouraged not only a remapping of the body but also established the foundations for modern medicine. Few would reject the idea that by the late eighteenth century pathological and clinical anatomy was to have a central role in reshaping medicine as theoretical and technical innovations were assimilated into a style of medicine labelled hospital medicine [see 'Hospitals']. Yet, it is possible to rethink this chronology and see how practice was more resilient to change than historians have traditionally assumed.

This chapter explores the history of anatomy from the Renaissance to the mid nineteenth century. It examines the emergence of new ways of understanding the body through anatomy and explores the various intellectual, philosophical and religious influences that influenced anatomical inquiry, and how anatomy and dissection became central to the training of licensed practitioners and to new forms of medical knowledge. Rather than seeing the period from the mid eighteenth to early nineteenth century as a decisive turning point, the chapter explores ideas of continuity and the impact of anatomical investigation on clinical inquiry, on doctors' training, and on the clinical encounter.

Anatomy and the search for meaning

Accounts of anatomy in the Renaissance (roughly from 1300 to the mid seventeenth century) have frequently stressed the triumph of observation over a style of university learning based around Classical texts to emphasize how ideas and techniques from Padua and Bologna were rapidly adopted in Northern Europe. Until the 1990s, there was widespread agreement that by the end of the sixteenth century the changes initiated by Flemish-born physician Andreas Vesalius had resulted in a transformation of ideas about the body as human dissection became commonplace in medical education. This embodied both a rediscovery and revival of Greek and Roman medicine – known as medical humanism – as part of the renaissance in Classical culture, followed by a shift away from the works of the Galen, a Greek-speaking physician who worked in imperial Rome. As sixteenth century anatomists challenged Galen, anatomists moved beyond demonstrating what was already known to conducting original observational research.

Whether or not there was a conceptual change in the nature of anatomy in the late fifteenth and sixteenth centuries, and in what ways anatomy was influenced by various intellectual, philosophical and religious ideas of the period is open to debate. Whereas anatomy in the medieval period had been relatively static and based around the dissection of animals to describe gross human anatomy, in the late fifteenth and sixteenth centuries there was a flourishing of interest in anatomy. Anatomy was important to all fields of medicine – it indicated the location of the disease, aided diagnosis, and influenced how diseases were described. It combined an investigation of both structures and action, or how the body worked (what would now be labelled physiology). However, anatomical inquiry was not just medical in nature: it was part of contemporary philosophical and theological discussions, and often used the same scholarly approach. It was encouraged by a flourishing humanist interest at the end of the fifteenth and start of the sixteenth centuries in rediscovering and reviving all aspects of Classical Greek and Roman culture, a movement associated with the Renaissance. Humanists believed that Classical learning, and especially that of the Greeks, represented the pinnacle of knowledge. The aim of early sixteenth century anatomy was therefore to achieve a better understanding of the Classical texts that provided the foundations of medical knowledge. The surge in interest in anatomy was sustained by a number of major Greek texts becoming available, notably a new translation of Galen's *On Anatomical Procedures* in 1531, which outlined procedures for carrying out dissection. A commitment to the critical assessment of Classical texts enhanced the prestige of anatomy as a branch of learning. The need to understand the human body was given a further rationale by the theological turmoil associated with the Reformation, a sixteenth century movement for the reform of the doctrines and practices of the Catholic Church. Anatomy offered a means to explore the work of God and the nature of Creation [see 'Religion']. Sixteenth century anatomy was therefore more than a practical art or a bloody exercise associated with dissection: it was shaped by the impact of the Renaissance and the Reformation on medicine.

Advances were also made in the technical skill of dissection. Although anatomy drew on Classical texts, the practice of dissection – and to a lesser

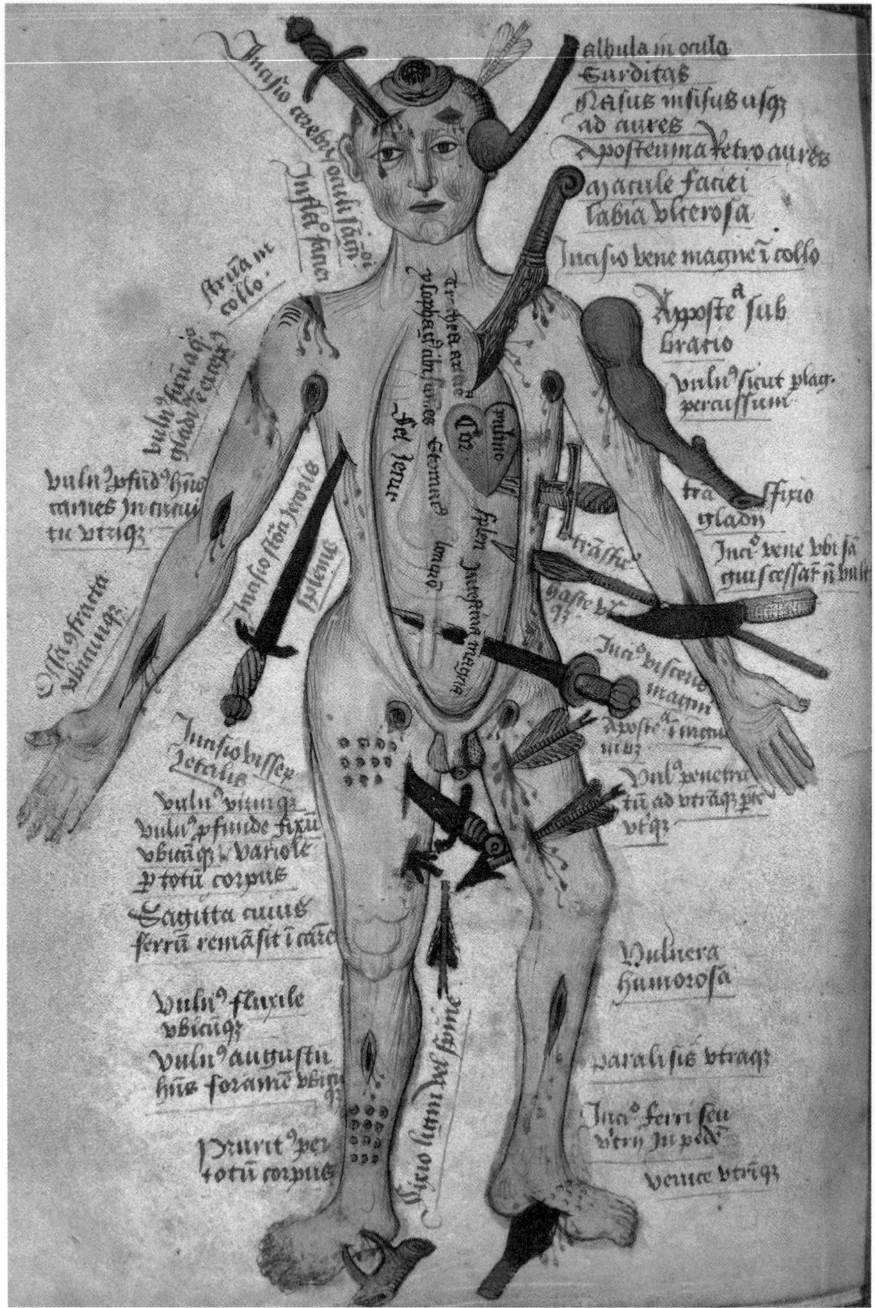

Figure 6.1 'Wounded Man'. Anatomical illustration from the mid fifteenth century.
Source: Wellcome Library, London.

extent vivisection – increasingly defined the work of sixteenth century anatomists. The teaching of human anatomy through dissection is thought to have originated in Bologna in the fourteenth century. During the fifteenth century, dissection for educational purposes extended to other European universities, and in the following century permanent anatomical theatres were built in universities and hospitals as attendance at dissections rose. These developments reflected the growing demand for licensed practitioners and a system of medical training in which students were expected to attend lectures, read Classical texts, and observe an annual dissection. Hung criminals were used as subjects for dissection: they tended to be young or middle aged and had not died of disease. This made them attractive to anatomists. Although criminals were not the only source of bodies for dissection – in Sweden, for example, the cadavers of suicides, the insane and beggars were used – the connection between dissection and punishment was to prove enduring.

Dissections in the sixteenth and seventeenth centuries were public events conducted in front of an audience, a fact that encouraged some anatomists to become increasingly theatrical. Normally held in winter over three days to ensure that the bodies did not decay too quickly, dissections served an educational, social and religious function, and became the means through which observations were confirmed and communicated. The aim was to reveal to students and practitioners the inside of the body and to display to a wider audience the workmanship of God in order to inspire admiration. Dissection and anatomy were hence a combination of ritual and teaching event. Their public nature allowed authorities to keep track of how many bodies were dissected and permitted physicians and surgeons to demonstrate their knowledge and acquire prestige. Dissection was problematic, however. On the one hand, it was a public spectacle; on the other, popular discomfort existed about the dangers of separating the body from the soul. Anatomy and dissection therefore had an ambiguous status in the sixteenth century.

Vesalian autonomy

Positivist studies of anatomy have emphasized the centrality (if not the sole role) of the Flemish-born Andreas Vesalius in the revitalization of anatomy in the sixteenth century. Upon taking up a post at the city's prestigious university, Vesalius began reorganizing the teaching program in Padua in 1537. He introduced demonstrations of human anatomy with the aid of bodies he had dissected himself. He also prepared anatomical illustrations to clarify his oral presentations to show how knowledge derived from Classical texts should be understood, and if necessary, modified. The conventional account asserts how in the process of translating Galen's work from Greek to Latin, Vesalius discovered errors and subsequently insisted that instead of looking at existing texts physicians and surgeons should study the body.

Vesalius certainly raised questions about Galen's work on anatomy and criticized his reliance on animal dissection, suggesting that his findings needed to be reconfirmed by observation. In addition, Vesalius's practice of performing all the parts of the dissection – the cutting, the showing and the teaching – that had traditionally been divided between the offices of *ostensor*, professor and surgeon, quickly became the standardized model of anatomizing across Europe. However, Vesalius's work was a complicated mix of critique and a reworking of existing knowledge. His early treatise, now know as the *Tabulae Anatomicae Sex* (Six Anatomical Tables), reflected the humanist tradition he had been trained in while a student in Paris. It depicted the ideas expressed in Galen's newly translated *On Anatomical Procedures* and was influenced by contemporary disputes about bloodletting. Like other contemporary works, it placed anatomy within the framework of natural philosophy (or the natural sciences). His *De Humani Corporis Fabrica* (On the Structure of the Human Body, 1543) was a lavishly illustrated anatomical narrative of an ideal version of the human body against which others could be compared. Having seen that his approach in the *Tabulae* was popular with students and colleagues, in the *Fabrica* Vesalius laid out the entire body. Throughout Vesalius stressed the importance of anatomy as the basis for medicine and asserted the value of public and human dissections as a way of learning what was normal and abnormal.

Vesalius did not see his work as anti-Galenic though: he emphasized how his anatomy was more accurate than Galen's as a way of reviving the practice of Galenic anatomy and presented a corrected Galenic anatomy. The disagreements were in the detail. In many ways, the poorly paid Vesalius was engaged in self-promotion. He glossed over how anatomy was taught elsewhere and took an extreme stance to assert his own position. This tendency was reflected in the language and images Vesalius incorporated. *Fabrica* was extensively illustrated so that the anatomical facts could be visualized, fusing science and art in the way the anatomy of the body was represented.

Historians have used the *Fabrica* to inform their views of anatomy prior to its publication, but contrary to the oft-received impression, Vesalius was not the only anatomist in the period. Anatomical studies were thriving in the new and growing print culture of the sixteenth century. Whereas these other texts have frequently been overlooked, they demonstrate how other anatomists were equally dedicated to the idea of *autopsia* – seeing-for-oneself – and to producing commentaries on anatomy as part of a wider attempt to revive the practices associated with Galenic anatomy. For at least fifty years before Vesalius, anatomists had been questioning the details in Galen, pointing out errors and making additions. For example, Vesalius was not the first to note that Galen had worked exclusively on animals and most anatomists and surgeons had already accepted that anatomy was best studied through human dissection. In their published works, and through their public anatomies, these other anatomists also helped to transmit a growing knowledge of anatomy.

The *Fabrica* had an immediate impact, however. Vesalius's controversial ideas

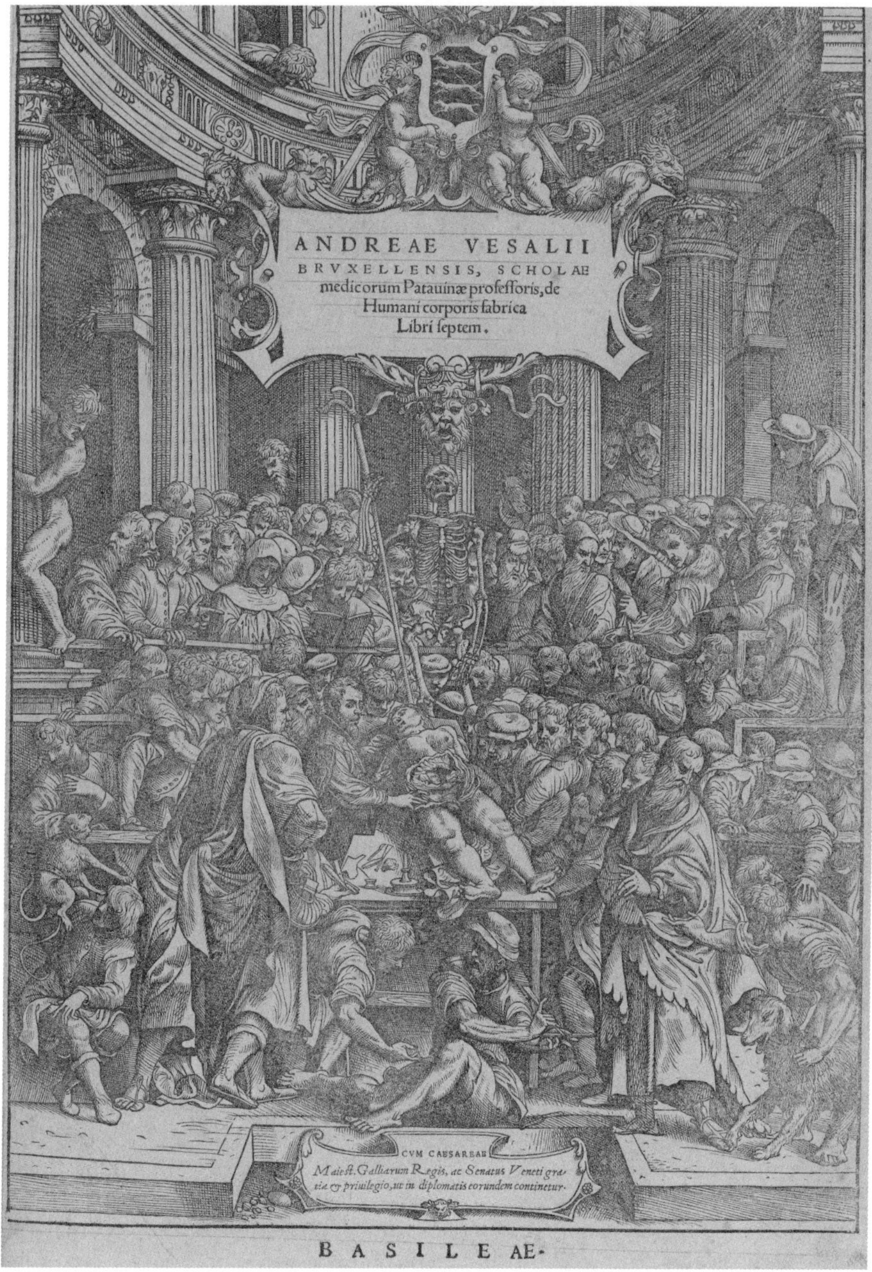

Figure 6.2 Title page of Vesalius's *De Humani Corporis Fabrica libri septem* (Basileae, 1555).

Source: Wellcome Library, London.

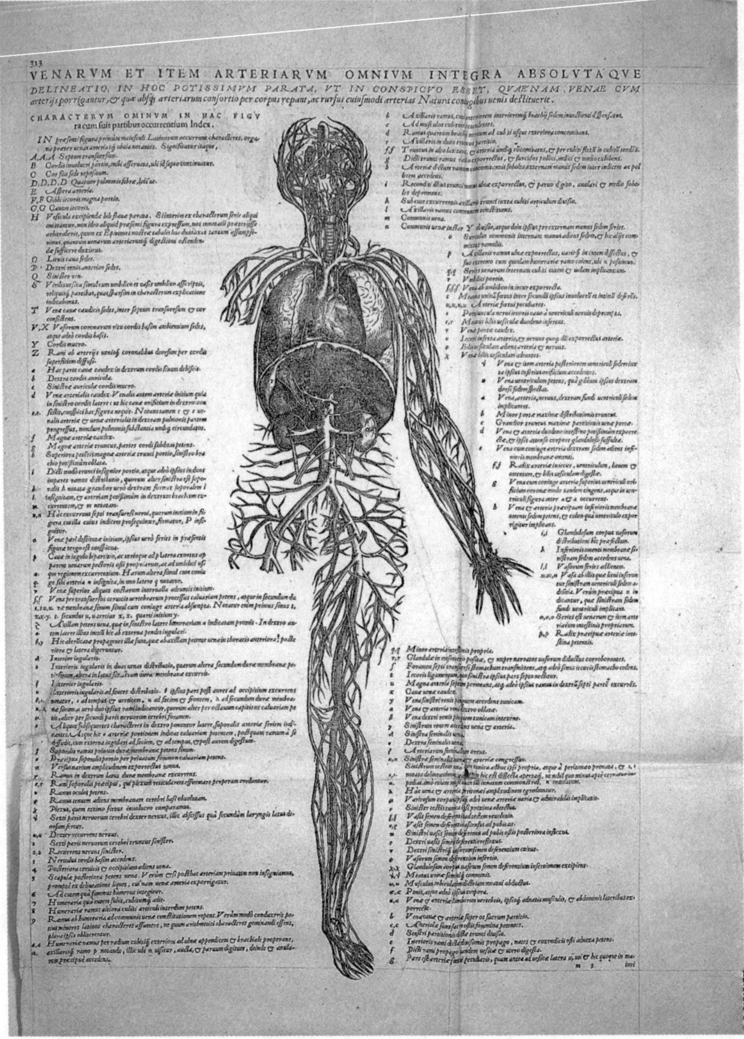

Figure 6.3 An illustration from Vesalius's *De Humani Corporis Fabrica libri septem* depicting the veins and arteries.

Source: Wellcome Library, London.

were hotly debated, and the *Fabrica* was pirated and widely emulated. Traditionalists attacked Vesalius for daring to correct Galen. These views were strongest in Catholic countries where scholars sought to defend the Catholic vision of anatomy that had been based on Galen's work. However, many contemporaries did feel that Vesalius presented a new start by daring to go beyond existing anatomical knowledge. Anatomy became central to the study of medicine as Vesalius's critics and supporters first followed his lead and then extended inquiry, often amending Vesalius's findings. Faith in Galen started to be superseded by the pursuit of universal principles as evident in the work of Fabricius (Girolamo Fabrizio), Vesalius's successor at Padua. Public anatomies became more frequent and the language of anatomy quickly permeated sermons, plays and other literary works. The process of looking inside the body became modern and exciting – albeit a form of excitement tinged with horror.

Although Renaissance anatomy remained theoretically conservative in its approach, and the study of anatomy continued to be largely book-based and delivered through lectures, the changes in the sixteenth century did increase the observational knowledge of the human body's structure. Following Vesalius, anatomists emphasized the worth of anatomy to the understanding of medicine, a move that was to gain momentum in the seventeenth century. Although this in part reflected a rhetorical slight of hand as anatomists emphasized the dignity of their work and downplayed the nature of dissection, anatomy was represented as a way of understanding Creation and as a subject that was modern and learned.

Anatomy and observation in the seventeenth century

Anatomy continued to grow in importance in the seventeenth century and helped shape a pathological tradition and approach as post-mortems and dissections were performed with increasing frequency. New philosophies about the body were put forward that owed more to new modes of inquiry than to the earlier emphasis on re-evaluating Classical texts. More standardized views of the body emerged as anatomists, surgeons and physicians discussed the body and the internal organs in new ways. These ideas were part of what has been traditionally labelled the Scientific Revolution with its emphasis on empiricism and observation.

Seventeenth century anatomy acquired a material space – the dissection room or theatre and the museum – and a wider audience through advances in printing. Most European universities built anatomical theatres and used anatomy as a bridge between natural philosophy (the natural sciences) and moral philosophy (or ethics). One consequence was a growing demand for cadavers for dissection. Some of this demand was met through post-mortems, but hospitals became important sites for anatomical demonstrations and research [see 'Hospitals']. This was evident in Rome where hospital dissections had become routine by the beginning of the seventeenth century. Public annual demonstrations continued, however. In these public anatomies the philosophical and theological implications of anatomy were discussed, while anatomical texts for professional and public consumption were published that met the demand for information about the inner secrets of the body.

Surgeons and physicians looked at the nature and actions of the body, seeing in anatomy an essentially experimental approach that reflected the values of empiricism and observation that was coming to shape inquiry during the seventeenth century. This approach has been associated with William Harvey, physician to St Bartholomew's Hospital from 1609 to 1643, and his work on blood circulation. Influenced by his training in Padua, and the anatomical investigations of Italian physicians, Harvey performed dissections and numerous vivisections on animals, concentrating on the heart's movement. Like sixteenth century anatomists, his work was experimental in nature although it dealt principally with physiology. He pointed to the value of observation and personal experience. Through dissection and vivisection, Harvey argued that the blood circulated in the body. In *Exercitatio Anatomica de Motu Cordis et Sanguinis* (Anatomical Exercise on the Movement of the Heart and Blood, 1628) he described a series of experiments in which he demonstrated the heart's role. He saw the circulation of the blood as an observable fact and placed circulation firmly within the realm of the anatomist.

It would be easy to assume that Harvey's discovery was modern, but if it was certainly far-reaching, his studies were driven by established concerns. Harvey was a traditionalist, well-versed in Galenism, and influenced by Aristotle's works on natural science. His observations about the circulation of the blood built on Aristotle's emphasis on the heart as the main organ in the body; on ongoing efforts to re-examine Classical texts; and on existing anatomical studies. Nor did his work mark a sudden break with existing ideas: the new doctrine he outlined in his books met with a mixed reception. However, his ideas and his support of observational knowledge contributed to new philosophical interpretations and inspired further experimental and anatomical investigations, including early (unsuccessful) experiments with blood transfusion.

Through the observational findings derived from dissections and post-mortems, surgeons and physicians asserted a rational basis for medicine. The seventeenth century saw a series of innovative models of the body put forward as physicians and surgeons responded to contemporary philosophical and theological issues, as can be seen in the anatomical work of the English physician Thomas Willis and his interest in locating the soul [see 'Medicine and religion']. Although the application of new tools (for example, the microscope) aided this approach, models of the body were influenced by broader debates associated with mechanical philosophy, which endeavoured to explain all natural phenomena by physical causes. These ideas have been associated with the mechanical and philosophical principles put forward by René Descartes and Isaac Newton. Much of this work was philosophical rather than medical and was heavily empirical and teleological in nature.

Why European learned culture embraced new philosophical ideas remains open to debate, but a combination of forces encouraged what can be seen as a 'New Science', which was influenced by new philosophical currents that stressed the importance of observation and experimentation [see 'Science and medicine']. In England, the philosopher Francis Bacon emphasized the need for an inductive and experimental method, while the French philosopher and physiologist Pierre Jean Cabanis and the Anglo-Irish natural philosopher Robert Boyle argued that true knowledge came from experience. These ideas influenced medical thinkers and supported a reassessment of anatomical and physiological structures. For example, the English physician Thomas Sydenham, although hostile to anatomy, agreed that observation was crucial to medicine. The Dutch physicians, Franciscus De la Boe Sylvius and Hermann Boerhaave, championed Sydenham's views on observation at Leiden where they taught. Influenced by mechanical philosophy, Boerhaave in his *Institutiones Medicae* (1708) argued for a systematic approach that placed knowledge of anatomy at the centre of understanding the body and disease. Under Boerhaave, clinical teaching and dissections were introduced at Leiden, which replaced Padua as a centre for medical education and exported a style of training and practitioners to other European medical institutions.

The process was not one way, however. Philosophical and political thinking were affected by new views of the body. The French natural philosopher and mathematician Descartes was influenced by anatomical ideas. He conducted a limited number of anatomical investigations and incorporated discoveries from anatomy and physiology into a philosophical framework that equated the body with a machine-like system. His clear distinction between body and soul – known as Cartesian dualism – suggested a controversial view of the body. For Descartes, mechanism was either an ontology of nature, whereby all natural things had only mechanical properties, or a method of explanation. His ideas offered a radical new way of looking at the body.

Following Descartes, many philosophers adopted mechanism or the metaphor of the body as a machine (or watch) as a method of explanation and his view of the body was incorporated into medicine. Boerhaave, for example, revised Descartes's explanation to show how the body represented a hydraulic system whereby the constant flow of the blood and other fluids kept it healthy. However, Descartes's notion of the body as a machine was not the only model. Some saw limitations in a mechanical approach, a concern that stimulated interest in what animated the body. Vitalists, who believed that the processes of life were not just explainable by the laws of physics and chemistry but that a vital force distinguished living from non-living matter, placed a different emphasis on the nature of functions. In doing so, they raised questions about what might be seen as physiological processes. The intricate interactions between such competing ideas suggests that a new language and understanding of the anatomical body was being worked out in the seventeenth century as medical theory was reformulated and medical debate about the body intensified.

Anatomy during the seventeenth century came to represent a dynamic field of medical inquiry. Investigators had increased the accuracy of anatomical knowledge, but, more importantly, anatomy had become a vehicle through which new views of the body were being developed. However, notwithstanding the contribution of anatomists to how the body was understood, anatomy did not significantly challenge learned medical theory or therapeutics. Medicine remained firmly rooted in traditional practices, and the connection between anatomy and practice was limited; something that contemporaries did not miss. Yet, if the ideas associated with anatomical and philosophical inquiry often had little effect on medical practice, medical practitioners were now turning to anatomy and dissections to understand how the body worked, and increasingly saw anatomy as the foundation of medical training.

Enlightened anatomy: 1700–1789

By the start of the eighteenth century, the knowledge of gross anatomy was well advanced and accounts of disease were informed by an anatomical understanding. Anatomy was firmly established as a progressive discipline and anatomists tackled important questions of morbid processes, the differences between male and female bodies, and between races [see 'Women and medicine'; 'Medicine and empire']. Improvements to microscopes permitted closer attention to the form and structure of the human body. Interest focused on localized disease as morbid anatomy and pathology came to overlap.

During the eighteenth century the value of observing disease and morbid anatomy encouraged anatomists to explore the connections between the body and the signs of disease. Curiosity about the possible organic sites for certain conditions, such as angina pectoris, inspired practitioners to undertake post-mortems. Changes to the status and nature of surgery, and how surgeons were trained, not only required new skills but also stimulated demand for anatomical teaching [see 'Surgery']. This combined with the changing role of the hospital in the delivery of healthcare [see 'Hospitals']. Often drawing on Boerhaave's teaching, practitioners increasingly asserted the need for post-mortems to view and comprehend disease. This emphasis on morbid anatomy challenged earlier humoral interpretations of disease as a result of a general physiological imbalance. The result was to make anatomy more relevant to medical theory and practice. This interest in morbid anatomy and the associated ideas about disease has been placed at the heart of a shift to modern clinical medicine.

Although this refinement of approach can be found in a large body of medical writing in the eighteenth century, it is encapsulated in the Italian anatomist Giovanni Battista Morgagni's *De Sedibus et Causis Morborum* (On the Seats and Causes of Disease, 1761). Well-placed in Italian society and medicine, Morgagni was working in the tradition of the Italian anatomists, but he aimed to reveal the clinical utility of anatomy and correlate symptoms to what was occurring inside the body. To do this he studied the course of the disease from its onset to death, establishing a chain of events between the symptoms and the pathological changes. In collecting hundreds of case histories together, *De Sedibus et Causis Morborum* represented disease in terms of where it was located in the body; showing what doctors should look for in the living and what they would find in the dead.

The ideas expressed by Morgagni, and his stress on correlating the signs of disease with their symptoms, were taken further by other doctors. In Britain, an important school of morbid and clinical anatomy developed around the work of the Hunters in London and Glasgow, and the Monros in Edinburgh. It was particularly visible in the studies of the Scottish physician and anatomist Matthew Baillie. In *The Morbid Anatomy of Some of the Most Important Parts of the Human Body* (1793), he asserted the power of the post-mortem in diagnostic terms and in clinical practice. In doing so, Baillie emphasized the structural changes caused by disease that would be found in the organs. Practitioners influenced by this approach started to produce precise descriptions of disease as a way of defining different morbid states. Their work contributed to the spread of ideas about morbid anatomy, but at a broader level the attention directed at morbid and clinical anatomy in eighteenth century medical writing provided the foundations for a style of medicine that suggested that a symptomatic approach was not always reliable; that disease should be understood in terms of its pathological changes.

These changing views of anatomy and the body were incorporated into how and where licensed practitioners were trained as demand for practical anatomy courses increased as physicians and surgeons stressed that experience was essential and as the market for licensed practitioners expanded [see 'Professionalization']. Medical entrepreneurs initially meet this demand, offering courses in anatomy as part of a growing culture of learning and interest in science that reflected the search for the rationale in the Enlightenment, and the value placed on observation and experience. In London, William Hunter, aided by his brother John, set the pattern through his private anatomy school in Great Windmill Street, with its emphasis on seeing and interpreting the morbid signs of disease so that the symptoms could be understood in patients. The Hunters' school confirmed a new way of looking at the body and disease through anatomical investigations that was instrumental in integrating medicine and surgery. Although opposition existed to these new ideas, such as in Catholic Spain where medical training and anatomy remained conservative in nature, the number of anatomy lectures and courses increased in Europe. If some anatomy lecturers aimed to entertain and educate the public in much the same way as in early modern public dissections, an increasing number of lectures and practical classes were aimed at apprenticed or young practitioners – proto medical students – as ideas about how licensed practitioners should be trained were revised. Distinctions were at first often blurred, meeting a desire for knowledge and for morbid voyeurism, but anatomy courses became increasingly vocational in nature. Many were designed to equip surgeons with a practical knowledge of anatomy as surgeons and anatomists, such as Domenico Cotugno in Italy and Pierre Joseph Desault in Paris, came to place knowledge of the human body at the centre of an approach to clinical training that was becoming increasingly institutionalized in anatomy schools and hospitals in the eighteenth century.

The resultant demand for cadavers for classes and schools was often difficult to fulfil. Although the Paris faculty had a traditional right to the bodies of deceased prisoners, while in England the Surgeons' Company, College of Physicians, and Royal Society could dissect the bodies of executed criminals, these legal arrangements proved insufficient for the growing number of anatomy courses and schools. Renaissance anatomists in Italy, for example, had engaged in grave-robbing, and by the mid seventeenth century these sources of supply were beginning to arouse public unease. More entrepreneurial solutions evolved in the eighteenth century to meet this demand as anatomy teachers, fearful of riot or damage to their reputations, delegated the task of supplying cadavers. In the early eighteenth century these practices took on the dimensions of trade and grave-robbing, bribery, and the theft of bodies from the gallows or hospitals became commonplace in Paris, London and other teaching centres. Mass graves and the poor state of most urban churchyards made the practice relatively straightforward. As Ruth Richardson explains in *Death, Dissection and the Destitute* (1989), the result was that the human body became a commodity. Scandalous stories circulated: for example, in 1783 it was claimed that anatomy assistants in Paris were keeping warm by burning fat from the dead. Bodysnatching and dissection aroused hostility and provoked violent disturbances as they violated ideas about how the dead should be treated. Rather than supporting ghoulish accounts of the horrors of dissection, the trade in cadavers did have an important effect on institutions and knowledge. How many bodies an institution acquired for dissection affected its reputation and the knowledge produced.

By the late eighteenth century, anatomy was firmly established as a discipline. It was institutionalized in how medical practitioners were trained and helped affirm the empirical and observational basis of medicine. In morbid anatomy, a tool was provided for understanding both the body and the disease. Less clear is how much these ideas initially influenced practice. Many medical practitioners continued to resort to traditional therapies to cure disease within a framework that supported a holist or whole-body approach. However, in the half century after 1794, pathological anatomy and clinical anatomy were to assume a new importance in medicine and clinical practice.

Anatomy in the age of Paris medicine: 1789–1830

The importance of pathological and clinical anatomy to the transformation of medicine in the last decade of the eighteenth and the early nineteenth centuries has been represented as a revolution and an example of modernization. This revolution has been associated with 'Paris medicine' and 'the clinic'. These terms became shorthand among historians for a new style of medicine that was characterized by pathological anatomy, clinical observation in the hospital, physical examination, and the use of statistics, which came to dominate medicine in the first half of the nineteenth century as the geography of reform and innovation shifted to favour North-western Europe. Although it is clear that the new pathological and clinical anatomy was different from the general or morbid anatomy that had preceded it, historians are divided over the issue of continuity. In this debate, the extent of the changes made to the structure of medicine in Paris following the 1789 revolution and rise of hospital medicine have become central. Although there can be no doubt about the contribution of Paris to reshaping medicine, it is the nature of that contribution that has been scrutinized by historians.

At the centre of this debate is the historical work of Erwin Ackerknecht and Michel Foucault. Ackerknecht's influential *Medicine at the Paris Hospital* (1967) located the birth of modern hospital medicine within the political and technological revolution in France after 1789. Concerned with political and social change, Ackerknecht argued that what was happening in post-Revolutionary Paris fashioned a distinct type of hospital medicine that was to dominate practice in the first half of the nineteenth century. In *The Birth of the Clinic* (first translated in 1973), Foucault drew on a different approach and asserted an interpretation of modern medicine that focused on the structures of medical perception and experience that emerged in the half century following 1794. Foucault was interested in systems of power and knowledge, and was concerned with the relationships between language, knowledge and experience. He used the anatomical and pathological ideas of Parisian clinicians as a model to reveal how the local pathology associated with post-Revolutionary Paris represented a radical break with the past. Foucault argued that in the work of Parisian clinicians disease was no longer the subject of deduction but something that was observed through dissection. This he believed created a new way of seeing disease – or a clinical gaze – that focused on organic changes. Unlike other historians, Foucault did not see this as essentially progressive: he contended that this clinical gaze objectified the patient and in doing so elevated the doctor's power over the patient. For Foucault, these discourses ushered in a new style of hospital medicine based around physical examination, post-mortem (if the disease proved fatal), and statistical analysis [see 'Hospitals'].

Despite their different aims and approaches, both Foucault and Ackerknecht focused on the same shift in medical ideas and methods. Both identified what was happening in Paris after 1794 as central to the shift from 'bedside medicine', in which the patient dominated the clinical encounter, to a style of 'hospital medicine' where the doctor dominated. Their work encouraged other historians to place Paris at the centre of a paradigm shift from theoretical studies of disease to their practical application in the dissection room and wards that characterized medicine in the half century after 1794. In this view, the post-Revolutionary reforms to French medicine and the changes that were played out in Paris created structures and arrangements that provided an ideal environment in which a new theoretical canon could flourish and in which pathological anatomy could move beyond a small elite and become a practical and professional project.

However, it would be unwise to separate the theoretical notions associated with pathological anatomy from the milieu within which they occurred. The political and social upheavals and ideological currents associated with the French Revolution of 1789 – liberalism, progressivism and the individual – affected most aspects of French society and reverberated across Europe. The revolution, in seeking to overturn established hierarchies, sought to do away with hospitals and old elites and restructure the physical and professional landscape of French medicine [see 'Hospitals']. New systems were imposed but, as we shall see in more detail below, rather than abolishing the hospital, they institutionalized training and realigned professional hierarchies. New regulations made hospital patients accessible to examination and, if they died, for dissection. This forced new ways of conceptualizing health and disease. Reforms reflected the revolutionaries' aspirations and the practical realities of protracted war between 1793 and 1814.

In 1794 a fundamental reform of French medical education, which was now free and open to all, saw *Ecoles de Sante* (Schools of Health) established. Of these *Ecoles*, Paris was the most distinguished and prominent. The reforms promoted freedom to examine and dissect the vast number of patients admitted to Paris's public hospitals. They created a climate in which René Laennec, inventor of the stethoscope, Jean-Nicholas Corvisart, who disseminated the value of percussion, and other Paris clinicians could develop new diagnostic and theoretical approaches. New diagnostic techniques both allowed practitioners to determine pathological changes in the body and organs and asserted the importance of understanding pathological anatomy: for example, the stethoscope offered a mechanism for revealing morbid changes in the lungs and became the symbol of Paris medicine. New theoretical approaches reinforced the clinico-pathological method associated with Paris. For example, as a result of his detailed work on anatomical descriptions, the anatomist and physiologist Xavier Bichat divided organs into membranes and tissues. His work focused attention on physiological processes and the internal manifestation of disease to assert the importance of tissue pathology. This style of pathological anatomy encouraged a more precise definition of disease that linked symptoms and lesions, which could be confirmed by physical examination or post-mortem. A new curriculum was introduced. Stress was placed on practical and empirical training and the importance of anatomy, observation and physical examination. Reforms to medical licensing broke down traditional hierarchies to merge the functions of the surgeon and physician and made it easier for French doctors to view disease in localized, structural and anatomical terms.

The concentration of so many talented and enterprising doctors in an atmosphere of socioeconomic and political change and medical reform encouraged innovation and created an unparalleled environment in Paris that did not exist elsewhere in Europe. Students from across Europe and North America flocked to Paris. Here they attended courses that emphasized practical instruction, observation and put forward the principle that each student should dissect. Paris had

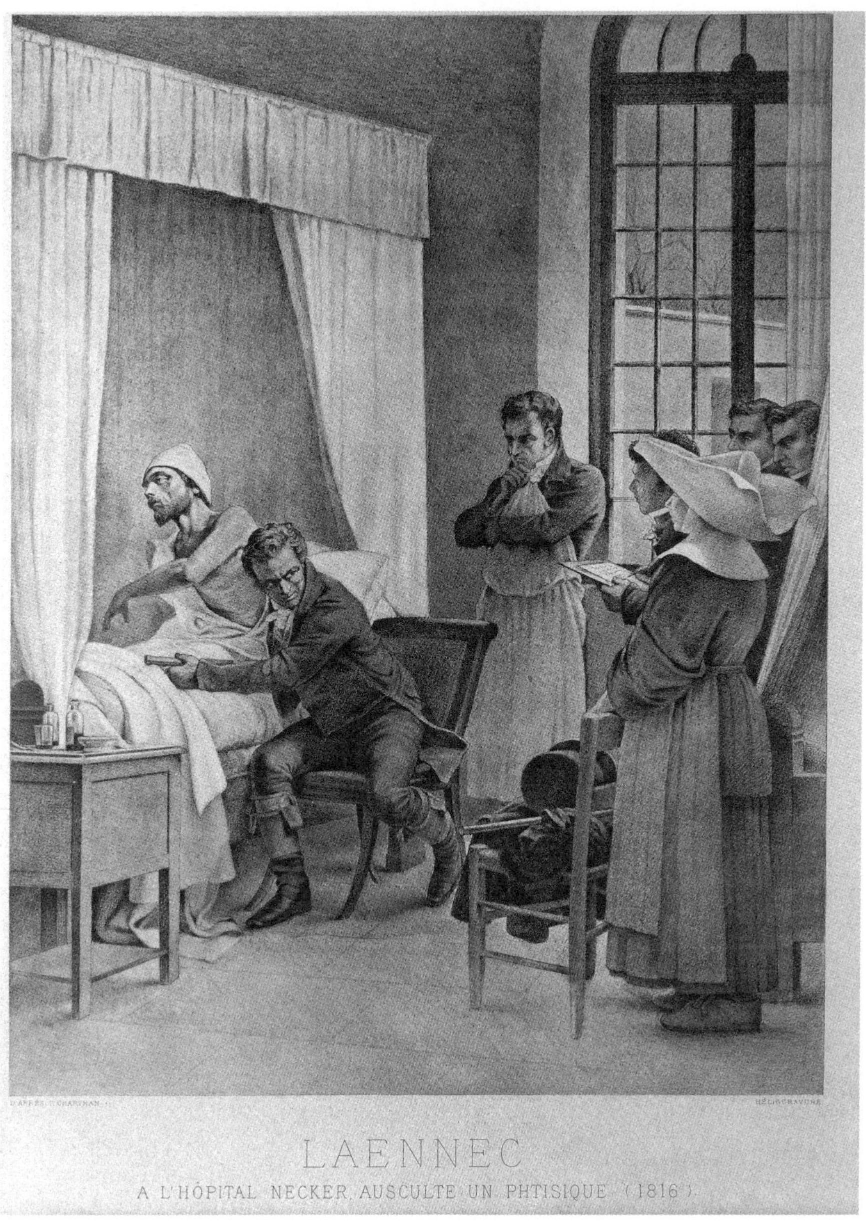

Figure 6.4 René Laennec and the use of auscultation on a patient at the Hospital Necker, Paris, 1816. This rather romanticized image associates Laennec with the stethoscope – a simple wooden tube – which he is holding in his hand while concerned doctors and a medical student look on.

Source: Wellcome Library, London.

other advantages: fees were low and students were invited *en masse* to the wards to view a new type of patient – which Dora Weiner has termed the 'citizen patient' – who provided the raw material for clinical examination and post-mortems. Public hospitals, an extensive supply of bodies, and reforms to the structure of teaching created an environment in which pathological anatomy could develop. Visitors to Paris brought the ideas they were exposed to back with them.

Although it is hard to escape the impact of Paris, questions need to be asked about just how important Paris was in championing a new style of hospital medicine. Research in the 1990s suggested that the uniqueness of Paris medicine at an institutional and individual level was a myth, part of a long-running construction by contemporaries and historians alike. If revisionists did not overlook the favourable milieu for change that existed in post-Revolutionary Paris, they did reveal more complex stories and chronologies.

Caroline Hannaway and Ann La Berge have shown in *Constructing Paris Medicine* (1998) how the primacy of Paris first emerged in the 1790s and gained momentum in the nineteenth century. As French clinicians strove to maintain their position in the face of the growing dominance of German medicine, they asserted the importance of Paris to medicine. In effect, Paris medicine was manufactured, a generalization that conceals both the disagreements and the diverse range of views that gave Paris its vitality and the practical realities of overcrowded ward rounds. By digging beneath the surface, it is possible to come to a view of Paris medicine that shows the difficulties of imposing a single, generalized view of the nature of medicine and anatomy in the half century following 1794.

Change was neither sudden nor as far-reaching as it is often suggested. Rather than being a fossil before 1789, Paris was already a centre for medical and scientific research, a place where medical, scientific and intellectual elites met and discussed their findings. The main components of the Paris school were all in place before the Revolution and existing medical institutions were coming under scrutiny in the last decades of the eighteenth century. What was happening in Paris after 1789 did not therefore mark a dramatic break with the past. The same was true of anatomy and its significance to understanding disease and its place in how doctors were trained. New ideas, techniques and currents do not form in a vacuum. The previous section has already suggested that changes were occurring to the role of anatomy in clinical medicine before 1789. Support for the teaching of morbid anatomy can be found in the sixteenth and seventeenth centuries, both in Paris and in London. In the second half of the eighteenth century, many European surgeons and physicians were, to varying degrees, interested in morbid anatomy. In London, private anatomy and hospital schools had started to offer medical training that integrated medicine and surgery and emphasized the importance of morbid anatomy and dissection. If problems were encountered in securing access to cadavers, practical anatomy classes were a common feature of medical education by the mid eighteenth century.

Nor was Paris alone in its emphasis on the anatomical localization of disease and pathological anatomy. From the mid seventeenth century onwards, doctors were searching for basic pathophysiological principles that explained disease. Physicians in seventeenth century London were already dissecting hospital patients on a regular basis. The same was true of Amsterdam where under the influence of Nicolaas Tulp and Franciscus Sylvius hospital patients were being autopsied. In the eighteenth century, physicians and surgeons increasingly saw disease in localized, structural and anatomical terms, and many felt that the 'frequent Dissection of Morbid Bodies tends greatly to ascertain the Diagnostic and Prognostic of Disease'.[1] Bichat's work had similarities to the ideas of eighteenth century vitalists and with the organ-based pathology of Morgagni and Baillie's interest in tissue pathology. In Britain, pathological anatomy and tissue pathology was attracting attention. For example, the Edinburgh physician William Cullen used gross pathological changes and the sequence of symptoms to build up his physiological ideas on the importance of nerves that had a marked impact on eighteenth century medical thought. In many ways, there was a cross-fertilization of ideas in the eighteenth century.

Parisian clinicians' stress on anatomy, pathological anatomy, observation and dissection were not novel therefore. They drew on ideas already current in the eighteenth century, and in doing so brought to fruition and gave practical form to established pathological ideas. Yet, a chronology that places what was happening in Paris in context should not diminish the role of Paris medicine. Post-Revolutionary Paris provided the political, material and socio-institutional framework for new ideas about pathological and clinical anatomy to flourish to an extent not possible elsewhere in Europe. Reforms in France and Paris fostered a climate in which pathological anatomy could find a receptive audience and become part of normal routine. These ideas gained purchase because of changes to how French clinicians were trained – changes that were replicated elsewhere in Europe. Therefore, rather than dismissing what was happening in Paris, or emphasizing its uniqueness, a different perspective which argues that continuities existed can be adopted to challenge the myth of Paris medicine.

Anatomy beyond Paris

Accounts of anatomy and the impact of pathological anatomy on medicine and medical education usually stop with Paris and the early nineteenth century. However, anatomy and pathological anatomy continued to underpin nineteenth century medicine and medical education. Anatomy schools flourished in the first decades of the nineteenth century. Although their fortunes started to wane with the rise of hospital schools and university departments, anatomy and pathological anatomy continued to be central to how licensed practitioners were trained. Anatomy departments institutionalized this knowledge and the ambitious used anatomy posts as stepping stones to senior positions. Pathological anatomy was seen to go hand-in-hand with bedside observation to represent a natural history of disease and a means to advance medical knowledge. This approach was particularly strong in Britain.

As more institutions offered anatomical lectures and dissections the demand for cadavers rose. Anatomists asked few questions about where bodies came from and the earlier trade in bodies reached new heights in Britain. The names of William Burke and William Hare have often been mistakenly identified with the practice of grave-robbing. Their activities were different, however. Between 1827 and 1828, Burke and Hare killed sixteen people, selling the bodies of their victims to an anatomy school in Edinburgh. After the Burke and Hare case, bodysnatchers started to be regarded as potential murderers.

The discovery of Burke and Hare's murders was merely the most public example of an established trade. The difficulties of procuring bodies for dissection were well known in Britain. Numerous schemes were proposed in the 1820s to improve the supply of cadavers, but it was the ideas put forward by the utilitarian reformer Jeremy Bentham that attracted most official attention. He borrowed from the Parisian model and outlined a system whereby bodies might be supplied from 'friendless' paupers – those without family or friends to claim them – dying in Poor Law workhouses. This established a link between dissection and poverty where previously one had existed with criminality. Notwithstanding the horror generated by Burke and Hare, legislation was delayed by the violent debates over parliamentary reform until further reports of bodysnatching reinvigorated public outrage and debates about grave-robbing. In 1832, an Anatomy Act was passed which encapsulated Bentham's ideas. It aimed to protect respectable families, halt the trade in cadavers, and increase the supply of bodies. In doing so, it turned the Poor Law into an official supplier of cadavers. In this way, the bodies of the poor were made to serve the needs of anatomists and medical education.

If the 1832 Act provoked outrage among the poor and bodysnatchers were marginalized, other arrangements emerged to overcome the continuing scarcity of cadavers as student numbers and demand for bodies rose. The national inspectorate worked to limit public scandal and it developed a number of subterfuges to supply cadavers. Evidence from medical schools shows how they competed for cadavers and regularly received bodies from unknown origins or exploited local arrangements with workhouses or asylums, overlooking breaches of decency and the Act's regulations to secure a stable supply of bodies. Historians have argued that limited supplies in Britain consolidated the position of the London schools as they had access to bodies from their own mortuaries. Certainly, some private schools failed to adapt, but this was not always the case and a metropolitan dominance should not be presumed.

Notwithstanding the place anatomy and pathological anatomy had secured as the backbone of medical and surgical studies, by the mid nineteenth century this position was being challenged. If new ways of understanding disease owed much to the emphasis placed by anatomists on localization in the late eigh-

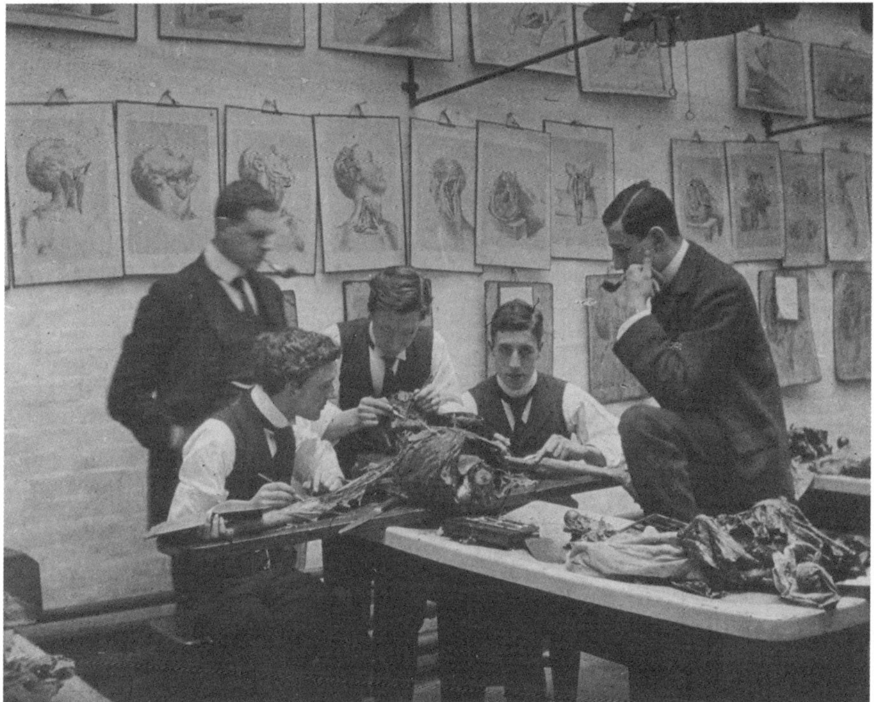

Figure 6.5 Interior of a dissection room.
Source: Wellcome Library, London.

teenth and early nineteenth century, the emergence of physiology as a discipline offered new ways of thinking about disease processes. Traditionally, interest in structure and function had been inseparable, but greater emphasis was gradually placed on the finer structures of tissues and cells and on physiological explanations. Initially much of this physiology was clinical and anatomical in nature and focused on the organs. By mid-century, however, many of the advances in medicine – for example, on digestion – were increasingly related to physiology and to creating an infrastructure in which physiological experiments could be undertaken. A more experimental approach was being asserted that emphasized the importance of the laboratory and the basic sciences to medical investigation where previously interest has been concentrated on anatomy theatres, museums and dissection rooms [see 'Science'].

However, although during the second half of the nineteenth century the major developments in understanding how the body and disease functioned took place in experimental physiology and bacteriology, this did not mean that anatomy or pathological anatomy was effectively marginalized. Investment continued to be made in the provision of anatomical theatres and teaching facilities as anatomy departments expanded. Many of the new diagnostic techniques developed during the nineteenth and twentieth centuries were based on the principles associated with pathological and clinical anatomy and the localization of disease. New instruments from X-rays to magnetic resonance imagining (MRI) developed from an anatomical perspective on diagnosis. Work with microscopes encouraged histological investigations, helping to advance a cellular model of pathology and the development of pathology as a discipline distinct from anatomy, a move associated with German investigators and in particular the work of Rudolf Virchow. However, it was not just in histopathology and cellular pathology that anatomical investigations continued to have an influence. An anatomical approach was crucial to neurologists and the development of neuropathology in the late nineteenth century [see 'Asylums']. New techniques of staining and serial sectioning, and the microtome or plastic reconstruction, encouraged new views of complex structures (for example, of the brain or embryos) to emerge. Close links were also forged between anatomy, zoology, embryology and pathology. Notwithstanding these contributions, anatomy was no longer the premiere science of the early nineteenth century. If this does not diminish its importance to medicine, it does show how the position of anatomy had once more been reconfigured.

Conclusions

Until the nineteenth century, anatomy occupied a dual position: it was both a spectacle and a means to explain how the body and disease worked. In the Renaissance it acquired a central position in how licensed practitioners were trained and in how disease was understood. If often controversial, anatomy became the knowledge of most worth, a way of asking wider theological and philosophical questions, which contributed to new views of the body. In the eighteenth century, a growing emphasis on the localization of disease stressed the connections between morbid anatomy and clinical practice, ideas that were to inform an approach to medicine associated with Paris and hospital medicine. Although as this chapter has shown the position of Paris as a centre for pathological and clinical anatomy should be questioned, the importance of this way of thinking should not. In the first half of the nineteenth century many of the advances in the understanding of disease were associated with pathological and clinical anatomy. By examining anatomy and dissection, it becomes possible to explore how the body and disease have been conceptualized and understood. As we shall see in later chapters, this is important to understanding the development of new systems of medical education that influenced professionalization, the role of hospitals, and the nature of surgery.

Further reading

There are a number of good studies of early modern anatomy. For a traditional assessment of the importance of Renaissance anatomy, see A.G. Debus, *Man and Nature in the Renaissance* (Cambridge: Cambridge University Press, 1978). Andrew Cunningham, *The Anatomical Renaissance: The Resurrection of Anatomical Practices of the Ancients* (Aldershot: Scolar, 1997) explores the links between Classical and Renaissance anatomy, and Roger French, *Medicine Before Science: The Business of Medicine from the Middle Ages to the Enlightenment* (Cambridge: Cambridge University Press, 2003) looks at how classical ideas were challenged. On the role of Vesalius, see Nancy Siraisi, 'Vesalius and the Reading of Galen's Teleology', *Renaissance Quarterly* l (1997), pp. 1–37, and Vivian Nutton, 'Wittenberg Anatomy', in Ole Peter Grell and Andrew Cunningham (eds), *Medicine and the Reformation* (London: Routledge, 1993), pp. 11–32, while on Padua see Cynthia Klestinec, 'A History of Anatomy Theatres in Sixteenth-Century Padua', *Journal of the History of Medicine* 59 (2004), pp. 375–412. A considerable body of literature exists on William Harvey, but a good starting point is Andrew Wear's *Knowledge and Practice in English Medicine, 1550–1680* (Cambridge: Cambridge University Press, 2000) which explores the wider milieu and the contribution of anatomy and dissection. For the importance of pathological anatomy and Paris to medicine, see Michel Foucault's seminal *The Birth of the Clinic* (London: Tavistock, 1973) and Erwin H. Ackerknecht, *Medicine at the Paris Hospital, 1794–1848* (Baltimore, MD: Johns Hopkins University Press, 1967). Dora B. Weiner, *The Citizen-Patient in Revolutionary and Imperial Paris* (Baltimore, MD: Johns Hopkins University Press, 1993) and Russell Maulitz, *Morbid Appearances: The Anatomy of Pathology in the Nineteenth Century* (Cambridge: Cambridge University Press, 1988) extend the analysis. For an alternative view, see the collection of essays edited by Caroline Hannaway and Ann La Berge (eds), *Constructing Paris Medicine* (Amsterdam: Rodopi, 1998) along with their excellent introduction which outlines the historiography. On dissection and bodysnatching, Ruth Richardson, *Death, Dissection and the Destitute* (London: Penguin, 1989) remains the key text. Elizabeth Hurren, *Dying for Victorian Medicine* (Basingstoke: Palgrave Macmillan, 2011) provides a nuanced reading of these themes after the 1832 Anatomy Act. Less has been written on anatomy in the nineteenth century, but Susan Lawrence, *Charitable Knowledge: Hospital Pupils and Practitioners in Eighteenth-Century London* (Cambridge: Cambridge University Press, 2002) and Thomas N. Bonner, *Becoming a Physician: Medical Education in Britain, France, Germany, and the United States, 1750–1945* (New York and Oxford: Oxford University Press, 1995) provide good starting points for understanding the central position of anatomy to medical education.

7
Surgery

It would be easy to write a history of surgery, with all its claims to a heroic status, as a story of empirical progress, manly surgeons, and the adoption of new techniques or technologies to create a narrative that emphasized breakthroughs. Such an approach would stress a transformation in surgery from the agony and speed of early modern surgeons to the heroic successes of the nineteenth century pioneers of anaesthetics and antiseptics. However, there is much more to the history of surgery. Historical research has come to reveal a more contested history; how complex relationships existed between technology, practice and professionalization, and how surgery reflected professional goals and theories of the body as well as the socioeconomic, cultural, political and institutional contexts in which surgical knowledge was constructed and surgery performed. This chapter provides an introduction to the history of surgery that explores how the nature of surgical knowledge and practice changed over the last five hundred years. In doing so, the chapter challenges the idea that surgery knowledge and practice progressed in a neat or linear fashion. It examines how changes in surgical knowledge and practices were neither inevitable nor even.

Understanding innovation and practice

Although few historians of medicine now see surgery as part of a positivist narrative, there has been a tendency to concentrate on successes, on elite surgeons, on the impact of technology, or on the introduction of new procedures. Consequently, relatively little is known about how new procedures were developed; why some were adopted and others were not. In *Medical Theory, Surgical Practice* (1992), Christopher Lawrence encouraged historians to examine how problems were defined as surgical, how surgeons discovered, improved or invented techniques, and how they were adopted. Thomas Schlich extended this approach. He argues that the history of surgery should be viewed as the 'interweaving of professional, conceptual and technical developments'.[1]

Schlich's approach offers a useful model for understanding how surgery changed over time, but his way of conceiving the history of surgery can be broadened to consider other factors. Surgical practices generated meanings – or more accurately multiple meanings – which not only informed how disease was viewed but also approaches to, and perceptions of surgery. At an individual level a surgeon's desire for fame and their individual skill influenced innovation and adoption. Nor should generational issues be underestimated. Older surgeons frequently stuck to the methods they knew. If this did not mean that they resisted new procedures, it did ensure continuities in surgical practice, which are often overlooked. Institutional contexts, especially with the growing importance of hospitals to medicine [see 'Hospitals'], had a further role in structuring surgery. Surgery's move into the hospital not only influenced how surgery was taught, but also how technologies and other innovations were introduced. Contexts influenced surgery in other ways. Warfare, for example, created new demands that necessitated new practices, some of which were translated into peacetime [see 'Medicine and warfare']. Through state-funded medical services, research and safety controls on medical innovations, twentieth century governments became more important in influencing surgical practice, and not just financially in terms of the resources available to surgeons and where surgery was conducted. Medical companies, such as those involved in the development of prosthetics, and the patients' rights movement, equally came to shape the surgeon's world.

The history of surgery can therefore be seen as an interaction between professional, conceptual and technical developments, and between these and individual and generational issues, institutional contexts, and external demands. The result is a series of overlapping and intricate relationships.

Status and training[2]

How surgery was perceived, and how surgeons were trained, influenced the type of surgery performed and the acceptance of surgical intervention. However, as Christopher Lawrence explains in *Medical History, Surgical Practice*, getting at these issues, and indeed the history of surgery, is complicated by the rhetoric surgeons adopted. Most of our evidence about surgery comes from elite surgeons who wanted to project surgery in particular ways. They embraced a language of progress that celebrated the achievements and surgical heroes of their age. The result was an overt link of surgery to modernity and breakthroughs.

The emergence of surgery as a distinct discipline had its origins in the thirteenth century. In 1215, the Fourth Lateran Council had insisted that priests in higher orders, who formed the main body of those studying medicine, could not shed blood. Surgery was hence to be the province of the laity and developed separate forms of organization, particularly in Northern Europe. Although distinctions at a practical level were blurred, divisions existed between internal medicine, as practised by university-educated physicians, and external manipulation, the realm of the surgeon. These divisions were embodied in how early modern surgeons were licensed to practice. Guilds had emerged in the medieval period to regulate trade, ensuring a basic level of competence through apprenticeship and granting licenses to practise [see 'Professionalization']. In this guild structure, surgery was linked with other crafts, such as barbers, bathmasters and grocers. These surgical guilds sought to assert codes of conduct and promote a corporate, respectable ethos, but an association with trade and manual skill was confirmed by how surgeons were trained. Unlike physicians, those wishing to become surgeons were first bound as an apprentice to a qualified master; for example, for seven years in Britain or three years in Württemberg. Whereas the very nature of how surgeons were training carried with it connotations of trade, critics further compared surgeons to uneducated butchers. Surgical practice was represented as demeaning and contaminating in part because surgeons worked with diseased flesh, and because many provincial surgeons also cut and shaved hair.

However, a simple lumping together of surgeons as a single occupational group conceals divisions. Hierarchies existed: early modern surgeons ranged from the village barber to the elite surgeon, which makes assumptions about the low status of the surgeon something of a generalization. Although many, if not all surgeons, were of a lower social status than physicians, many master surgeons were learned men. Elite surgeons distanced themselves from the taint of manual labour and trade by stressing experience and learning as the hallmarks of a surgeon, and by limiting the surgical activities of barbers. They sought to bring surgery closer to book-learning and physic by emphasizing the value of regimen and pharmacy. The surge in interest in anatomy in the sixteenth and seventeenth centuries encouraged new ways of looking at the body that benefited surgeons, as experience and observation became highly regarded sources of knowledge [see 'Anatomy']. War further extended the realm of surgery. Naval and army surgeons devised new techniques to deal with more complicated wounds and as surgeons assumed a new role in military medicine their status rose [see 'Medicine and warfare']. These trends aided the emergence of a new class of learned surgeon who based his practice on anatomy, regimen and medicines, and encouraged a surgical perspective on internal disease that was to dominate medicine in the late eighteenth century.

Surgeons themselves stressed improvement to emphasize their status and win cautious patients fearful of the pain involved in surgery. Although fame came from the association individual surgeons had with particular operations, eighteenth century surgeons emphasized how surgery was a respectable profession. One way they did this was to claim that whereas early practices were crude, surgery in the eighteenth century had become a science and an art that embodied Enlightenment values of experience and observation.

Key to this transformation was the growing influence of surgical thinking in medicine. Although holistic views of the body were maintained, in the eighteenth century the understanding of disease was increasingly associated with a new way of seeing disease based on localized, structural and anatomical terms. Morbid anatomy and the changing function of the hospital provided medical practitioners with new forms of power and ways of seeing disease [see 'Hospitals'], and the surgical elite used morbid anatomy and the hospital to assert their theoretical and scientific credentials. Eighteenth century surgeons like Jean-Louis Petit in France and the Hunters in London emphasized the scientific nature of surgery and exerted a considerable influence on contemporary surgeons. In constructing their professional identity, these elite surgeons distanced themselves from empiricism and used the surgical theatre and dissection room to display their knowledge. They exploited the hospital's potential for clinical training and stressed the vital role of observation and experimentation in constructing surgical knowledge to strengthen the image of surgery as a science.

This shift in the nature of medicine not only enhanced the status of surgery but also influenced how surgeons and physicians were trained as elite surgeons and placed greater emphasis on formal instruction. During the eighteenth century, new centres of surgical training and private schools were established, such as by the Hunters in London and Pierre-Joseph Desault in Paris, and quickly acquired important reputations. They took advantage of the growing demand for lectures and practical demonstrations in anatomy as practitioners endeavoured to improve their opportunities in an increasingly competitive medical marketplace [see 'Professionalization']. Even in Catholic and conservative Spain, where medical reforms were slower to take hold, there were moves to found new colleges of surgery. These institutions represented a considerable departure from previous methods of training. As demand for surgical courses increased, a number of surgical schools were opened, such as the Royal College of Surgery in Madrid in 1788. This in turn accelerated the decline of apprenticeship and the links between surgery and trade.

Increasingly these schools were linked to hospitals, with Leiden, Edinburgh, London and Paris providing major centres for surgical education. By the late eighteenth century, hospital schools had become the foci for the formulation of medical and surgical knowledge [see 'Hospitals'; 'Anatomy']. Here medical students walked the wards, observed patients and dissections, and attended lectures. Hospitals had advantages for students and surgeons alike: they offered major sites for accident and emergency cases, which were amenable to surgical intervention, a ready supply of cadavers for dissection, which provided lessons in manual dexterity and operative technique, and patients for observation and demonstration. Such opportunities were not available in private practice or through an apprenticeship. Surgeons successfully gained control of hospital schools to give them access to these resources and increasingly argued that theirs was not a mere empirical craft but a science rooted in anatomy and physiology, the new pillars of hospital-based training and the understanding of disease [see 'Anatomy'].

By the beginning of the nineteenth century, elite surgeons had come to vie with physicians in terms of status and learning. In Britain this change was symbolized by the renaming of the College of Surgeons as the Royal College of Surgeons in 1800. Increasingly, surgery and physic were taught alongside each other in hospital schools as a style of morbid anatomy asserted by surgeons became the foundation for understanding disease and for medical education. By merging physic and surgery in institutional training, as in Paris after 1794, surgeons asserted a way of looking at the body that both extended what they were able to do and added to their status as rational and scientific practitioners. Progress was slower in the German-speaking states where the traditional trade of the barber-surgeon ran in parallel to university-based surgery.

The shift in medical education and medicine in the late eighteenth and early nineteenth century ensured that old distinctions between practitioners broke down. Whereas they had previously been radicals and reformers, such as in Spain, surgeons were now moderates, part of the elite, with some early nineteenth century surgeons, such as John Abernethy or Astley Cooper in Britain, acquiring celebrity status. A number of technical advances and the redefinition of internal disease in the nineteenth century as a surgical problem further enhanced surgeons' status. Through anaesthetics and antiseptics, surgery became associated with science, heroics and the hospital operating theatre. Successful surgeons attained a social prestige that was equal to that of the upper classes, amongst whose ranks elite surgeons considered themselves.

By the 1930s, surgery had entered a 'golden age'. The manual dexterity involved in surgery was downplayed and the science of surgery was emphasized to distinguish surgery from merely operating. Surgeons were acknowledged as doctors and scientists, and were associated with modern, sophisticated hospital medicine. The elite surgeon's position as hero was assured; a status reflected in the media after 1945 and in operations on the heart and transplantation. Pioneering (and successful) surgical techniques contributed to the general prestige of medicine and public confidence. Increasing specialization created new types of heroic surgeon – the brain surgeon, the heart surgeon, etc. This optimism encouraged ambitious surgeons to become the first to pioneer new techniques. At times this led to an almost reckless approach, but for the most part, surgery was associated with quick cures and lifesaving.

The apparently unassailable position of the surgeon was not to last. In the last decades of the twentieth century this optimism and heroic image of surgery was challenged. Surgery came under increasing scrutiny. The work of individual surgeons was attacked in the media, whilst the growth of malpractice suits fuelled anxiety amongst surgeons. Surgery was still cast as offering medical miracles, but surgeons felt themselves increasingly under threat. Over the last five hundred years therefore surgeons had moved up the medical hierarchy to become modern heroes but as the events of the last decades of the twentieth century reveal this position was not a secure one.

The surgeon's art: 1500–1700

One view of sixteenth and seventeenth century surgery suggests that there were few significant changes to surgery. The nature and organization of surgery remained closely related to medieval practices. Few surgical texts were published and medieval Italian texts, such as that by Roger Frugard, continued to influence practice. What evidence we have from elite surgeons indicates that early modern surgery tended to be conservative and concentrated on the physical manipulation of the body's exterior to repair or maintain. However, rather than surgery being brutal, surgeons and their patients were conscious of pain. Most surgery was therefore minor surgery given the absence of adequate methods of pain control and often involved extended pre- and postoperative treatments. Although this did not mean that ambitious or extensive operations were avoided if vital for the patient's survival – for example, gangrene or serious injury – the limited evidence available suggests that surgeons generally treated common, acute but rarely life threatening conditions. They dealt with accidents, set fractures, stitched and bandaged wounds, let blood, and dealt with renal stones – a widespread condition before the nineteenth century. As the skin was also the province of the surgeon, they treated burns, lanced and dressed boils. Manual dexterity and anatomical knowledge were essential, but the range of conditions that could be treated discouraged many from technical or theoretical elaboration.

Although differences existed between the realm of the surgeon and that of the physician, the lines separating physicians from surgeons were not clearly drawn. There were similarities in how surgeons and physicians understood the body and disease. Both shared a common Classical tradition of knowledge based around the humors, albeit with surgeons adopting a more localized understanding. As we have seen in the above section, elite surgeons were keen to stress this common heritage and make links with physic to improve their status. If it is difficult to determine the practical impact of these ideas, surgeons were the most widely available medical practitioners in early modern Europe and performed a range of medical tasks, many of which were non-surgical. Many surgeons dealt with the external manifestations of disease, administered oral remedies, and were actively involved in hygiene and the medical treatment of venereal disease. Their involvement with physic modifies perceptions that strict divisions existed between different types of early modern practitioner.

Nor was early modern surgery stuck in the past. The introduction of gunpowder in the fifteenth century necessitated changes, but after 1500 there was also a renewed emphasis on making surgery learned. Surgeons borrowed from physic to stress the value of regimen and medicines, and exploited the printing press. Vernacular surgical texts, such as Peter Lowe's important *Discourse of the Whole Art of Chyrurgerie* (1597) were published, although it was only from the seventeenth century onwards that detailed accounts of operations, such as by the celebrated French surgeon Ambroise Paré, became common. Surgeons were also involved in the revitalization of anatomy and the philosophical debates in the seventeenth century [see 'Anatomy']. They observed dissections and undertook post-mortems as a way of learning about the consequence of injuries and disease, associating their work with new forms of knowledge. Limited changes were made to surgical

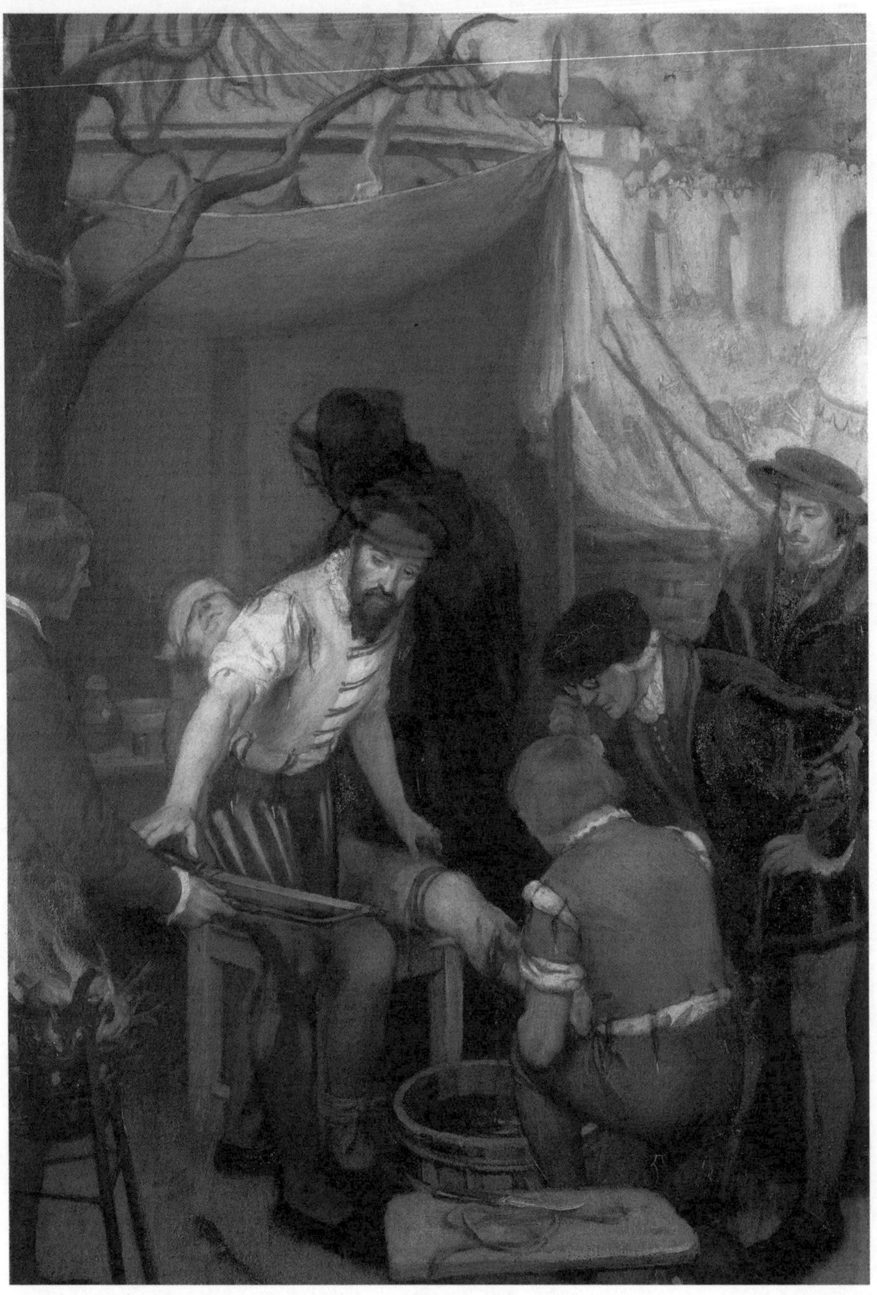

Figure 7.1 Ambroise Paré using a ligature when amputating on the battlefield at the siege of Bramvilliers. Oil painting by Ernest Board, c.1912.

Source: Wellcome Library, London.

techniques as surgical intervention became more active. French and Italian surgeons, such as Paré, Santo and Tagliacozzi, played a prominent role in innovation. For example, the use of boiling oil for cauterizing wounds gradually fell into disuse, largely in response to objections from patients. Cataract surgery and operations to remove bladder stones were perfected. Other innovations, including the invention of forceps by the Chamberlain family or the Colot family's procedure for removing bladder stones were, however, kept secret. Innovation and improvements to existing operations were in part the result of a surgical rhetoric that emphasized experience and practicality, but they were also driven by the need to attract patients.

However, although surgeons contributed to the revitalization of anatomy, and shared common boundaries with physic, surgery was constrained by the need for caution and the problem of pain. The relationship of anatomy to practice is hard to decipher and most surgical practice was conservative in nature. The need to avoid censure and protect reputations ensured that surgeons kept away from dangerous or complicated operations unless necessary. It is perhaps here that early modern surgery deserves its reputation for being cautious.

An 'age of agonies'? Eighteenth century surgery

Eighteenth century surgery is often characterized as a brutal and bloody art – a view nineteenth century surgeons endorsed to emphasize how far they had come. This image distorts the view of eighteenth century surgery. Certainly, some surgeons continued to shave and cut hair, perform heroic operations, and regularly bled their patients. However, as the boundaries between surgery and physic became increasingly blurred, professional roles overlapped. Surgeons had a central role in the provision of general healthcare in most European states and studies of surgeons' accounts and institutional records point to the broad range of their work. Most surgeons were involved in cleansing wounds, treating inflammations and abscesses, applying ointments or bandaging. Bloodletting and treating leg ulcers and chronic infections were the mainstays of surgical practice, whilst cures for venereal disease represented a highly profitable branch of surgery. In a period when wounds and broken bones were common, surgeons were required to treat fractures and attend accidents. Through such simple procedures, surgeons could relieve or cure many common complaints.

Surgery was not all about the surgeon, however. Patients would often first seek assurances that non-surgical treatment would alleviate or cure their condition. The result was that some conditions would keep getting worse until surgery was necessary. Surgeons were affected by their responsibility and tended to be cautious. Even when surgery could not be avoided, what could be achieved was limited. Speed was vital to limit blood loss and trauma. There were certain parts of the body, like the abdomen, where the risk of infection was so great that an operation was considered too dangerous. Major surgery therefore often tended to be a last resort: amputations were undertaken only to combat gangrene, or when serious injury meant no other option was available. By steering clear of difficult and involved operations, surgeons avoided high fatality rates that were bad for business.

This is not to suggest that the eighteenth century was a sterile period for surgery. Surgery was a discipline in transition as new techniques were introduced. This is evident from the publications emanating from the French Royal Academy of Science. Although the Academy represented the French surgical elite, its publications celebrated new operations, reconstructive surgery and the development of new surgical instruments. New surgical disciplines started to emerge, based around a combination of new instruments, practices, and models of the body that combined with growing demand for medical care. French surgery came to be revered, particularly by English surgeons who were keen to emulate the inductive scientific method embodied by Parisian surgeons. For example, Petit developed a new practice of amputation, which involved an effective tourniquet to limit blood loss, whilst his countryman Jacques Daviel devised a way to extract the lens of the eye once it had become opaque. Progress was also reported in England, where new techniques and operations were reported. A large literature on curing bladder stones appeared as epitomized by William Cheselden's *Treatise on a High Operation for Stone* (1723). Existing operative procedures were refined. Better methods were devised for common complaints, such as for the treatment of fractures by Pierre-Joseph Desault, or for dealing with hernias. The result was the gradual rise in the professional status of the surgeon and the emergence of new surgical disciplines, such as obstetrics or ophthalmology.

However, as already noted, the growing authority of surgery was not just the result of technical skill or technical innovations. Surgery aligned itself with new ideas about the body [see 'Anatomy']. Advances in anatomy provided surgeons with an intellectual rationale, while anatomical demonstrations strengthened their collective identity. As morbid anatomy became the key to understanding disease, European surgeons were at the forefront of asserting this new conception of disease and provided the basis for the reform of how regular practitioners were trained.

Making modern surgery: 1800–1900

The nineteenth century has been portrayed as central to the evolution of modern surgery. This interpretation not only favours a model of progress, but also focuses on hospital-based practice and the intimate relationship established between hospitals and surgery in the nineteenth century. For individual surgeons, a hospital post did come to confer professional status. Facilities for operating were improved and by the start of the twentieth century the hospital had become the desired location for patients and surgeons for more complex or hazardous operations. In many ways therefore, hospitals provided the context

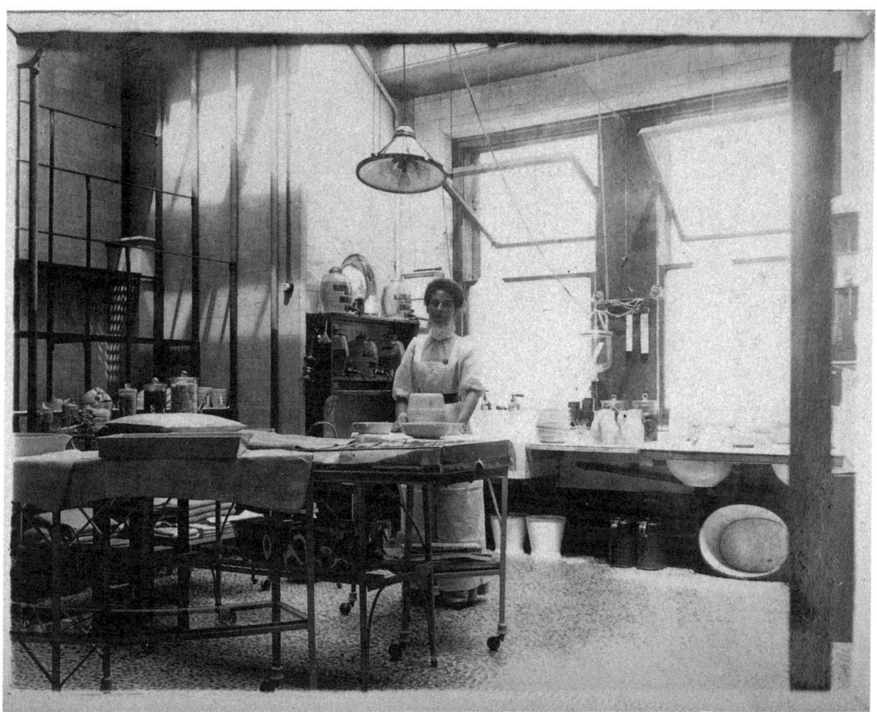

Figure 7.2 Operating theatre at St Bartholomew's Hospital, London, c.1890.
Source: Wellcome Library, London.

for the introduction of new techniques and surgical specialities. How healthcare was organized in the hospital, its links with medical education, and how it was funded, were crucial to innovation.

With the hospital becoming increasingly important to surgical innovation, historians have tended to focus on the surgical developments associated with them. This has been seen as a reciprocal process: if the hospital was key to technical advances that revolutionized surgery, surgery contributed to the re-conceptualization of the hospital as a medical space, a move that elevated its status and created demand for institutional care [see 'Hospitals']. Accounts have hence concentrated on the advent of new procedures and technologies that resulted in new operating theatres equipped with the necessary technical infrastructure. Anaesthesia and antiseptics have been held up as key elements of this progress, marking heroic landmarks in surgery. Anaesthesia made longer operations and more intricate procedures possible. Antiseptics allowed the innermost parts of the body to be operated on without fear of infection. This narrative has lent itself to a positivist view that emphasized the work of great men. However, although anaesthesia and antiseptics did make surgery less dangerous and more reliable, and allowed surgery to emerge as a realistic therapeutic option, their impact and adoption is far from straightforward. Rather than representing a single event or breakthrough, they were contested and underwent a process of modification. In the next section we will explore this process and how surgical practices could be contested.

Revolutions in surgery: anaesthesia and antiseptics

Chloroform anaesthesia has been represented as the cornerstone of modern surgery that contributed to nineteenth century surgeons' claims to competence. Prior to its introduction in the 1840s, speed had been essential in operations to minimize pain, shock and blood loss. This placed limitations on surgery. However, the impression that surgeons before 1840 were brutal and insensitive needs to be revised. Eighteenth century surgical writers discussed the necessity of minimizing pain and suggested practical methods to reduce its intensity or duration. Various agents were in use before the 1840s to manage pain, including opiates and alcohol, although the latter was employed mainly to fortify patients. None proved satisfactory or predictable in their results. Historians have therefore asked why anaesthetics emerged in the 1840s. Whereas the possibility of surgery without pain had been discussed, for example by French surgeon Velpeau, and chemists and medical practitioners were aware of the analgesic properties of certain substances (including ether), the historian Stephanie Snow argues in *Operations Without Pain* (2006) that it took a paradigm shift to make anaesthesia possible as surgeons changed their attitudes to pain. For Alison Winter, mesmerism – the practice of producing a hypnotic state in a patient by the exercise of animal magnetism – and its potential to relieve pain drew attention to suffering. Winter argues in *Mesmerized* (1998) that in doing so mesmerism created a threat to orthodox practitioners that encouraged medical men to turn to the chemistry of gases and pain relief. This is not to downplay the practical need to limit pain: early nineteenth century surgeons were already expanding their operative skills and performing operations that required longer periods on the operating table. Under these conditions, some form of effective pain relief became increasingly desirable.

It was two operations in 1846, both performed with ether – the first at Massachusetts General Hospital, Boston, and the second at University College Hospital, London – that have been credited with introducing painless surgery. Competing claims as to the discoverer of anaesthesia quickly ensued. Within a matter of months, the new technique was used in Paris, Bern, Berlin and Australia, and doctors and the public were debating pain control. New anaesthetic agents and methods were sought. Practice shifted from light anaesthesia (in which the patient was often conscious) to deep anaesthesia. Techniques for local anaesthesia and spinal application were devised. Anaesthesia allowed surgeons to rethink their methods: instead of speed and dexterity, surgeons had greater freedom to be more systematic.

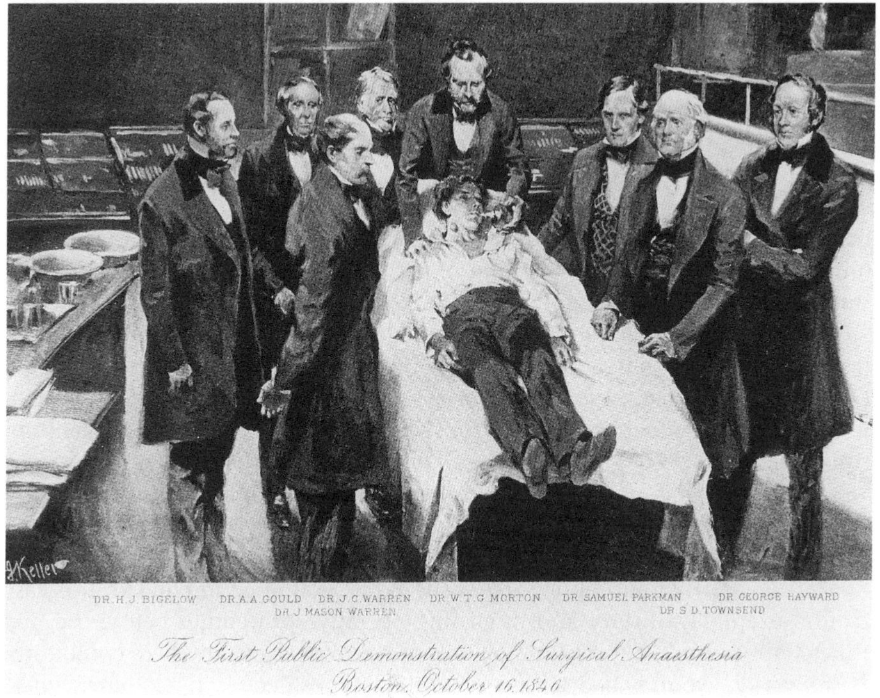

Figure 7.3 Artist's impression of the first demonstration of surgical anaesthesia at the Massachusetts General Hospital, Boston, in 1846. Painting by Washington Ayer, 1897.

Source: Wellcome Library, London.

Anaesthesia has often been presented as a natural and inevitable phenomenon of modern medicine; one that was immediately welcomed. This was not the case. Anaesthesia did not suddenly solve the problems facing surgeons: fear, skill, practicality, cost and postoperative management remained important concerns. Evidence from individual hospitals reveals neither a dramatic increase in the number of operations performed after 1846 nor that all operations were henceforth undertaken with an anaesthetic. Medical journals contain numerous examples of major operations going ahead without ether or chloroform. Their use was determined by convenience, the patient's age, sex and occupation; by the severity of the operation, where it was performed, and the cost.

The slow adoption of anaesthesia reflected generational differences, but anaesthesia was also controversial, especially between 1846 and 1860 when debate over its risks exceeded the discussion of its benefits. Mesmerism and numbing with cold initially offered viable alternatives that were openly debated. Opposition was expressed to chemically-induced insensibility. Questions of the risk to patients were raised, especially following reports of sudden death from cardiac arrest. Some doctors worried that anaesthesia might prejudice wound healing. Others feared that it somehow emasculated their work. Critics were apprehensive that the use of anaesthesia would increase the power of the surgeon over the unconscious patient, leading to excessive or unnecessary operations. Other concerns were voiced, particularly on the use of anaesthetics in childbirth as it was feared that it would hinder what was seen as a natural function. By the 1860s, opposition had begun to subside. Rather than anaesthesia being accepted uncritically therefore, its introduction was problematic, at least until the 1860s when a combination of patient demand and support from elite surgeons reduced opposition.

Whereas anaesthesia has been represented as heralding the start of modern surgery, antiseptic surgery has been portrayed as the final breakthrough. Combined with anaesthesia, antiseptic surgery is frequently presented as providing the unprecedented opportunity for safe and unlimited surgical intervention. Antiseptic practices did bring changes. Postoperative infections became less of a certainty, and the nature of operations and the environment they were conducted in altered. Surgeons became more ambitious; some experimented and evolved new methods, others were more cavalier.

The evolution of antiseptic surgery should be examined in context. It is easy to find examples of dirty and disgusting operative procedures before the mid nineteenth century, but it would be unwise to over-exaggerate these conditions. Postoperative wounds had always presented a considerable risk of cross infection. Surgical texts at the start of the nineteenth century frequently began with the problem of infection and methods were introduced to limit gangrene. By the 1840s, surgeons were being urged to adopted clean practices and use treatments that would assist healing, but by the 1860s levels of postoperative infection had become a major concern. In Britain, hospital mortality – often referred to as hospitalism – appeared out of control. Several solutions were advanced that broadly reflected the two opposing explanatory theories of how infection was acquired and spread: contagion theory and miasma theory. Although in practice these ideas about infection overlapped, each theory presupposed a different solution to preventing postoperative infection.

Surgeons influenced by contagion theory worked on the assumption that contact with the source of infection spread disease. They therefore believed that infected material needed to be removed. This approach lay behind the observations of Ignaz Semmelweis of Vienna of how puerperal fever was transmitted between women after childbirth. He argued in 1848 that the fever could be prevented if doctors scrubbed their hands in soap and water between examining women. Although Semmelweis's approach is often cited as the first example of aseptic practices, at the time his observations had a limited impact.

Those swayed by the rival miasma theory argued that infection was spread by the presence of poisonous particles in the air and an unsanitary environment. Here the solution was an improvement in the environment. Sanitarians had already noted the nauseating smells similar to rotting meat that permeated many hospital wards, associating them with unhealthy conditions, lack of air, and overcrowding. One solution – popularized by the British nursing reformer Florence Nightingale in her *Notes on Hospitals* (1863) – was to build hospitals around the pavilion principle to allow the better circulation of clean air. Others looked to improved cleanliness and hygiene to prevent postoperative infections. Support was expressed for whitewashing and the more rigorous cleaning of everything associated with the operating environment.

Yet despite the discussion generated by the cleanliness school it was the methods associated with the British surgeon Joseph Lister that has dominated narratives of antiseptics. For the historian W.F. Bynum in *Science and the Practice of Medicine in the Nineteenth Century* (1994) this was because Lister, more than his predecessors, built his antiseptic principle on medical science, but Christopher Lawrence and Richard Dixey are perhaps closer when they suggest that Lister's reputation was constructed by Listerian propaganda.[3] The story is a familiar one. Lister devised his antiseptic methods – the killing of infective agents present in the wound with disinfectants – in Glasgow and performed his first antiseptic operation there in 1865. It built on the principle of excluding microbes from the wound by using an antibacterial agent (carbolic). Lister's system (first published in 1867) therefore aimed to exclude germs, although it was only later that Lister used Pasteur's germ theory to justify his action. By making these claims, historians have associated Lister's methods with the application of germ theory to surgery.

Lister's approach did attract considerable attention. Through his teaching, he created disciples who went out and spread antiseptic practices. Surgeons from Britain and Europe visited Lister to see his practices at first hand. German surgeons were particularly taken with his methods and developed new operations that entered areas of the body previously associated with high mortality. For example, the development of gastrointestinal surgery by Thomas Billroth was strongly dependent on Lister's methods. Abdominal and thoracic surgery became more common. Traditional operations became safer. Nor was it just in hospital operating theatres that antiseptics influenced practice. Chemists from the 1880s started to sell topical antiseptics, which could be used in general practice or in the home. Manuals directed at general practitioners explained how antiseptic procedures could be performed.

There are several problems with the conventional account. Lister's reputation and contribution is a complex construct and his work needs to be placed in the context of what other contemporary surgeons were doing, and how antiseptics evolved in terms of the rationale behind it and the methods employed. In many ways, rather than being a pioneer or a great innovator, Lister was a transitional figure. For example, his use of carbolic was not revolutionary: turpentine, alcohol and carbolic were already being used to fight wound infection. Nor were Lister's methods uncontroversial. Lister was attacked for concentrating on local wound treatment and his approach was considered too complicated for practical use. The cleanliness school claimed that they achieved comparable results with simpler methods. Although this debate stimulated improvements in surgical care, opposition proved longstanding. Nor did Lister pave the way for the acceptance of germ theory: doctors were initially suspicious and it was only in the 1880s that bacteriology gained ground. A more sophisticated approach – as proposed by Michael Worboys in *Spreading Germs* (2000) – suggests that Lister's ideas were more closely connected to germ practices. It was around these practices and the experimental approach Lister adopted that a theory of germs was introduced.

Listerians projected a particular narrative that celebrated Lister's role and allied their version of antiseptics with a powerful language of science and hospital-based medicine. However, antiseptics were not a single event or the responsibility of one man. Lister's system evolved over time. Antiseptic methods and the rationale for them were therefore different in 1900 from the approach Lister had announced in 1867. For example, if Lister initially made reference to the germ theory of putrefaction and Pasteur's experiments, by the early 1880s putrefaction had become subordinate to a German germ theory of infection. As bacteriologists identified species of bacteria that caused wound infection, Listerians modified their views.

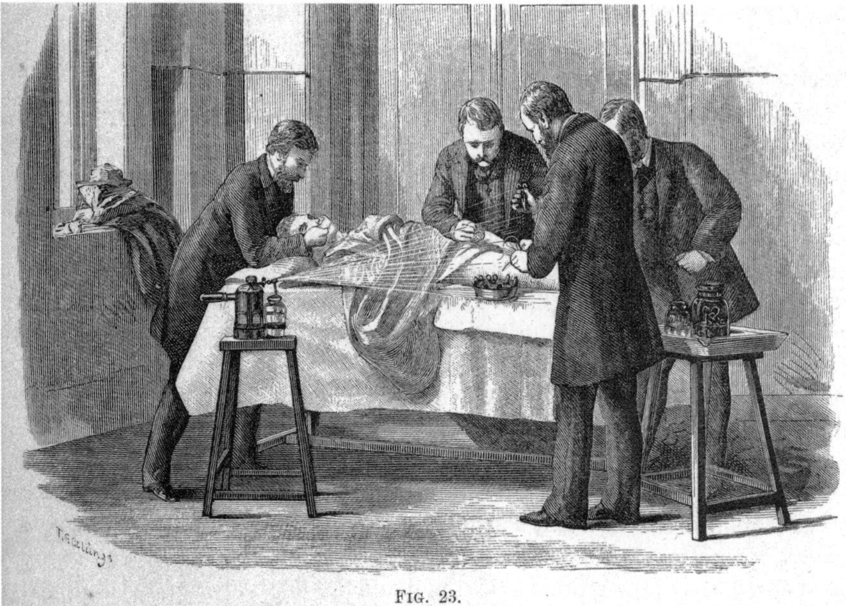

Figure 7.4 Use of Lister's carbolic spray.

Source: Wellcome Library, London.

The methods employed equally changed, broadening from a concern with local conditions to a more general environmental emphasis. This was part of a general process: all surgeons modified and improved their techniques. Lister constantly adjusted his antiseptic practices as he tried and discarded a range of methods. At first he was unconcerned about cleanliness: Lister would operate in his street clothes and merely dip his hands in carbolic instead of scrubbing them. In the early 1870s, he refined his method and added a machine to spray a mist of carbolic acid in an attempt to keep the whole atmosphere sterile. This was gradually abandoned. The spray was difficult to work with and later studies revealed that it was not very effective, findings that encouraged the introduction of new antiseptic compounds and an interest in sterilization.

Nor should Lister be viewed in isolation. The assault on wound infection did not derive from a single or sudden innovation by a small group (the Listerians). Rather it was the product of numerous small intellectual and practical deviations and developments. Lister's methods were adapted by his former students and adherents, often to make them easier. During the 1870s and 1880s, surgeons developed a variety of routines (or rituals) to prevent wound infection. Compromises were made as a general interest in cleanliness merged with a desire to prevent contamination with infectious agents to overcome deficiencies in antiseptic practices. Asepsis hence emerged in the late 1870s in parallel to refinements in antiseptic practices. It reflected moral and medical notions of cleanliness, and required everything coming into contact with the wound to be sterilized, through either washing or heat.

German surgeons and bacteriologists quickly acquired pre-eminence in this new style of surgery. They built operating rooms that utilized innovations, such as disinfectant sprays and large and easily washed amphitheatres, and adopted new techniques derived from laboratory culture: for example, the Pasteur oven and later the Chamberland autoclave were used to sterilize instruments. Other surgeons refined the aseptic technique. For example, the American surgeon William S. Halsted introduced rubber gloves in 1890 after his fiancée, a theatre nurse, developed a reaction to the antiseptics used, while in Breslau, Johann von Miculicz-Radecki claimed in 1897 that speaking during an operation enhanced droplet infection and argued that the risks were reduced by wearing facemasks. By the late 1890s, the familiar ritual of sterilized gowns, masks and gloves was beginning to be established, and hospitals invested in new operating theatres. Antiseptics and asepsis came to be viewed as a single doctrine and provided surgeons with a new set of craft skills and equipment.

Surgery in the nineteenth century

To see anaesthetics and antiseptics as marking the start of a modern era of surgery ignores what was happening before the 1840s. The popular view that surgeons were only able to perform a small number of procedures before the introduction of anaesthesia conceals the large number of major and minor operations surgeons were undertaking with growing competence and confidence. Between the 1790s and 1840s, there was an accumulation of anatomical and physiological knowledge that encouraged changes to surgical practice. Experiences during the Revolutionary and Napoleonic wars (1792–1814) not only stimulated demand for surgeons but also saw them modify and refine existing operations and gain confidence [see 'Medicine and warfare']. Surgeons embraced experimentation and sought professional benefit by devising new operations. As surgeons made assaults on the body, the province of surgery expanded. For example, new methods of amputation were devised and new techniques were adopted. Many of these new operations were initially controversial because they challenged orthodox practices.

Nor was surgery after 1840 solely about anaesthetic or antiseptic procedures. New forms of medical and laboratory technology extended the surgeon's realm. Instruments offered new forms of knowledge and techniques that were absorbed into surgical practice. They encouraged the emergence of a number of surgical specialities and new ways of seeing. Improvements in microscopes and histological techniques, for example, aided surgical diagnosis. The introduction of the laryngoscope in 1854–55 permitted observations of the interior of the larynx, while the otoscope provided the basis for ear, nose and throat surgery. Other diagnostic tools, such as the gastroscope and later X-rays, allowed surgeons to explore other areas of the body.

Changes in surgical practice were not just limited to new diagnostic technology or procedures. Shifts in the understanding of disease, influenced by physiology and pathology, and the broad shift in medical gaze from the whole person to individual organs or systems, influenced surgical treatments. Although surgeons were not primarily concerned with disease theories, and often had a practical approach, they benefited from changes in disease concepts. The importance of localized anatomical change in the early nineteenth century offered surgeons greater potential for intervention and encouraged an organ-based approach that made surgery on internal organs a therapeutic option. The growing emphasis on cellular pathology in the mid nineteenth century gave surgery a further rationale that favoured the removal of diseased organs or structures. This approach is evident in surgeons' move to adopt a more interventionist approach in the treatment of cancer.

The relationships between context, innovation, technology, resistance and conceptual changes in the understanding of disease point to a more complex history of nineteenth century surgery in which operations and operative methods were resisted and progress was by no means inevitable. It is possible to go further and argue that there were practical barriers to the adoption of new techniques or technologies. Although this is not to deny that important changes occurred in surgical practice in the period, there were practical limitations on the nature of surgery performed which an emphasis on elite or hospital surgery frequently overlooks. The realities of surgery covered a diverse range of practitioners from elite hospital surgeons to regimental surgeons and general practitioners, and an equally diverse range of contexts. Although European surgery shared many similar problems and practices, surgery differed according to the individual, the location, and the local and national context. For example, British surgeons in the first half of the nineteenth century were more accepting of German innovations than French practices, while French surgeons believed that British treatments for fractures were sloppy. Nor was hospital surgery the dominant arena of surgical practice until the late nineteenth century. It might have attracted professional and public attention, but hospital posts were limited and a considerable amount of minor surgery was conducted outside the hospital. General practitioners would, for example, dress wounds and remove stitches, as well as lance boils, set fractures and reduce hernias. In those regions where access to hospital care was limited, more ambitious procedures were attempted. For wealthy and middle-class patients, surgery performed in the home was the norm, at least until the 1890s. Most surgical lecturers assumed that the majority of their students would work in private practice and told them how to adapt their surgical practice accordingly. The nature of this surgery in a domestic setting is difficult to recapture, but if this did not preclude innovation, day-to-day practice changed less dramatically than hospital-based surgery.

Even in hospitals the speed of innovation varied. Surgeons were encouraged to be cautious and the decision to operate was rarely a straightforward one. The realities of funding, the practicalities of space, and generational differences all influenced the nature of surgery. Older procedures continued to be used by older surgeons and it took time for diagnostic tools to influence patient care, especially away from teaching hospitals. In the case of cancer this meant that many preferred radical solutions as to wait for tumours to be diagnosed clinically often meant they were inoperable. New methods were often time consuming and expensive and hence not always possible. Established procedures or standards were yet to be developed. New surgical practices, rather than being adopted uniformly, therefore tended to be diffused, creating differentials in success rates. As the case of anaesthetics, antiseptics and operations like abdominal hysterectomies reveal, opposition was encountered from within the profession. It was also encountered from patients: fear and pain deterred many.

By 1900, the practice of surgery had shifted from an emergency measure to become increasingly interventionist and reconstructive. Anaesthesia, asepsis and pathological anatomy aided the development of new operations, reduced surgical mortality, and increased confidence in the value of operations. Hospital surgery and innovations attracted popular attention, but as argued above, change was not universal or inevitable. Although in the 1860s and 1870s there was considerable excitement about advances in surgery, not all surgery conformed to ideas of modernity, especially outside the hospital. Traditional practices remained. Lessons learned during medical training were often modified or discarded. What might be seen as innovations were often contested, evolved over time, or were slow to take hold.

A 'golden age' of surgery?

Although the rapid growth of surgery in the late nineteenth and early twentieth century has attracted more attention than any other period, how to generalize these accounts is problematic. Part of the problem comes from the fact that modern surgery is a diverse field. Specialization, which became a feature of German and French medicine, created different surgical specialties with their own cultures and practices. Not all surgeons saw surgery or the surgeon's role as meaning the same thing. Although surgery after 1900 continued to be associated with technological progress and modernity, some surgeons remained anxious about moves to scientific and standardized surgery. They protested against what they saw as the reduction of surgery to a mechanical application of standard treatments.

Yet, contemporaries readily associated twentieth century surgery with progress. Interest in the removal of pathological matter and structural questions, as seen in the treatment of cancers, was slowly replaced after 1914 by greater concern with restoration and the adoption of other therapies to extend the range of operations. Development came in stages and often relied on the activities of individual operators, as evident in the treatment of heart disease. Successful procedures were modified and standardized and surgery was extended to treat many familiar and life threatening conditions. Although private practice remained important, surgeons increasingly worked in a hospital setting aided by improved ambulance services. In this institutional setting there was a move to teamwork and further specialization, a shift encouraged by experiences during the First World War (1914–18) and interwar technical advances. Neurosurgery, cardiology and plastic surgery offered opportunities for the ambitious, and special surgical clinics for these and other conditions were established in most hospitals.

Given the above changes, it has been argued that the first half of the twentieth century marked a 'golden age' for surgery. As German surgical pre-eminence declined, the emphasis in innovation shifted to the United States. Existing operating theatres were renovated or were replaced with new operating suites. Operations were refined and greater attention was directed at patient comfort. New procedures were introduced – often in rapid succession – and conditions previously defined as medical, such as gastric ulcers, became the subject of operations. Routines of hand washing and barrier methods became established to prevent infection and evolved into complex procedures of scrubbing up, donning gloves, masks and protective clothing. New medical technologies and the greater use of laboratory tests to assess, for example, heart, kidney or liver functions, not only required institutional treatment, but also influenced the nature of operative procedure and diagnosis, and became important symbols of medical power. Advances in pathology provided a way of determining if tumours were cancerous or not, shaping surgeons' clinical judgement. Other technologies, such as the early use of radiotherapy in the treatment of cancer, helped surgeons extend the field of operability.

The First World War forced the introduction of new surgical procedures to tackle postoperative infections in an environment laden with bacteria [see 'Medicine and warfare']. Surgeons turned to more drastic solutions: debridement, or the cutting out of the damaged tissue, which was a breeding ground for bacteria, was adopted. The war also contributed to the development of several surgical specialties, notably orthopaedics, plastic or reconstructive surgery, and cardiology. Individual surgeons were encouraged by their wartime experiences and in the 1920s and 1930s they went on to perform difficult procedures on the brain, lung, heart and other organs. Surgical interventions in the treatment of tuberculosis were developed, and new operations, such as tracheotomy or for the relief of intestinal obstructions, were devised. Appendectomies became fashionable in the 1920s and 1930s, as did hysterectomies and tonsillectomies. Surgeons started to work on the abdomen and the head. As their confidence grew, surgeons became more ambitious. Only slowly did surgery enter a new phase, with a shift from a preoccupation with removal to a concern with restoration and transplantation – a transformation that was to come to the fore in the 1950s and 1960s.

Despite improvements in surgery, change was uneven. Although antiseptic and aseptic procedures ensured that epidemics of postoperative infection did not occur in institutions, infection remained a problem. Many surgeons were complacent, especially after the First World War where experiences on the battlefront prompted questions about medicine's ability to tackle infection. Problems were encountered in operations, which did not always go well. Surgeons made mistakes, but a proportion of patients did not recover, even when no mistakes were made. Much depended on the surgeon's skill and the patient: older patients and those undergoing difficult operations were most at risk of complications. With few restrictions on surgical practice, standardization was problematic and many surgeons were actively engaged in the process of innovation, either devising or modifying operations or introducing new instruments or other surgical tools. The majority rejected some procedures because they proved beyond their skill, while surgeons distrusted published results if they did not conform to their own experiences. Personal preference was important: individual surgeons modified operations as they adjusted procedures, instruments and the nature of pre- and postoperative care provided. Disputes occurred over which operations were best or had the lowest surgical mortality, and between general surgeons and new surgical specialists. Not all surgical specialties had the same status, and some, like trauma surgery, struggled to assert their position. Surgeons also had to be convinced of the efficacy of new procedures, as can be seen in their resistance to the use of radium therapy in the treatment of cancer.

The institutional settings also need to be taken into consideration. Surgical facilities were limited outside the major metropolitan and teaching hospitals. Operative technology remained at a minimum until the 1950s and the daily life of most surgeons revolved around dressing wounds, draining abscesses and routine surgical procedures. In Britain, this was revealed by the outbreak of war in 1939 and the creation of the Emergency Medical Service. A review of hospitals quickly exposed a shortage of modern equipment and facilities in many provincial institutions. Outside metropolitan hospitals, therefore, surgery did not always conform to its image of entering a 'golden age'. Surgery was changing but not always quickly.

Surgery and technology: 1945–2000

The period after the Second World War (1939–45) to the end of the twentieth century has been associated with rapid advances in surgery. It has been characterized by a growing emphasis on replacement and technological innovations, as well as by the use of biochemical and immunological knowledge. Increasingly complex procedures were developed in orthopaedics, neurosurgery, cardiac, thoracic and eye surgery. Surgery, which before 1940 had a predominately generalist ethos, became more fragmented and specialized. Professionals and patients increasingly talked about brain surgeons, heart surgeons or orthopaedic surgeons, and new specialist surgical departments were established as part of hospitals. Changing disease patterns, particularly those related to more affluent lifestyles, made new operations necessary, and others, such as cosmetic surgery to enlarge breasts or to reduce obesity, culturally desirable. The introduction of antibiotics, immunosuppressive drugs, new anaesthetic compounds and technical innovations allowed surgery to expand into new areas considered impossible in the 1920s and 1930s, such as heart surgery, and made other previously dangerous operations routine. For example, a better understanding and improved methods of blood transfusion made many surgical treatments involving substantial blood loss viable, while the growth of intensive care medicine from the 1960s widened the field.

New methods – including computerized axial tomography (CAT), magnetic resonance imaging (MRI), nuclear isotopes, and fibre optics – in visual diagnostics allowed surgeons greater precision in determining the presence and extent of disease. This new diagnostic technology created a resource for surgeons to extend their professional credentials and realm and was used in much the same way as science had been used as a resource to assert medical practitioners' authority in the nineteenth century [see 'Medicine and science']. Keyhole surgery was made possible using fibre optics and instruments that could pass down a small tube into the body. Such procedures were less invasive and required less time in hospital, which made them popular with patients and hospital administrators. However, the positive impact of these developments should not be overstressed. New technology and procedures could come at a cost, which was not just financial. They brought with them new problems – particularly in terms of postoperative infection – and increased the cost of healthcare, imposing a growing financial burden on state medical services that forced changes to the structure of healthcare [see 'Healthcare and the state'].

Rather than the second half of the twentieth century seeing linear improvements, the adoption of many new operations and procedures was not always smooth. Just as with anaesthetics and antiseptics in the nineteenth century, the acceptance of certain operative procedures had a more complicated history than is immediately apparent. The history of organ transplants provides one such example.

The principle of organ transplantation was accepted in the 1880s through the work of the Swiss surgeon Theodor Kocher on thyroid transplantation for goitre, the pathological enlargement of the thyroid gland. The principle was applied to other organs as surgeons sought new techniques to replace diseased organs and tissue. However, although the technique for organ transplant was perfected by the French-American Alexis Carrel, who won the Nobel Prize in 1912 for his work on blood vessel surgery and organ transplant, problems with organ rejection saw surgeons abandon transplant surgery in the 1920s. The practice was revived in the 1950s, initially with kidney transplants, but problems with organ rejection remained. It was only with the development of immunosuppressive drugs that transplantation became a practical reality. Successes with kidney transplants encouraged surgeons to consider transplanting other organs.

The publicity generated by the first heart transplant by the South African surgeon Christiaan Barnard in 1967 concealed serious early problems. High fatality rates – the first heart transplant patient died within days – saw the operation abandoned after initial enthusiasm. Improvements were made to the procedure. Research was undertaken into the selection criteria for patients; into tests to assess rejection criteria and how to prevent rejection. Heart transplants were gradually reintroduced, and by the 1980s the survival rate had risen to 80 per cent. However, the operation remained a last resort and, as with the transplantation of other organs, continued to generate new concerns from the ethical problems in relation to organ donors to problems with the supply of organs.

Nor was new technology always enough. Just as with Lister's antiseptics, in the twentieth century the adoption of new procedures or technologies also involved questions of efficiency, utility, standardization, success, and the practicable nature of a procedure, and patient support or compliance. To this might be added a further economic dimension, especially in state-funded healthcare. New surgical spaces and procedures were designed to prevent infection, but funding and existing hospital infrastructures ensured that these were slow to be implemented. Cooperation was also required, often between surgeons, but also increasingly between surgery and business, surgeons and other medical and paramedical specialties, and between surgeons and hospital administrators. This cooperation was not always harmonious and the resultant inter- and intra-professional tensions should not be ignored.

Conclusions

Rising costs in the 1990s and early twenty first century undermined mid twentieth century optimism that surgery could cure all ills. Questions of cost-effectiveness started to impose limits on surgical practice. New technologies and ways of managing disease, such as through chemotherapy, saw surgical solutions replaced by other forms of treatment. Although the history of surgery in the late twentieth and early twenty first century became increasingly subject to external economic and state forces, the *long duree* of the history of surgery equally reveals how surgery was shaped by professional, conceptual and technical developments; by institutional contexts and by external demands. Development was by no means natural, inevitable or always self-evident. By thinking about surgery as a series of overlapping narratives and changes, a better picture can be produced: one that acknowledges the important practical, technical and intellectual changes being made, but also recognizes surgery outside the hospital and how generational and other forces ensured that change was uneven. Hence, rather than a progressive narrative, a more contested history of surgery is revealed, one that helps question our assumptions about progress, breakthroughs and the adoption of new ideas or methods in medicine.

Further reading

One of the best accounts of the historiography of surgery can be found in Christopher Lawrence, 'Divine, Democratic and Heroic', in his *Medical Theory, Surgical Practice. Studies in the History of Surgery* (London: Routledge, 1992), pp. 1–47, with the volume also offering essays on surgical techniques and practices. There are few good general narratives, although Owen Wangensteen and Sarah Wangensteen, *The Rise of Surgery from Empiric Craft to Scientific Discipline* (Folkestone: Dawson, 1978) is an exhaustive survey. Early modern surgery has attracted relatively little attention but readers should see Vivian Nutton, 'Humanist Surgery', in Andrew Wear, Roger French and Iain Lonie (eds), *The Medical Renaissance of the Sixteenth Century* (Cambridge: Cambridge University Press, 1985), pp. 75–99, for a comparative study of Renaissance surgery. Andrew Wear, *Knowledge and Practice in English Medicine, 1550–1680* (Cambridge: Cambridge University Press, 2000) discusses the nature of surgery in early modern England, while David Gentilcore, *Healers and Healing in Early Modern Italy* (Manchester: Manchester University Press, 1998) and Margaret Pelling, *Medical Conflicts in Early Modern London: Patronage, Physicians, and. Irregular Practitioners, 1550–1640* (Oxford: Oxford University Press, 2003) address the surgeon's position. A larger literature exists on the eighteenth and nineteenth centuries. Toby Gelfand, *Professionalizing Modern Medicine: Paris Surgeons and Medical Science and Institutions in the Eighteenth Century* (Westport, CT: Greenwood Press, 1980) shows how surgeons came to dominate the hospital, while Susan Lawrence, 'Medical education', in W.F. Bynum and Roy Porter (eds), *Companion Encyclopaedia of the History of Medicine*, vol. 2 (London: Routledge, 1997), pp. 1151–79, and Thomas N. Bonner, *Becoming a Physician: Medical Education in Britain, France, Germany, and the United States, 1750–1945* (New York and Oxford: Oxford University Press, 1995) examine medical education and the importance of surgery. There is a substantial literature on anaesthetics and antiseptics. On anaesthetics, see Peter Stanley, *For Fear of Pain: British Surgery, 1790–1850* (Amsterdam: Rodopi, 2003) and Stephanie Snow, *Operations Without Pain: The Practice and Science of Anaesthesia in Victorian Britain* (Basingstoke: Palgrave Macmillan, 2006) for a revisionist assessment. Studies by Christopher Lawrence and Richard Dixey, 'Practicing on Principle: Joseph Lister and the Germ Theories of Disease', in Christopher Lawrence (ed.), *Medical Theory, Surgical Practice* (London: Routledge, 1992), pp. 153–215, and Lindsay Granshaw, 'Upon this Principle I have based a Practice': The Development and Reception of Antisepsis in Britain, 1867–90', in John Pickstone (ed.), *Medical Innovations in Historical Perspective* (Basingstoke: Palgrave Macmillan, 1992), pp. 16–46, offer detailed re-assessments of Lister and antiseptics, with M. Anne Crowther and Marguerite Dupree, *Medical Lives in the Age of Surgical Revolution* (Cambridge: Cambridge University Press, 2007) examining Lister's students and how Listerian ideas spread. For the day-to-day nature of nineteenth century surgery, see Anne Digby, *The Evolution of British General Practice 1850–1948* (Oxford: Oxford University Press, 1999), while Christopher Lawrence and Tom Treasure, 'Surgeons', in Roger Cooter and John Pickstone (eds), *Medicine in the Twentieth Century* (London: Routledge, 2000), pp. 653–670, gives an excellent overview of twentieth century surgery. Less has been written about individual surgical specialisms, but Roger Cooter, *Surgery and Society in Peace and War: Orthopaedics and the Organization of Modern Medicine, 1880–1948* (London: Macmillan, 1993) provides not only an account of orthopaedics, but also raises questions about the nature of surgery and medical expertise.

8
Hospitals

From their medieval and Christian origins, hospitals came to stand at the apex of medical science and training in the nineteenth century. By the start of the twentieth century, hospitals had become not only key sites for research and new technologies, and the desired location for surgical care, but also had acquired a central importance in the professional structure of medicine. During the following century, the hospital's position was consolidated as it became the epitome of modern, high-tech medicine.

To understand this process, historians have asked what drove these changes. Whereas early accounts outlined a view that saw the hospital as a natural response to developments in medicine, since the 1980s there has been a considerable shift in the ways in which historians have approached the subject of the hospital. The publication of *The Hospital in History* (1989) embodied this new approach to show how the hospital was 'a microcosm of society'. By placing founders, patrons and the wider socioeconomic and political contexts at the centre of hospital history, contributors to the volume revealed how the growth of towns, social mobility, charity, and the pursuit of status by donors and doctors, were crucial to explaining the growing importance of the hospital. A doctor-centred approach was shown to be inadequate as non-medical factors were balanced against professionalization and medicalization to reveal how the hospital was a social *and* medical institution.

Research in the early twenty first century suggested new directions in hospital history. Drawing on trends in welfare history, a new generation of scholars examined the role of patients in negotiating care. Other types of institution – children's hospitals, sanatoriums, maternity hospitals, etc – and functions – for example, the hospital's liturgical or educational roles – were explored to illustrate the uses hospitals had to patrons, practitioners and communities. Studies began to look beyond the nineteenth century to examine the nature of hospital provision in the twentieth century as a way of questioning narratives of state welfare [see 'Healthcare and the state']. In this historiography, the hospital was no longer a discreet institution, but as this chapter shows, the hospital existed at the centre of much wider social, political, professional and medical narratives.

A religious and social institution: 1500–1700

Traditional views of sixteenth and seventeenth century hospitals have represented them as pre-modern institutions that served a limited medical role acting as 'gateways to death' or, following Michel Foucault's characterization, as essentially repressive institutions. Such accounts, which stressed the changes to hospital medicine in the eighteenth and nineteenth centuries, overlook what was happening in early modern Europe and how hospitals came to perform an increasingly complex role. Rather than being marginal or instruments of repression, early modern hospitals became important institutions in the delivery of healthcare.

Although the sixteenth century was a turbulent period – encompassing wars in Italy, the Reformation and the Counter-Reformation with its consequences for poor relief, and the civil war in Britain – the century witnessed an expansion of hospital provision. The term hospital covered a variety of institutions from hospices for travellers and pilgrims, to places to isolate the infectious and institutions for the indigent, but increasingly emphasis was placed on ministering to the sick poor. Although many small medieval institutions closed, especially in rural areas, prominent medieval hospitals were refurbished: in the Imperial towns of southern Germany, for example, new buildings were added to the existing Holy Spirit hospitals. Population growth and migration, urbanization, rising demand for institutional care, and the growing problem of urban disease, created favourable conditions for expansion, as well as resources to fund new hospitals, particularly in those regions (like Italy) that saw notable urban and commercial growth. In Florence, a wealthy merchant community provided the resources for the city to become a leading centre for hospital provision, while Naples had eleven hospitals by the seventeenth century. Expansion was not limited to Italy. In Paris, the Hôtel-Dieu doubled in size, remodelling its wards, and opening satellite hospitals for infectious and incurable patients. Away from the major urban centres, hospital provision remained sparse, however.

Early modern hospitals were shaped more by religious, charitable, socioeconomic and political factors than by medicine. Like their medieval predecessors, many were founded and managed by religious orders. The Christian emphasis on charity and healing remained strong and contemporaries widely regarded hospitals as pious works. The Reformation and Counter-Reformation reaffirmed the hospital's spiritual functions, and the emergence of new Christian and nursing orders devoted to the care of the sick, particularly in sixteenth century France, served to revitalize local institutions. Most European hospitals were therefore as much houses of God as institutions for healing, but they were also conduits for patronage and had important political or socioeconomic functions. Prominent citizens and confraternities established hospitals with the aim of improving healthcare for the sick poor, but their ongoing involvement in how they were managed also ensured that hospitals were often significant political institutions that offered a power-base for local elites. Hospitals helped enforce traditional social hierarchies and the elite saw them as vital to maintaining the prestige of their towns, their personal status, and their influence.

Although religion, local patronage and charity were crucial to the expansion of hospital provision in sixteenth and seventeenth century Europe, municipal authorities also cultivated hospitals. As greater emphasis was placed on welfare and poverty in the seventeenth century, the hospital acquired a growing significance to municipal authorities. Italian princes and city councils started to intervene in welfare and rationalize charitable resources, while in the German-speaking states, city councils funded small institutions that offered specialized treatment. Although only partially successful, municipal authorities wanted to make sure that hospitals were well-managed, and that the right patients were admitted. Involvement could extend to the purging of hospitals of political opponents, as apparent in Britain during the Restoration, or attempts to rationalize charitable institutions by closing inefficient or corrupt foundations and appropriating their resources. Whereas in France this saw a substantial number of small provincial hospitals close, more often, as in Verona, cities and states intervened only when the economic resources of a hospital were threatened.

New types of hospital were established by the state in the sixteenth and seventeenth centuries. In France, following Louis XIV's order in 1676, cities opened *hôpitaux-généraux* to house and police the indigent and disorderly poor. Other European states established similar institutions – for example, *Zuchthäuser* in German-speaking territories, the workhouse in Britain, or *ospedali di carità* in Italy performed similar functions – although they did not offer the systematic repression and control that might support Foucault's ideas of a 'great confinement' [see 'Asylums']. Military hospitals were opened, such as the Hôtel des Invalides (1640) in France, to serve other functions. They not only treated sick and maimed soldiers, but also trained medical practitioners for the army and navy. The importance of medicine in military hospitals highlights how hospitals were beginning to take on more medical functions in early modern Europe.

Voluntary hospitals: 1700–1800

Although the growth of hospital foundations was uneven – Moscow, for example, had only one hospital for a civilian population of some 200,000 people – the eighteenth century witnessed a marked growth in the number and type of hospitals. If these institutions did not met the medical needs facing many communities, new hospitals were established: for example, general hospitals were opened, such as the Charité in Kassel or the *Allgemeine Krankenhaus* (General Hospital) in Vienna. There was also a growing differentiation between institutions: whereas some institutionalized teaching, new smaller specialist hospitals also opened, such as the Hôpital des Enfants Malade (1778) in Paris. Existing institutions were expanded or rebuilt. Hospitals became increasingly for the care of the sick poor as other inmates were segregated into different institutions, such as the workhouse or asylum. Hospitals acquired clearer medical functions and took on a growing role in the training of licensed practitioners through bedside teaching, lectures and opportunities for dissection [see 'Professionalization'].

Demographic or socioeconomic factors have been put forward to explain this renewed interest in hospitals. Although there was no simple link between charity and the economy, commercialism and industrialization in the eighteenth century new groups were created and resources for supporting hospitals. Growth also reflected the religious revivalism of the period, and Enlightenment and mercantilist thinking, which emphasized the importance of social progress and prosperity linked to population, and provided a rationale that suggested that curing illness would prevent poverty, return the labourer to work, and contribute to national wealth. The problems associated with urbanization stimulated redefinitions of poverty and welfare, and encouraged civic responsibility. These ideas were manifested in hospital foundations. Local resources and networks were important, as evident in Hamburg or London. Elsewhere hospital foundation was shaped by state initiatives. In the German-speaking states, for example, the foundation of *Allgemeine Krankenhaus* was driven by Joseph II's plans for reform and administrative centralization. Existing institutions were attacked as 'gateways to death' and critics called for sweeping reforms of existing hospitals which resulted in experiments in hospital planning and forms of medical care.

Nowhere was this growth in hospital provision more apparent than in Britain, as first London and then the rest of England went mad for hospitals. This wave of hospital foundation – referred to as the voluntary hospital movement – was underwritten by the economic and social transformations associated with industrialization and by a growth in charitable contributions. The foundation of the Westminster Infirmary in London in 1719 saw a shift in the nature of the hospital, and began a new and rapid phase of hospital foundation. The Westminster was a hospital by accident, however. Those behind the institution had not initially intended to establish an infirmary. Instead, they had sought to promote a Christian and charitable spirit of relief to educate the children of the poor. The idea for a hospital only emerged in 1719, but then quickly gathered momentum. The Westminster set the pattern for other hospitals by creating a new conduit between patron and patient that represented a new space for medicine. London provided the focus, although hospitals followed in prosperous towns, such as in Edinburgh (1729) and in Winchester (1736). These new hospitals were clones of existing institutions and were often little more than houses or big mansions rather than purpose-built institutions. This allowed their rapid spread spurred on by urbanization, a booming economy, the growth of an urban middle-class, an upsurge in charitable effort, and an expanding medical marketplace: whereas no provincial hospitals had existed in 1735, twenty-eight had opened by 1800 as part of an urban renaissance.

Although the voluntary model was not uniformly adopted – for example, in the German-speaking territories and Sweden it was the state that had the main role – similar institutions were founded almost everywhere in Europe and the voluntary model travelled to North America. As public and participatory institutions, voluntary hospitals in Britain quickly acquired an important charitable and medical role and embodied contemporary values of voluntarism and distinctive social and hierarchical arrangements. The charitable impulse to found and support them came from a number of motives that ranged from guilt to gratitude; from worries about the state of society to a desire for social emulation at a time when stress was being placed on a mercantilist approach in which the population was a source of wealth. Many of these new institutions became a focus of civic pride and local charity as the wealthy and aspiring gave their support, establishing networks that aided benefactors and displayed their social position. It helped that these new hospitals were relatively easy to establish – requiring only a group of like-minded supporters, a doctor, some nurses and a building – and delivered clear benefits to subscribers. Voluntary hospitals institutionalized and democratized patterns of paternalism and reflected social rather than medical needs. This complex interaction of socioeconomic and political forces helps explains why British hospitals became so effective at soliciting charity. They were expressions of a new type of charity that promoted the idea that the benevolent had a duty to oversee where and how their money was spent. Eighteenth century charity in effect stressed a duty to give as the emphasis shifted from moral good and saving souls to social and material aid, or saving bodies. Hospitals benefited.

If the example of Britain highlights the complex factors that shaped the foundation of hospitals in the eighteenth century, not all were convinced of their worth. This was apparent in Germany. Here debate centred on whether or not the sick would be better served by domiciliary care in which the patient was treated at home or in a hospital. Cost was an important concern. Support was not always forthcoming as shown by the failure to establish hospitals in Düsseldorf and Münster. Even where hospitals were established, many struggled to raise funds. However, a reconfiguration of the hospital and its supporters in the eighteenth century underwrote a period of rapid expansion in hospital provision and established a type of hospital that was to be replicated throughout the nineteenth century.

Hospital growth: 1800–1945

The nineteenth century saw a further phase of hospital growth. New general hospitals were founded, greater numbers of specialist institutions, such as for children, opened (see below), and hospital medical schools were established, with teaching hospitals (or university clinics in Germany) quickly emerging as prestigious institutions. In Poland, for example, twelve hospitals were opened between 1832 and 1834; in Norway, the number grew from eighteen in 1853 to over thirty-six hospitals in 1900, with the number of hospital beds tripling in

Britain between 1861 and 1911. Existing institutions were improved or modernized. Hospitals were remodelled and expanded to cope with the changing demands of education and research, new technologies, nursing reforms, and changes in medical and surgical practice and ideas about hygiene – changes that were reflected in hospital design. Whereas previously inpatient care had dominated, the growth of outpatient departments and specialist clinics extended the utility of the hospital as greater numbers could be treated. The growing role of the hospital in medical education, their material environment in terms of space and resources, and how they were funded, were all crucial to innovation so that by the end of the nineteenth century healthcare was increasingly organized in the hospital.

Some historians believe a significant difference existed between these hospitals and their predecessors. Post-Revolutionary Paris has been at the centre of these accounts and what has been labelled the 'birth of the clinic'. Influenced by the work of Erwin Ackerknecht in *Medicine at the Paris Hospital 1794–1848* (1967) and Michel Foucault in *The Birth of the Clinic* (translated 1973), historians have focused on changes in medical ideology and medical authority encouraged by the social and political upheavals generated by the French Revolution (1789–99). These upheavals and reforms undermined some of the fundamental features of the Old Regime and allowed new social relations and institutions to emerge. Whereas the revolutionaries had ironically sought to abolish hospitals because of their associations with Catholicism and corruption, their medical reforms had the effect of inventing the hospital as a medical institution. French hospitals were nationalized and secularized; the medical curriculum was revised; the importance of pathological anatomy was stressed; greater emphasis was placed on hospital attendance; and the professional structure of medicine was reformed to break down divisions between physic and surgery. The social, political and medical reforms associated with post-Revolutionary Paris placed the hospital at the heart of medicine and medical education, creating centralized institutions that acted as training centres. Many of the clinical advances, such as René Laënnec's introduction of the stethoscope at the Necker Hospital or Corvisart's dissemination of percussion at La Charité, came to be associated with Paris. The result was a new style of reductionist and analytical medicine based on observation, hospital wards, and the post-mortem room [see 'Anatomy']. Hospital patients, Foucault argued, came to provide both resources for the construction of medical knowledge and for medical education as doctors gained control over the hospital and the clinical encounter and became key actors driving hospital provision. These processes ushered in a style of hospital medicine typified by observation, physical examination, pathological anatomy, the use of statistics, and hospital-based training that was to dominate medicine in the half century following 1794.

Although few historians disagree that the above changes and the ideas associated with Paris had a significant impact, the timing, nature and extent of this transformation can be questioned. As discussed in Chapter 6, revisionists have argued that the model associated with Paris built on existing trends and even supporters of Paris medicine as epoch making recognize pre-cursors. The features associated with Paris medicine – hospital-based training, pathological anatomy, bedside diagnosis – were not unique to Paris. The conditions associated with the 'birth of the clinic' were already present in mid eighteenth century London. Professionalization, developments in pathological anatomy and clinical observation, and the institutionalization of training – for example, in Vienna, Paris, Edinburgh and London – during the eighteenth century were already making hospitals important sites for practitioners and in the construction of medical knowledge before 1789 [see 'Professionalization'].

Whilst not denying the importance of changes to the understanding of disease, and the growing centrality of hospitals to medicine and professional structures, social factors linked to urbanization, social mobility and bourgeois identity, industrialization and migration, continued to be crucial in shaping hospitals in the nineteenth century. Religious concerns equally remained important: hospital foundations were supported by the religious revivals of the early nineteenth century and by the growth of religious orders, such as the Sisters of Charity in Ireland. Whereas these factors suggest greater continuity with the eighteenth century, different patterns of industrialization helped determine hospital foundation. Non-industrialized societies, such as the Netherlands, were slower to open general hospitals, while in more industrialized regions the problems created by industry, migration, overcrowding and urbanization, with its attendant impact on ill health, created demand for hospital services. Local communities responded as best they could.

Yet it was faith in charity that continued to underpin nineteenth century British general and specialist hospitals. Benevolence in cooperation with local government were the desired agencies through which institutional healthcare was to be provided, and hospitals represented an important conduit for charity. This was not just evident in Britain, but also in Austria, France and Poland. Although not free from conflict, supporting a hospital helped bring old and new elites together by renegotiating social, political and religious interests, and by offering common ground for civic pride and for action to tackle disease or social issues. Links between charity, civic pride, and the social utility of hospitals for the middle classes and businesses saw the number of hospitals mushroom in Britain as the population grew, urbanization increased, and the extent of disease multiplied.

In other European countries, a mixture of state and voluntary provision was more characteristic [see 'Healthcare and the state']. In Ireland, committees of local subscribers managed hospitals with additional funds from grand juries or municipal corporations. A similar pattern existed in the German-speaking states where charity and mutualism was mixed with public support. Although mixed economies of care were important, an active investment was made in municipal medicine; for example, in Naples hospitals were rationalized and placed under the control of a general council in the early nineteenth century. Efforts to coordinate medical welfare in France saw hospitals in Paris placed under the control of the *Conseil supérieur de l'assistance public* in 1888. A decade later, many municipal authorities had started to invest heavily in institutional healthcare.

A bleak view has been adopted of hospital provision in the 1920s and 1930s, an approach shaped by traditional accounts of health policy in Britain and the perceived failure of the pre-National Health Service hospital sector. This approach overlooks the continuing growth in hospital provision, which was shaped by a mixture of charitable, mutual, private and government support. The exact mix varied: whereas in Germany, hospitals were funded largely through national and municipal support and state insurance schemes, in Britain a more pluralistic system developed [see 'Healthcare and the state']. A substantial investment was made in hospital facilities in Germany and France, with the latter seeing considerable reforms as effort and money was invested in a much needed modernization programme. In Lyon, for example, new facilities were built and thousands of beds were added along with new operating facilities, better kitchens and more comfortable wards so that by the 1930s Lyon had some of the best hospital facilities in Europe. Elsewhere in Europe, more local and community hospitals were opened, and university hospitals and medical schools assumed a prominent role in influencing the structure of local or regional health services. Existing institutions were extended – Britain saw a doubling in the number of beds in voluntary hospitals in the interwar years. Hospitals became increasingly subdivided as new specialist departments were created. Access to hospital care was extended; for example, through the new relations being developed in Britain between hospitals and local working-class communities through workplace contribution schemes. At the same time, local hospitals developed closer relationships by sharing patients and fundraising activities, or by coordinating services, often for financial reasons. One consequence of this growth, and the increasing importance of the hospital to the delivery of healthcare, was that the nature of provision and the relationship between hospitals and the state became a source of recurring debate.

Although charitable hospitals remained wary of government, state subsidies became progressively more important to shaping hospital growth in the 1920s and 1930s [see 'Healthcare and the state']. This was clear in Ireland and France. The virtual collapse of the charitable hospital system in the face of increased demand, new technologies, and rising poverty as a result of the First World War (1914–18) overstretched charitable resources. In response, French municipal authorities were forced to fund an increasingly large proportion of healthcare. State subventions (amounting to over 43 million francs in grants by 1933) not only allowed a programme of modernization, but also saw new municipal hospitals opened. Grants provided the state with a means to influence, and in some cases dictate the nature of hospital services. In Britain, despite the addition of new forms of funding through contribution schemes and municipal support, voluntary hospitals faced increasing financial difficulties that eased the acceptance of state funding and nationalization under the National Health Service. A similar pattern was repeated elsewhere as post-1945 welfare programmes endorsed the hospital's position at the centre of healthcare [see 'Healthcare and the state'].

Specialization

As we have already seen, hospitals varied by type and function. At a basic level, distinctions were made in the sixteenth century between hospitals with a medical function, and those that provided other services for the poor. Provision was made for isolating plague patients through the pesthouse or lazaretto; for incurables; for treating new diseases, such as syphilis, and for specific groups as reflected in the foundation of foundling hospitals. Military hospitals were opened in the late sixteenth century and in the following century a reorganization of poor relief saw new institutions established, such as the *hôpitaux-généraux* in France.

The move to open specialist institutions accelerated in the eighteenth century. The growth of specialist hospitals not only benefited from the same range of factors that drove the foundation of voluntary hospitals, but also from demand for specialized care from patients, growing specialization in industry, which provided a model, and by philanthropic and administrative moves to isolate certain groups of patients defined as immoral or dangerous. Other factors were at work that combined sentimentalism and morality with concerns about the strength of the nation during a period of industrialization, war and colonial expansion. Provision therefore initially focused on institutions for pregnant women, as in the Rotunda Hospital, Dublin (1745); for venereal disease, such as the Hospice of Vaugirard, Paris (1780); or for the insane, such as St Luke's Hospital, London (1751). These hospitals offered opportunities for the understanding of particular diseases and reflected shifts in medical thinking. This is apparent in the provision of maternity hospitals; institutions that in part owed their opening to a growing interest in obstetrics [see 'Women and medicine']. Other institutions, such as St Louis Hospital, Paris, were built for pragmatic reasons to isolate the infectious.

During the nineteenth century, specialist hospitals were established in greater numbers, at least in those cities, such as London, Paris or Berlin, that had a breadth of medical practitioners and a dense enough population to support them. Although specialization generated professional opposition [see 'Professionalization'], new institutions were opened. For example, in the first wave of foundation, children's hospitals were established in Paris (1802), Berlin (1830) and London (1852) along with hospitals for treating diseases of the eye. Other specialist hospitals followed, for a particular organ or system (heart, lung, skin), disease (tuberculosis, cancer), category of patient, such as the German Hospital in London, or to offer a form of treatment like the Sea Bathing Hospital in Margate on the south coast of England.

Historians have traditionally pointed to how changes in medical knowledge, growing patient demand, and the development of new instruments, such as the ophthalmoscope, encouraged particular fields to develop and specialist institutions to be founded. These factors all helped, but other forces were at work as specialist hospitals frequently emerged before the development of specialist fields or instruments. In a comparative study of Paris and London, the historian George Weisz suggested how specialization was shaped by doctors' collective desire to expand medical knowledge, and a result of institutional pressures and administrative reforms (see Further Reading). These processes were most visible in Paris: different groups of patients were grouped together in dedicated institutions, such as the Maternité de Paris or the Hôpital des Vénériens (for venereal patients), and from the 1870s the Parisian hospital administration invested more heavily in specialist facilities. The foundation of specialist hospitals in Britain was influenced by a further set of concerns closely associated with the professional structure of medicine. Lindsay Granshaw in her influential study shows how specialist hospitals not only provided an institutional focus for the creation of specialist knowledge, but also were an outcome of the professional monopoly of general hospitals and an overcrowded medical market (see Further Reading). For Granshaw, specialist hospitals were a mechanism for the excluded or marginal to advance their careers through an institutional appointment. Other reasons might be added. Specialist hospitals were also social institutions and like general hospitals served non-medical functions that were appealing to subscribers. For example, children's hospitals not only aimed to provide medical care, but also to educate working-class mothers in middle-class values of maternity.

Although specialization remained contentious until after the First World War [see 'Professionalization'], specialist hospitals were popular with patients and gradually became an accepted feature of the hospital system. New institutional types were created: cottage hospitals served rural populations in Britain, while sanatoriums emerged in the late nineteenth century as the focus for the institutional treatment of tuberculosis, enjoying popularity throughout the interwar period until their utility was superseded by penicillin and new forms of diagnosis. Nor was specialization just limited to specialist hospitals. Although the culture of general hospitals was slow to adjust, many established specialist clinics or outpatient departments in the nineteenth century, with specialization in teaching hospitals driven by the need to train practitioners and attract students. In many cases, eye departments were the first to be opened followed by departments for ear, nose and throat, and obstetrics wards. In Paris, the Assistance Publique and its support for specialist wards, and the growing recognition of specialist practitioners, aided this process. Electrical departments were increasingly common from the 1880s, while the introduction of new technology, such as X-ray machines, saw the creation of further specialist departments to provide diagnostic services. In the 1920s and 1930s, new specialist departments were created around particular medical and surgical specialities, or were formed around new technologies or scientific disciplines. By the 1930s, specialization and specialist services had become a key feature of medical practice. Some historians have suggested that specialization and the development of specialist clinics provided an impetus to the hospital's medicalization.

Medicalization

Hospitals can be represented as paradigms of medicalization and their role in the development of modern medicine is undisputed. Accounts of the rise of the hospital have put forward a chronology of modernity that traces the process of medicalization and an apparent shift from a social to a therapeutic function. Early modern hospitals are depicted as primarily religious institutions or places designed to control the destitute that offered limited medical care. Often the impression of these institutions is a poor one, the product of contemporary attacks or Foucaultian characterizations of them as instruments of repression. The common assumption is that hospitals underwent a process of medicalization from the mid eighteenth century onwards, a process driven by medical practitioners. Although there has been a growing sensitivity to the process of medicalization among medical historians, hospitals have often been presented as sites in which experiments and discoveries were made, rather than institutions that provided both the location and the resources that facilitated medicalization and innovation. Yet, medicalization was a more multifaceted and gradual phenomenon than the above account would suggest.

If medicine was frequently subordinate to religious concerns in the early modern hospital, this did not mean that they were backward institutions dominated by suffering, superstition or repression. Medical treatment was an important feature of the early modern hospital. Hospitals could be grim places, but sixteenth and seventeenth century accounts also point to institutions offering sophisticated medical facilities, especially in northern and central Italy. During the fifteenth and sixteenth centuries, Florentine hospitals acquired features associated with the modern hospital, with lay control, physicians in attendance, and pharmacies for the preparation and storage of drugs. This model spread to other parts of Europe as hospitals took on clearer therapeutic functions. By the standards of the time, many of the institutions provided good levels of care. Bed rest, clean linen, and a supportive diet were essential components of care, along with mild medicines and nursing, with the latter provided by religious orders like the Daughters of Charity [see 'Religion']. This represented a system of medicine that does not match the image of a heroic regime traditionally associated with the early modern period.

During the seventeenth century, general hospitals became more medicalized as surgeons were employed and daily visits by medical practitioners were arranged. Hospitals offered limited sites for therapeutic innovation. For example, in Rome investigations into the effects of the mineral vitriol and mercury were carried out, while the Santo Spirito hospital acquired a reputation for the manufacture of a drug based on chinchona bark used in the treatment of fever. Hospitals also became sites for the production and dissemination of knowledge. This was apparent in Padua where by the seventeenth century dissections were being routinely carried out for teaching and study and practical classes were being taught in the wards. This approach spread to Utrecht and Halle, but it was in Leiden under Herman Boerhaave that clinical instruction regularly appeared as part of the curriculum. Boerhaave became known as the 'teacher of all Europe' and inspired others to establish clinical teaching. Clinical instruction was at first sporadic, but from the mid seventeenth century hospitals were slowly being used for medical training and research.

Although the medical functions of early modern hospitals should not be dismissed, or their growing importance to professional structures underplayed, it was in the eighteenth and early nineteenth century that the hospital's medical and administrative functions developed beyond the traditional institutional arrangements designed to provide relief to the sick poor. During the eighteenth century, general hospitals extended their medical and teaching functions. In Edinburgh, clinical teaching began in 1748, in Vienna in 1754, and in Prague in 1786, although it was in Paris following the 1789 revolution that this common pattern was given systematic form [see 'Anatomy']. Hospitals moved into the mainstream of medicine in the nineteenth century as the ideas associated with clinical observation, physical examination and pathological anatomy were disseminated and a generation of doctors trained in the late eighteenth century took up hospital posts [see 'Anatomy']. Hospital care emerged as distinct from domestic practice. As institutions, they became central to the training of doctors and in the construction of medical knowledge, with teaching hospitals emerging as prestigious institutions associated with advanced (and increasingly academic) medicine. By the 1890s, hospitals were firmly established as expensive institutions for treatment, research and medical education.

This transformation has been connected to changes in medicine and surgery, the institutionalization of training, and nursing reforms [see 'Nursing']. For many historians the medical reforms in Paris transformed the hospital into a site for a new style of medicine based around the bedside and local pathology. However, change was not just limited to the understanding of disease processes or to new diagnostic approaches and tools, such as percussion or the stethoscope. Nourishing and stimulating treatments started to replace older, lowering therapies, such as bloodletting. New methods of local wound treatment were employed, along with more liberal diets and greater use of stimulants. Changes in surgery associated with the introduction of effective pain control (anaesthesia) and wound management (antiseptics), and the growing importance of the laboratory, have been identified as at the heart of a revolution in hospital medicine [see 'Surgery']. Historians have detected a shift from the early nineteenth century, when very few operations were carried out, to surgical intervention dominating the hospital by the early twentieth century as new procedures were introduced and as medical practitioners attached importance to the conditions under which operations were performed. During the same period, hospitals became sites in which new diagnostic services were employed. Although some like the stethoscope were used in private practice, other new technologies were so large, complex or expensive, such as X-ray machines, that they could only be used in a hospital. Whereas some of these diagnostic facilities – often in the form of bacteriological or chemical analysis – provided services for general practitioners, hospitals became synonymous with laboratory medicine. The effect was to institutionalize medicine.

Swayed by a language of science, and changes to surgery, patients started to feel that hospitals were the best place to receive treatment. This change was reflected in the growth of pay beds, a process evident in England and France. By 1914, if patients, no matter what their social class, wanted to undergo sophisticated medical examinations or surgical procedures they needed to go into hospital. One result was a decline in patients' autonomy.

The extent and speed of medicalization should not be overstated. Often historical accounts have focused on the experiences of leading or teaching hospitals. If these institutions had a disproportionate impact, their experiences should not be generalized. Institutional cultures and practices were slow to change. Hospitals in the late eighteenth century were more often characterized by their unruly nature than by their medical care. Existing buildings created a material environment that had to be adapted. Outside the major metropolitan centres, changes in medicine and surgery did not immediately or radically alter the treatments available. The process of medicalization was also uneven. French hospitals remained behind their German and British counterparts, constrained by old buildings and city-centre locations. New procedures or technologies were slow to filter through, especially to small or rural hospitals. The drug treatments provided in many European hospitals remained simple and surgical procedures limited. Hospital care frequently meant bed-rest and nursing care rather than therapeutic intervention. Despite the impression and rhetoric of progress, hospitals in the closing decades of the nineteenth century could still be basic, unruly institutions.

Experiences during the First World War underscored the need for better-equipped hospitals and revealed the necessity of improving operating theatres, laboratories and clinics. The 1920s and 1930s consequently saw a substantial investment in hospitals as they became cathedrals of modern medicine, with the university hospital the key site for academic medicine and medical education. The growth of ambulance services helped make hospitals the focus for casualty care. Specialization encouraged the inclusion of further specialist clinics and wards. The high cost of complicated medical and surgical interventions – for example, radium therapy – and new therapeutic or diagnostic technologies, such as ECG (electrocardiogram) machines or biochemical tests, served to concentrate certain services in the hospital. Procedures and interventions, such as blood tests, became routine. However, even in the 1930s it would be unwise to overestimate the extent of medicalization. Outside of large cities, progress was slow. Although larger hospitals were able to invest in new equipment, small or rural hospitals were in a poorer position.

Notwithstanding the limits of medicalization, by 1939 the hospital was widely seen as the loci for medical advances and research, and central to the delivery of medical care. A different way of seeing medicalization would therefore be to think in terms of a more uneven process that takes into account local factors and contexts in shaping innovation and medicalization.

Doctors and hospitals

For those influenced by Michel Foucault's interpretation of the 'birth of the clinic', the processes of medicalization meant that doctors gained greater control over the hospital, a view firmly established in the historiography which suggests that the rise of hospital medicine saw the power relationship moved decisively in favour of the doctor. In this interpretation, the hospital became a vehicle through which licensed practitioners were able to assert their influence and advance their professional status, making doctors the driving force behind the increase in hospitals and their medicalization. However, to see the end of the eighteenth century and the reforms that took place in Paris as marking a break with the past and ushering in greater medical control ignores what was happening earlier; how from the sixteenth century doctors were becoming increasingly active in the hospital.

Physicians, surgeons and other medical practitioners started to be consistently attached to hospitals in the sixteenth and seventeenth centuries. At the Paris Hôtel-Dieu permanent paid positions for both physicians and surgeons were created and ancillary unpaid appointments were made as medical care was extended. Hospitals, especially in major urban centres, started to be regarded as professional vehicles for physicians and surgeons, offering them income and status. Yet if physicians and surgeons assumed a more prominent role in managing medical care, hospitals remained controlled by lay boards of governors or religious orders. This was clear in early modern France: at a local level the organization of admissions, the upkeep of the institution and the provision of food and treatment in French hospitals were in non-medical hands. It was only with the growth of hospitals in the eighteenth century that they became 'houses of care' with doctors in charge.

During the eighteenth century, hospitals acquired a growing prominence in medicine's professional and intellectual hierarchy. Demand for new forms of medical education based around pathological anatomy and observation merged with the growth in the number of hospitals. As institutions, hospitals became places where reputations were made, and where the orthodox knowledge that underpinned licensed practitioners' status was constructed and disseminated. Large metropolitan hospitals, like Vienna's *Allgemeines Krankenhaus* or St

Bartholomew's in London, were fashioned into educational and experimental sites. Although as discussed above, reform was most visible in France, where medical education was overhauled and structured around hospital wards and post-mortem rooms, across Europe hospital experience became linked to pedagogy, professional identities, and the production of knowledge [see 'Professionalization']. During the nineteenth century, the hospital became central to medical education and research and the construction of knowledge, and to the careers of elite practitioners even if this did not mean that standards of care or conditions in them were good.

It was not only the hospital's growing importance to medical knowledge and education that benefited practitioners. By giving their services to a charitable hospital, medical practitioners were able to display themselves as benevolent and genteel citizens. Such an investment in civic culture not only allowed them to discharge their responsibilities but also to acquire social capital and patronage in an increasingly competitive medical marketplace. Hospital attendance provided opportunities for conspicuous services and lucrative practices as the hospital emerged as a symbol of medical power and prestige. By the 1850s, the hospital had firmly established itself as the basis for the medical elite's authority: they invested more heavily in hospital work, and became closely identified with institutional appointments.

Although these changes did make hospitals important for doctors professionally, in terms of the hospital becoming a medical space the impact was not as extensive as might be assumed. As we have already seen in a previous section, social reasons rather than medical arguments were central to the foundation of hospitals. Even in specialist hospitals, which were often founded by ambitious doctors, the medical staff still had to rely on lay supporters to fund and manage their institutions. In Germany, where the majority of medical practitioners continued to emphasize the importance of home not hospital treatment, they placed greater emphasis on public health improvements than hospital care. This ensured that doctors played a relatively limited role in hospital reforms in the German-speaking territories until the 1860s. Nor was the hospital's importance for practitioners immediately reflected in how much influence they had. Older hospitals were run like landed estates with staff viewed as servants. New charitable hospitals fitted a pattern common to many voluntary organizations. Founded by small groups within the urban elite, or by doctors working with them, power was given to those who contributed to their up-keep; that power was limited to small cliques of male supporters who dominated how they were run. This had an impact on doctors' authority.

In many institutions, doctors hence had limited control over admissions, the wards, or treatments, and less control over how the hospital was managed. Benefactors and administrators placed limits on what their medical staff could do. From the mid nineteenth century, they also had to vie with a new breed of lady superintendents for control over nursing and the wards [see 'Nursing']. Although hospital staff had freer reign over outpatient admissions, it was not unknown for doctors to be summoned before the lay governors to explain a particular type of treatment, or for those running the hospital to insist that certain patients be discharged whether or not the doctor felt they had recovered. In response, doctors repeatedly asserted the need for greater medical influence as the nature of medicine and their professional aspirations changed. To support their claims, hospital staff employed a scientific rhetoric in their bid to gain autonomy from lay control and banked on the increased status laboratory medicine and surgery gave them [see 'Medicine and science']. However, those running hospitals were reluctant to cede responsibility to a group of men they saw as rising but still socially inferior. These conflicting ideas resulted in tension: admissions, attendance and nursing arrangements invariably became flash points as doctors struggled to assert their control over the inner workings of the hospital.

This situation had begun to change by the late nineteenth century. Senior staff were invited to serve on management committees, and a greater proportion of funding was directed to supporting the hospital's medical and surgical functions as new equipment was purchased, wards were added and specialist services were developed. Exactly why this shift occurred is unclear. Growing public faith in the effectiveness of medical science helped modify doctors' position in society and within the hospital. Doctors used this along with rising patient demand for institutional care to show that they had a right to influence how the hospital was run. The therapeutic breakthroughs in the first half of the twentieth century further enhanced the hospital's position as a medical and scientific space. Administrators increasingly found that they had less to say about how the hospital was organized or over what patients should be treated. Advances in medicine required them to cede more authority to their medical staff as management became more bureaucratic. Rather than conforming to the conventional chronology, it was therefore in the late nineteenth century as medicine became more effective at treating disease that the medical profession started to assume a more influential position in how hospitals were run and managed.

Hospitals and patients

Patients have frequently been silent in hospital histories, appearing as objects of control or medical procedures. Most accounts have focused on the literate or middle classes, or have provided breakdowns of the diseases treated or hospital mortality. Although interest in patients is growing, few historians have attempted the type of patient-centred history that Guenter Risse adopted in *Hospital Life in Enlightenment Scotland* (1986). The main picture to emerge from the early historiography is that until the nineteenth century hospitals were insanitary institutions and 'gateways to death' that patients actively avoided unless desperate. Studies in the 1960s revealed how the dismal representation of the hospital owed much to the negative views of eighteenth century critics and the appalling conditions that existed in the Paris Hôtel-Dieu. Revisionists suggested that rather than hospitals being 'gateways to death', mortality in them was relatively low. For example, between 1518 and 1522, the average death rate in Santa Maria Nuova in Florence was just over eight per cent, while mortality was under 10 per cent in the best run French hospitals by the eighteenth century. In the nineteenth century, an attempt to combat epidemic outbreaks in the wards (often referred to as hospitalism) and the gradual introduction of antiseptics served to reduce postoperative mortality and improve the image of the hospital as a curative environment.

Although the evidence does not support the image of hospitals as 'gateways to death', questions remain about who exactly hospitals treated. Different hospitals had their own patient base, differences that varied between institutional type (charity v. state) and between institutions. State institutions, for example, provided a greater level of care for the infirm or incurable. A number of factors shaped admissions, however. Charitable and social networks, patient demand, the extent of ill health in the population, the nature of the condition, the attitudes of those running the hospital and their medical staff, financial resources (of the institution and the individual), and medical knowledge and technology, were all important. Patients also made choices about when and where to seek treatment: hospitals until the end of the nineteenth century were seldom their first choice, but access to institutions varied. With many hospitals located in towns, access to institutional care in rural areas was limited. For the very young and the old, and for women, accessing care remained problematic until specialist and maternity hospitals were opened in larger numbers in the mid nineteenth century.

Although some early modern hospitals had a wide remit, others, especially those in the Italian states, had strict admission policies that excluded the contagious or incurable. Most patients were admitted for relatively short periods for acute illnesses that could be cured or remedied, criteria that accounts for the favourable mortality rate in many early modern hospitals. Although the focus on the curable remained important, admission criteria were strengthened in the eighteenth century as the hospital's function altered. General hospitals aimed to exclude the incurable (such as the physically handicapped), the infectious, the insane, the venereal, pregnant women and children. These cases were to be treated in specialist institutions. Ideally, most hospitals aimed to care for the deserving poor who were acutely ill. Although this group remained ill-defined, it included the respectable poor who were trying to support their families. In theory, better-off patients were to be treated privately, or in separate institutions, while the destitute or undeserving were to be provided for by the state in separate institutions, such as the workhouse. However, admissions did not follow rigid guidelines. Often a gap existed between the declared aims of an institution and actual practice. Medical staff were able to exert some control over outpatient cases: their interest in rare or complicated conditions, or in teaching, ensured that the rules governing admission were often bent.

Research on Victorian asylums suggests that individuals, families, communities and public welfare agencies were important in negotiating relief, and in determining admission and discharge [see 'Asylums']. The same was true of hospitals. Although their choices were not as wide-ranging as those of the moneyed classes, the poor were resourceful in negotiating care. Hospitals were strategic resources that could be used in some phases of illness, or during particular periods of hardship. For example, maternity hospitals offered poor women free access to a level of obstetrics care unavailable in the home. Hospitals were also part of a multilevel system of healthcare. Although this system was haphazard, local welfare agencies negotiated arrangements or subscribed to local hospitals. Churches, other charities, workplaces and employers also subscribed, as did local doctors and municipal agencies. This created a more complex pattern of admissions than the rules governing admission might suggest.

Hospital patients mainly came from those who fell into dependency, or who lacked local networks of family or community support. For example, most patients admitted to the Nîmes Hôtel-Dieu in the eighteenth century were unmarried individuals who had migrated to the region. In the nineteenth century, enormous social changes – industrialization, migration and urbanization – increased the numbers who lacked traditional networks of support. Consequently, demand for hospital care rose. The Lariboisière Hospital in Paris, for example, served a relatively young working and lower middle-class population. Although most patients had work, many were new to Paris or lived alone. Evidence suggests that in most countries demand for hospital care outstripped provision. Casualty cases were always treated and although certain classes of patients, such as the infectious or the venereal, were ideally to be excluded, they were often not.

In the nineteenth century, new procedures, technologies and nursing reforms altered the nature of hospital care and the perceptions of hospital medicine. For example, new operating theatres and the adoption of aseptic techniques offered better and safer facilities for surgery than domestic environments. Changing professional structures and links between students and their teachers encouraged a system of referral to develop. These changes served to refashion the hospital into more ordered, disciplined environments as shown in the photograph of Pitcairn ward at St Bartholomew's Hospital, London. Hospitals built on and manipulated their new popularity. At the same time, social change created new social groups and increased the numbers who lacked support networks, or were in real need of institutional healthcare. The result, as illustrated for London in Table 8.1, was a boom in inpatient and outpatient admissions as hospitals became more visible and viable locations for medical or surgical care.

Changes in how institutional care was perceived served to broaden the geographical area and social profile from which hospital patients were admitted. Many urban hospitals in Europe responded by adding new wards and larger outpatient facilities to cope with rising admissions. New hospitals emerged to cater for growing middle-class demand for institutional care. In Britain, cottage

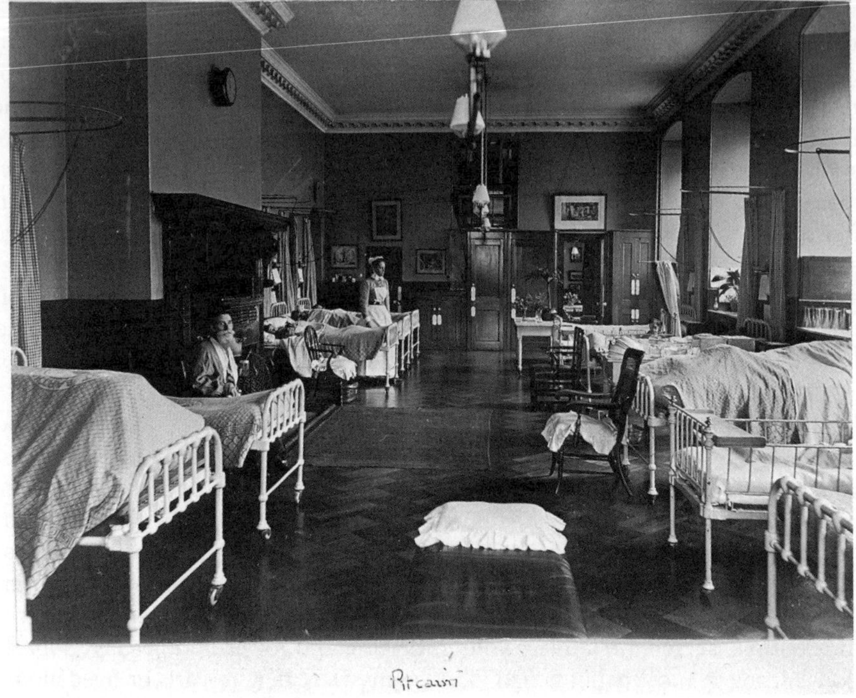

Figure 8.1 Pitcairn ward at St Bartholomew's Hospital, London, c.1908.
Source: Wellcome Library, London.

hospitals staffed by general practitioners were established in rural areas. In France, the traditional hospital started to be replaced with institutions that provided care to both the poor and the middle classes. A further, less popular response was to establish private beds and wards in general hospitals. Greater demand for hospital care and the creation of pay beds also encouraged the development of insurance schemes in Britain, France and Germany. The impact of

Table 8.1 Admissions to the principal London general hospitals, 1809–95

Hospital	*Inpatients*		*Outpatients*	
	1809	*1895*	*1809*	*1895*
London	1,406	10,599	877	152,411
Middlesex	555	3,404	522	41,707
St Bartholomew's	3,849	6,674	45,410	59,063
St George's	1,450	4,191	1,211	28,392
St Thomas's	2,789	6,150	4,322	112,056
Westminster	627	2,934	687	24,247

broadening the social base of hospital admissions was clearest in Germany where 65 per cent of patients were partially paid for through insurance funds by the end of the nineteenth century.

Demand for hospital care rose during the first three decades of the twentieth century. Scientific developments, the professionalization of hospitals (including nursing), and moves to medicalize childbirth, had further eroded the image of hospitals as primarily for the deserving poor. The extension of insurance schemes and social welfare provision confirmed this trend and changing social relations. In France, the near financial collapse of the hospital system saw greater municipal involvement and funding. Hospitals were required to take new types of patients. In some areas, free hospital care was provided, and in 1928 legislation extended hospital insurance to a third of the French population. The global depression of the 1930s deprived many people of resources and restricted traditional networks of support, encouraging them to seek hospital care where they might have previously paid for private care. In Britain, hospitals struggled to keep pace with rising demand. The growth of hospital contributory schemes, whereby workers paid at least a penny in the pound of their wages to support local hospitals, raised expectations. In exchange for regular contributions, members received free treatment at local hospitals without being subjected to a means test. Contributory schemes helped to empower patients and created a quasi-insurance system that was part of a broader move to coordinate healthcare [see 'Healthcare and the state']. In France, state subsidies encouraged a transformation in the social profile of admissions. More and more middle-class patients sought hospital care, and not just for casualty or emergency care. New hospitals contained more private beds and the number of private patients rose dramatically. This trend towards the democratization of hospital care was consolidated in France by the Vichy regime (1940–44), which in 1941 decreed that public hospitals be opened to all French citizens. In the following year, the publication of the influential Beveridge Report in Britain assumed a system of free healthcare. Although the reality of post-war welfare reforms was different, the principle was firmly established that hospitals by the 1940s were for all classes [see 'Healthcare and the state'].

Conclusions

By the 1920s and 1930s, the position of the hospital in medicine was unassailable. Hospitals had become associated with medical intervention, technology and progress and their central role in the delivery of healthcare was reflected in the welfare systems established after the Second World War (1939–45). In the decades after 1945, length of stay fell with the development of new producers, such as keyhole surgery, and a greater dependence was placed on medical technology. Yet, the optimism that had surrounded the hospital started to be eroded as criticism focused on the nature, alienation and effectiveness of institutional care. A growing emphasis started to be placed on the importance of primary care, while the rising cost of hospital treatment created problems for beleaguered welfare programmes [see 'Healthcare and the state']. Questions over the value or nature of hospital care show both their importance in the delivery of healthcare and how their position at the centre of medicine should not simply be assumed. The process by which hospitals have come to dominate the medical landscape, how medical practitioners are trained, and medical research has been a complex one. Rather than sudden breaks with the past, the history of hospitals suggests greater continuities in terms of their social and medical roles. Although institutional cultures and charity proved resilient, it was in the twentieth century that the hospital increasingly departed from the institutional arrangements originally developed to deliver care to the sick poor as the hospital moved into the mainstream of medicine, but as this chapter has shown, even this process of medicalization should not be taken at face value.

Further reading

The best overview of hospitals from the medieval period to the twentieth century remains Lindsay Granshaw and Roy Porter (eds), *The Hospital in History* (London: Routledge, 1989), with Guenter Risse in *Mending Bodies Saving Souls: A History of Hospitals* (New York and Oxford: Oxford University Press, 1999) offering an ambitious account of a broad range of institutional forms, putting forward a story of the innovative aspects of hospital life that stresses the experiential even if the breadth of the study make it problematic as an overview given the focus on case studies. The introduction to John Henderson, Peregrine Horden and Alessandro Pastore (eds), *The Impact of Hospitals 300–2000* (Bern: Peter Lang, 2007) shows how revisionist studies have developed and provides a lively account of hospital development. For early modern France, see Laurence Brockliss and Colin Jones, *The Medical World of Early Modern France* (Oxford: Clarendon Press, 1997) or Colin Jones, *The Charitable Imperative: Hospitals and Nursing in Ancien Régime and Revolutionary France* (London: Routledge, 1989). John Henderson, *The Renaissance Hospital: Healing the Body and Healing the Soul* (New Haven, CT: Yale University Press, 2006) examines Renaissance Florence, while Annemarie Kinzelbach, 'Hospitals, Medicine and Society', *Renaissance Studies* 15 (2001), pp. 217–28, looks at sixteenth century Germany. There is a substantial literature on the voluntary hospital movement: John Pickstone, *Medicine and Industrial Society: A History of Hospital Development in Manchester and its Region, 1752–1946* (Manchester: Manchester University Press, 1985), Hilary Marland, *Medicine and Society in Wakefield and Huddersfield, 1780–1870* (Cambridge: Cambridge University Press, 1987) and Keir Waddington, *Charity and the London Hospitals, 1850–1898* (Woodbridge: Boydell, 2000) provide revisionist interpretations, while Guenter Risse, *Hospital Life in Enlightenment Scotland: Care and Teaching at the Royal Infirmary of Edinburgh* (Cambridge: Cambridge University Press, 1986) offers a patient-centred account. An obvious starting point for any reading on nineteenth century hospitals and their position in medicine is Michel Foucault, *The Birth of the Clinic*, trans. A.M. Sheridan (London: Tavistock, 1973) and Erwin Ackerknecht, *Medicine at the Paris Hospital 1794–1848* (Baltimore, MD: Johns Hopkins University Press, 1967), with Mary Fissell, *Patients, Power and the Poor in Eighteenth Century Bristol* (Cambridge: Cambridge University Press, 1991) examining the 'birth of the clinic' in a British context. An overview of growth of specialist hospitals in Britain is covered by Lindsay Granshaw, '"Fame and Fortune by Means of Bricks and Mortar": The Medical Profession and Specialist Hospitals in Britain 1800–1948', in Lindsay Granshaw and Roy Porter (eds), *The Hospital in History* (London: Routledge, 1989), pp. 199–200, while George Weisz, 'The Emergence of Medical Specialization in the Nineteenth Century', *Bulletin of the History of Medicine* 77 (2003), pp. 536–75, provides a comparative study. The literature on hospitals in the twentieth century is more limited: most of the literature concentrates on the municipal or state medicine, though for Britain see Martin Gorsky, John Mohan with Tim Willis, *Mutualism and Health Care: British Hospital Contributory Schemes in the Twentieth Century* (Manchester: Manchester University Press, 2006) or Steve Cherry, *Medical Services and the Hospitals 1860–1939* (Cambridge: Cambridge University Press, 1996) for an overview, and for France see Timothy Smith, *Creating the Welfare State in France, 1880–1940* (Montreal: McGill-Queen's University Press, 2003). Given that the history of hospitals and that of medical education overlap, Thomas N. Bonner's *Becoming a Physician, Medical Education in Britain, France, Germany and the United States, 1750–1945* (New York and Oxford: Oxford University Press, 1995) provides a comparative study. Hospital architecture is addressed in a classic study by John Thompson and Grace Goldin, *The Hospital* (New Haven, CT: Yale University Press, 1975) and more recently by Christine Stevenson, *Medicine and Magnificence: British Hospital and Asylum Architecture, 1660–1815* (New Haven, CT: Yale University Press, 2000).

9

Practitioners and professionalization

One of the key concerns that has shaped the history of medicine is the concept of professionalization. For contemporaries, who was a member of the medical profession and who was not were crucial issues bound up with concerns about status, competition and the nature of medical knowledge. Historians have equally been concerned with this process of professionalization and have widely applied the concept to studies of medical practice, nursing, hospital medicine and psychiatry. Rather than supporting a single model of professionalization, this chapter outlines ways of thinking about what it meant to be a 'doctor'. It evaluates different approaches to professionalization and shows how concerns about competition and status, licensing, a move to institutionalize training, and inter- and intra-professional conflict, were all important in structuring professionalization.

Models of professionalization

There have been fundamental disagreements over what constitutes a profession and how professionalization occurred in a given occupation. Historians have recognized that definitions of a profession are problematic and, reflecting the influence of the social sciences on the discipline, have turned to sociology for explanations. Until the 1970s, sociologists broadly associated the rise of the professions with social progress as a way of explaining modernization and identified professionalization with the accumulation of traits, which distinguished professions from other occupational groups. A profession was defined as involving: the possession of specialized knowledge, formalized training, a code of ethics or conduct, regulation by a professional or government body, a monopoly of practice, high social prestige, and considerable autonomy. It was an attractive model, one that offered sociologists and historians a way of measuring professionalization.

The 1970s not only marked the highpoint of post-war professional power but also saw new formulations of professionalization put forward. Heavily dependent on Anglo-American experiences, these new models distanced themselves from earlier, uncritical abstractions that had been informed by professionals' definitions of themselves as possessing distinctive characteristics. Radical critiques of medicine created more pessimistic views of medicalization that made strong connections between knowledge and power [see 'Historiography']. Encouraged by these trends, sociologists turned away from the trait approach. As attention was directed at the relationship between the professions and class structure, sociological approaches were recast to emphasize how a profession exerted a high degree of autonomy – economic, political or technical – and collegial control. By using concepts of occupational closure and monopolization, sociologists relabelled professions as inherently self-interested and elitist. Professionalism came to represent an occupational strategy in which knowledge, training and professional bodies were used to secure and justify a market monopoly.

Aware that professional cultures developed in particular contexts, historians did not take these sociological interpretations of professionalization at face value. For example, scholarship on Germany and France pointed to the greater role of the state in professionalization. Studies of alternative medicine and the medical marketplace highlighted problems with using occupational closure as a model by illustrating how boundaries between different types of practitioner were often arbitrary. Research on medical education questioned assumptions about a single portal of entry into medicine, whilst work on licensing in Britain and France exposed how regulation often failed to establish a monopoly. More generally, historians questioned professionalization as a simple power relationship in which doctors increasingly dominated their clients. Although the idea that the authority of medicine increased during the nineteenth century was widely accepted, the extent of medical influence was shown to be more limited than traditionally assumed, particularly at an institutional level. Professionalization came to be defined not as a static attainment of rigid criteria, but as a rhetorical device. What emerged was a view of professionalization based around ideas of expertise and licensing.

If the chronology of professionalization often depended on local and national contexts, a concentration on the canonical settings of medicine – the hospital or university for example – has meant that attention has frequently overlooked the other actors involved, or made them into marginal figures. For example, those labelled alternative practitioners also pursued a professionalizing agenda. They established hospitals, societies and journals, and equally assimilated a scientific rhetoric to enhance their status. Whereas the experiences of alternative practitioners suggest how those deemed 'orthodox' did not have a monopoly on pursing professional aims, attention to the gendered nature of professionalization illustrates the importance of exclusion and segregation in delimitating medical roles; how credentialist, legalistic tactics of occupational closure were pursued in the nineteenth century to define who was part of the medical profession.

The above approaches to professionalization can be extended to include questions of identity, socialization, and practice to cover less tangible criteria. A simple model of identity, which suggests that groups identify with each other through a common collective interest, can be useful in thinking about how practitioners defined themselves and others, and how this bound particular groupings together. This identity was partially fashioned through medical societies, institutional training and journals, which created sites around which practitioners could develop a visible community of interests. A model of socialization can further suggest how the common experiences of medical education represented an important vehicle through which this identity and the values associated with it were transmitted. So-called alterity studies supplies a further analogy by pointing to the role of an outside 'other' in shaping identities. For physicians and surgeons this 'other' was the quack. Taking this further it is possible to borrow from social psychology and social anthropology to examine professionalization in terms of the creation of in-groups and out-groups, and how the definition of these groups contributed to collective identities. Practices or activities also had their role. Practices not only generated meaning but also shaped identities as illustrated by the process of specialization.

Notwithstanding their limitations, sociological models offer ways into thinking about professionalization rather than what constitutes a 'profession'. Professionalization was a flexible process. It was shaped by local and national contexts, and was bound up with questions of identity, medical knowledge and practice, status and authority, competition, and training. Above all, professionalization should be seen as historically determined.

An early modern profession

For Margaret Pelling and Charles Webster the sixteenth century was 'a particularly significant phrase in the development of the medical profession in England'.[1] If England lagged behind Italy, here and elsewhere in Europe, it is possible to identify the existence of professional groups in medicine. Of these, physicians and surgeons were the most clearly defined. New professional structures and identities, often based around practice and corporate structures, were beginning to emerge. Did this mean that professionalization was occurring? An approach that points to the acquisitions of traits, or one that draws on ideas of power and a monopoly of practice, would suggest not, but what was happening in the sixteenth and seventeenth centuries should not be measured against modern criteria. Although medicine was neither well organized nor firmly controlled in early modern Europe, it was already more than an occupation.

Three distinct groupings of 'official' medical practitioner – physicians, barber-surgeons and apothecaries – represented a differentiated medical community. During the sixteenth and seventeenth centuries, physicians, surgeons and to a lesser extent apothecaries organized themselves into medical corporations, such as the Rome College of Physicians, or the surgeon's Collège de Saint Côme in Paris. These bodies attempted to control particular areas of practice, promote a corporate ethos, and protect the economic and political interests of their members. Membership required proof of training or proficiency. In return members were granted licenses to practise, which established what type of treatments or medical practice the holder was allowed to dispense and where, as most corporations were responsible for limited geographical areas. Although this structure was replicated across Europe, there were important differences. For example, in Spain and the Italian states medicine was strictly regulated by the crown and municipalities, whereas in England few controls existed. Notwithstanding these differences, licensing bodies ensured that members had specialized knowledge, met certain training requirements, and sought to control practice.

One way to answer whether or not these licensed practitioners formed a profession is to examine the divisions within medical practice. Physicians saw themselves as the medical elite. They broadly dealt with the inside of the body; for example, diagnosing and treating disease and fevers. At least until the eighteenth century, they primarily based their knowledge on a university education. However, physicians were not a homogenous group. Although successful practice depended on acquiring wealthy patrons and patients, those practising in small towns mainly dealt with the poor or those of modest means. Nor did all physicians have university degrees, while intense rivalry often existed between them. Yet notwithstanding these differences, physicians self-consciously considered themselves as belonging to a profession. All identified physic as something more than an occupation and claimed a privileged role. They based their authority on their judgement and advice, which they argued came from their university training in learned medicine. They collectively used this authority to make claims that they could judge other practitioners. As the example of the *protomedicati* in Spain and the Italian states illustrate, they were often successful in securing crown or municipal support in their efforts to control the medical system.

The attention directed at physicians in the historical literature might suggest that they dominated medical practice. However, although physicians strove to maintain their elite status, they did not want to monopolize practice. They left certain medical activities – surgery and dispensing drugs – to other practitioners provided they maintained their position. These practitioners far exceeded physicians in number – for example, in France there were an estimated 3,086 surgeons to 643 physicians by the 1590s – and had their own corporate structures, specialized knowledge, and patterns of training. Surgeons – or barber-surgeons – dealt with the outside of the body; for example, treating wounds, fractures and skin diseases, and carrying out manual procedures, such as bloodletting. Because of their associations with trade and apprenticeship training, surgeons have been characterized as ill-educated and often hardly differentiated from barbers or craftsmen. As Chapter 7 demonstrates, these caricatures are often inaccurate and surgeons had an essential role in providing medical care, as did the apothecary. Apothecaries prepared and sold medicines prescribed by physicians and those remedies that could not be made in the home. Popular with patients, and widespread, they organized themselves into guilds – for example, the Communauté des Marchands-Apothicaires et Epiciers in France – and claimed a monopoly in the production and sale of drugs.

Despite physicians' attempts to police the boundaries between practitioners, distinctions between healers were fluid. Even the most rigorous licensing bodies, such as the Medical Faculty in Paris, were unable to impose total control. Jurisdiction was often unclear and licensing was more about maintaining boundaries than it was about establishing monopolies. All types of medical practitioner sold advice and some form of medical care. Apothecaries were consulted by patients and prescribed remedies independently of physicians; surgeons also practised physic, especially in rural areas. The methods used by different types of practitioner equally overlapped: surgeons and physicians both drew on lengthy discussions of the patient's history, made physical examinations, and advised regimens to promote health. For many the term apothecary or surgeon probably therefore referred to any medical practitioner.

If an understanding that the boundaries between licensed practitioners were fluid introduces one level of complexity, this does not capture the nature of medical practice in early modern Europe. Licensed practitioners did not have a monopoly, and it was normal for patients of all social classes to seek cures from a range of different sources [see 'Self-help']. Many contemporaries did not appear to make rigid distinctions between licensed or unlicensed (irregular) practitioners. Most towns had a number of practitioners, and whereas some were little more than swindlers, others were skilled practitioners. Pelling and Webster estimate that London in 1600 had 250 licensed and 250 unlicensed practitioners for a population of 200,000.[2] With ill health widespread, and with many sufferers experiencing prolonged periods of sickness, the sick were often proactive in their search for care and maintained control over their treatment. Many in need of medical care often consulted several practitioners and were rarely satisfied with one opinion. Given this heterogeneity, a medical practitioner covered any individual whose occupation involved care of the sick.

Historians have used the idea of a medical marketplace to explain this diversity of practitioners. The marketplace model rejected a hierarchical view of early modern medicine and pointed instead to a diverse, plural and commercial system of healthcare [see 'Historiography']. In approaching medical practice in this way, historians highlighted the economic dimension of medical encounters. Patients became active agents and medical practitioners entrepreneurs in an environment in which regulation and professionalization had limited success. Although the idea of the medical marketplace drew attention to the importance of socioeconomic forces and competition in shaping access to care, it does have limitations. The concept is vague and ill-defined. It tends to emphasize conflict and the economic rather than the practical aspects of care assuming as it does that a market model dominated clinical encounters often without attention to how early modern economies or societies functioned. Why particular healers were consulted was not just economically driven. Decisions were informed by the perceived seriousness of the condition, a perception of the ability of the healer, cost, fashion or fads, and the healer's position in the community.

Early modern medicine was therefore characterized by a wide range of practitioners – rather than a medical profession – that operated within a marketplace for medicine in which patients could pick and choose, and in which consulting a variety of healers was the norm. The position of practitioners in this market depended on their reputations and patronage, on personal qualities, rather than on therapeutic ability. Competition and the need for collaboration prevented any one group from establishing a monopoly. Although only physicians could lay claim to a self-conscious professional identity, it is possible to see not one medical profession but a range of professional groupings and practitioners involved in medical care. Distinctions between professionals and empirics were blurred, ensuring that two arenas of medical practice existed – licensed and unauthorized – both of which were disorganized and disunited.

Gender and practice: women and early modern medicine

A concentration on physicians and male practitioners ignores the important role of female healers in early modern medicine. Studies initially branded women, and especially midwives, as ignorant or dangerous, and failed to examine the activities of female healers, unless it was to chart a separate process whereby women were excluded from medicine. Often accounts have taken late sixteenth and seventeenth century attacks on female healers at face value. Recent research has questioned these claims to demonstrate how women had an extensive role in the delivery of healthcare. Caricatures of them as ignorant or dangerous were part of wider discourses of power and efforts by male physicians to limit competition, rather than representing a prohibition on female healers or a purely gendered attack.

Certainly, gender divisions existed. Few women held medical licences, and in the seventeenth century, women's freedom to practise medicine was curtailed. Women's access to education was limited, preventing them from acquiring a style of university education associated with physicians, while early modern surgery was a particularly masculine field. Female practitioners were equally subject to legal regulation and harassment. In Bologna, for example, women could only officially practise as midwives or as permit-holders for the sale of over-the-counter medicines. However, an emphasis on licensed practitioners or on midwifery obscures the position of female healers in the medical marketplace. Although women often did not have recognizable medical titles, they occupied a wide spectrum of healing roles and dispensed medical care on a formal and an informal basis. Given women's importance in the domestic sphere, they were expected to practise some form of medicine as a domestic art and had an active role in looking after the sick [see 'Self-help']. Healing was not always waged work and was often too unremarkable to be recorded: familial or community care was important and was based on a system of reciprocity. Women, either as wives, mothers and daughters or as domestic servants, performed much of this work. Women were hence important medical agents at home and in the community.

However, the assumptions that women's healing work was limited to the domestic sphere, or that women were little more than unofficial village doctors, does not hold up to scrutiny. Women did practise as a variety of medical practitioners and had positions of relative acceptance and security. Midwifery was an important area of female practice, and in the sixteenth century, a number of cities started to require midwives to attend formal courses. Yet it would be wrong to limit female practitioners to midwifery. Although women were encouraged to enter low-paid medical posts, such as those available through the parish, there were substantial numbers of female practitioners working at a local level. Nor were they always limited to low status posts: in Elizabethan London, female practitioners were employed in hospitals alongside male physicians and surgeons. Women were hence not confined to nursing, midwifery or maintaining household health, but were active participants in all levels of medicine and provided an important range of medical services.

Status, power and authority: 1700–1800

The tradition view of professionalization suggests that before the French Revolution (1789–99) qualified medical care was available from three distinct groups – physicians, surgeons and apothecaries – each with their own training and position in the medical hierarchy. By 1900 the situation had changed. This chronology emphasizes how during the nineteenth century old divisions were swept away; how new identities and patterns of training emerged, and how clear distinctions were established between licensed practitioners and other types of healer. Industrialization, Enlightenment ideas, medical reforms in France, and the growing role of governments in licensing were shown to be crucial in restructuring professional hierarchies. The result was that medicine became a single, relatively homogenous professional group characterized by a division between general practitioners and hospital consultants. Hence, it was not until the nineteenth century that medicine emerged as a profession in the modern sense.

Whilst a hierarchical view highlights the relative social status of the different medical occupations, it ignores the complexities of eighteenth century medicine. Medical practice was more multifaceted than the above account would suggest. Clear professional identities were beginning to be forged in the eighteenth century as the idea of a profession became more defined and as the numbers associated with medical care and with particular professional groups rose. For example, by 1809–10, David Gentilcore in his study of Italy suggests that more than 10,000 people practised the 'healing arts' of which 3,000 were physicians (see Further Reading). The growing number and diversity of medical practitioners reflected rising demand for skilled services, which was driven by growing consumerism, industrialization, urbanization and the emergence of more bureaucratic states. This combined with Enlightenment pragmatism and individualism to help define specialist groups. Professional men came to be seen as specialists who had expertise in particular fields, a position reinforced by their relative scarcity, and by the efforts of these proto-professional groups to organize and assert their identity.

Central to accounts of eighteenth century medicine are the changes that were occurring in the medical marketplace. The growth of a dynamic consumer culture encouraged and sustained a commercialization of medicine, which resulted in rising demand for medical care [see 'Self-help']. Rising disposable incomes, the growth of the press, a dramatic rise in the size of towns, and the growing strength and confidence of the middling orders, created an ideal environment to promote the business side of medicine. Although these explanations have tended to simplify local contexts and assumed that all sections of society benefitted in similar ways, the greater demand for medicine, and the resulting opportunities, stimulated an expansion of the medical marketplace and a rise in the number of licensed and unlicensed healers, intensifying competition. For example, by the 1770s there were roughly 159 physicians, 206 surgeons, 123 apothecaries and an estimated 1,778 empirics in Paris alone.[3] One consequence of this expansion was that the boundaries between licensed practitioners became less meaningful as distinctions between practitioners were increasingly blurred to take account of changing conditions and demand. A growing proportion of practitioners, particularly among the rank-and-file, came to be defined as surgeon-apothecaries – practitioners who provided treatment for a range of medical, surgical and obstetric complaints. By combining medical and surgical qualifications their work had more to do with the nature of medical practice than it did with licensing. This made good business sense.

This more generalist approach was influenced by changes in medical thought and in how licensed practitioners were trained. Although personal and gentlemanly qualities continued to be prized, practitioners began to draw on values that stressed their expert knowledge and a growing unity between surgery and physic as support grew for a localized model of disease [see 'Anatomy']. At the same time, Enlightenment ideas emphasized the value of practical education and empirical research to progress. As traditional patterns of training based around university study (for physicians) and apprenticeship (for surgeons and apothecaries) broke down, more entrepreneurial and institutional training was developed around private and hospital schools. Attendance at a private or hospital school presented clear market benefits for practitioners: it distinguished them as experts with particular claims to knowledge. As clinical training was institutionalized and formalized after 1750, surgeons and physicians were increasingly taught side-by-side. As a result, traditional hierarchies became more meaningless and more and more practitioners became *de facto* general practitioners.

New professional identities were also being fashioned in the eighteenth century as medical institutions and groups sought to assert their authority during a period when anti-doctor satire and growing competition drew licensed practitioners closer together. The creation of local and national medical societies and journals helped foster a sense of group identity. For example, Edinburgh's Medical Society, founded in 1737, aimed to build and support professional ties. These societies provided important professional voices and spaces, while national organizations, like the Fédération Médicale Belge in Belgium, vigorously promoted reforms to the licensing system. At the same time, practitioners capitalized on contemporary interest in health and used the press to assert their identity.

Notwithstanding the growing market for medicine and the assertion of a professional identity, licensed practitioners were seldom in a strong position. Changes to the nature of medical knowledge and training did not provide a clear basis for professional power. Doctors faced difficulties in terms of their status, with many remaining isolated from traditional structures of male authority. Studies have pointed to the dominance of bedside medicine and the power of the patient in shaping medical encounters to emphasize the demand driven nature of eighteenth century medicine. In two influential articles published in *Sociology* (1974; 1976), the sociologist Nicholas Jewson argued that what English physicians did at the bedside reflected their status and power, as well as the social context in which medical knowledge was produced. For Jewson, the nature of early modern English society, in which deference was praised and medicine was a commodity, ensured that power rested in the hands of the patient who decided where to get care and what type of care was received. This created a system of patient patronage in which the technical authority of the doctor was minimized. Although Jewson's work was on England, patronage was an important socio-political phenomenon in eighteenth century Europe and responsibility for consulting a medical practitioner and taking his advice rested with the patient or their family. Medical care often involved a process of active decision-making and negotiation between the patient and practitioners contracted to provide specific advice or a cure. Agreements and payment invariably depended not on any professional criteria, but on the patient's satisfaction. Practitioners were therefore keen to adapt their practices to patient's demands or to fashion. Hence, medicine was often patient-centred and a practitioner's business depended as much on their personal qualities, image and commercial flair as it did on their therapeutic ability.

This is not to suggest that eighteenth century practitioners were always second to the patient. Although most medical encounters were negotiated, the status of individual doctors depended on a range of factors, including birth and cultural attainments, as well as their patient-base, ability and entrepreneurial skills. Class and gender equally altered the power relationship between patient and practitioner. A growing emphasis from the mid eighteenth century on the localization of disease added to the authority of the doctor [see 'Anatomy'] and a new breed of licensed practitioner trained in the hospital (see below) were able to wield greater authority. Holding a post at a medical school or university, publications, political or religious affiliation, or municipal responsibilities all enhanced a doctor's reputation. If licensed practitioners were starting to assert their position, many were conscious of their relative social and political marginality and worked to cultivate their status and conform to social and civic expectations. Although this was linked to training and knowledge, and efforts to promote an image of licensed practitioners as experts, enlightened pursuits, such as botany or antiquarianism, along with regular attendance at church were also used to acquire social capital. In times of epidemics, heroic service stored up this capital, which could then be used to attract patients or acquire status. In France, for example, the official service of physicians in the Marseilles plague of 1720–21 was used to strengthen professional authority. By becoming involved in local charitable institutions, such as hospitals, or by contributing to civic organizations, medical practitioners were able to present themselves as benevolent and genteel citizens and acquire social capital and networks of patronage.

The eighteenth century was therefore a period in which professional identities were being reformulated. The period saw the emergence of various groups of medical professionals whose training and practice were shaped more by consumer demand and the growing medical marketplace than by traditional licensing regulations. Patronage and status often mattered more than skill, but the creation of professional organizations, increasing demand for expert services, and more unified patterns of training, if not creating a single profession, did begin to fashion a self-conscious professional identity and structures that started to be accepted by patients and the state.

Knowledge, power and the hospital

As discussed in the previous chapter, the creation of a new style of medicine – hospital medicine – in the late eighteenth and early nineteenth century based on observation and the dissection room – exemplified by the reforms associated with France following the revolution (1789–99) – has been identified as central to defining a professional ideology and linked to the growing authority of doctors. In this account, knowledge, power and the hospital became inseparable as new theories of disease based on pathological anatomy offered a means to discipline and control patients. The argument goes that whereas in bedside medicine practitioners had to cultivate personal qualities, in the hospital the patient ceased to be a patron and became an object of charity and the site of disease. Practitioners used the hospital and hospital-based training to link theory to practice and assert a scientific body of knowledge that was distinct from a lay understanding of disease. This allowed them to assert their influence and advance their professional status as a reconfiguring of the doctor-patient relationship resulted in a shift in power relations to favour the practitioner.

Historians have come to favour this account, but in asserting an idealized view of the transition from 'bedside medicine' to 'hospital medicine', they often overlook the fact that private patients were treated differently in favour of a view that puts forward an argument of growing medical dominance. Most medical care was domiciliary in nature and most hospitals sought to admit the sick poor at least until the 1890s. If in the hospital attempts were made to discipline patients, outside the institution patients remained clients who sought out medical attendance and often questioned both the diagnosis and the treatment. Old and new practices therefore coexisted, creating greater continuities between eighteenth and nineteenth century medical practices than a simple model of transformation suggests.

If doctors' professional authority over the patient cannot be assumed, the hospital did have an impact on professional structures by becoming a symbol, by strengthening a sense of identity, and by defining a body of knowledge around common courses. Although change was not uniform, by the first decades of the nineteenth century training in a hospital had become an accepted part of licensed practitioners' professional, intellectual and financial hierarchy in most European states. Hospitals, as places where experience was gained, ideas were disseminated and teaching was delivered, meet the needs of clinical instruction and knowledge, and undermined the power of licensing bodies. They also provided practitioners with shared experiences: training on the hospital wards, in lecture theatres and post-mortem rooms helped socialize students and equip them with corporate values. This strengthened professional identities. In the mid nineteenth century, medical schools worked to instil further values to reinforce patterns of work, whilst the development of a corporate life around sport in the late nineteenth century gave this further form. Hospital training equally helped foster professional networks, either around the school or around influential teachers like Joseph Lister at Edinburgh. As hospitals became centres of learning and centres for the production of knowledge, hospital appointments conferred status, both within medicine and with the public. Hospital physicians and surgeons began to see themselves as a new medical elite, further eroding traditional hierarchies and replacing them with more binary divisions between hospital consultants and general practitioners.

Whereas hospitals provided an arena through which medical authority was extended and offered a mechanism for socialization that strengthened professional ties, there were limits. Power was never one sided. Patients retained agency and were not always willing to obey institutional rules. Nor were hospital staff able to wield total authority. In many hospitals, there were limits on their authority and influence, at least until the twentieth century. Although there is no simple link between hospitals and power, the growing value of the hospital to medicine created an institutional setting through which professional identities were confirmed and new hierarchies were established.

Competition and regulation

Andrew Abbott in his *The System of Professions* (1988) emphasized the degree to which professionalization is structured by inter-professional competition and conflict. What happened in medicine in the late eighteenth and nineteenth centuries appears to conform to Abbott's ideas. Growing demand for medicine created new opportunities, but as the numbers entering medicine increased, so too did competition. By the start of the nineteenth century, licensed practitioners bemoaned that medicine had become grossly overcrowded.

Although licensed practitioners adopted individual strategies to cope with competition – for example, by taking on a range of institutional or municipal appointments – concerns about overcrowding were structured around the perceived threat from quacks and alternative practitioners. Whereas in the sixteenth and seventeenth centuries such healers had been a nuisance, after 1750 they represented serious competitors against which licensed practitioners defined themselves. The expansion of medical consumerism and national markets for medicine saw the number of unlicensed healers soar [see 'Self-help']. Although continuities can be detected, irregular practitioners took on new personas and forms to exploit the growing demand for medicine, new marketing opportunities, and lay scepticism of learned medicine. Patent medicines – effectively over-the-counter drugs – and quack cures offered popular sources of relief for all classes. Quacks proved a highly flexible group, but were often associated with secret remedies and were the most entrepreneurial sector of the medical marketplace. Alternative medical systems, such as mesmerism or homeopathy, were different. They represented an attack on the perceived therapeutic excesses and failures of mainstream medicine. Alternative medical systems gained support (and clients) in the late eighteenth and nineteenth centuries as the market for medicine grew and offered practitioners a means to distinguish themselves. Homeopathy, for example, had a large following in Germany, England, France, Belgium and Italy. Although there was a strong degree of overlap between regular and irregular practitioners, alternative medical systems represented an intellectual and commercial challenge to medicine.

During the eighteenth and nineteenth centuries, licensed practitioners struggled to create and then maintain economically viable practices. They invested heavily in hospital training and actively developed self-conscious professional identities to assert their positions. Competition from quacks and alternative practitioners were seen as a major obstacle to securing status and income. Like other professionals, licensed practitioners responded to competition by trying to create a monopoly and pursued what sociologists have referred to as occupational closure. Ferocious attacks were launched on informal and unlicensed medicine as licensed practitioners struggled to assert their professional credentials and limit competition. The effort spent reflected how central income and status were to late eighteenth and nineteenth century medicine. Moves to professionalize medicine can therefore be viewed as an attempt to limit competition by pursuing credentialist tactics – education and training – that defined who could practise medicine, tactics that stressed the link between education and occupation.

Numerous strategies were used. Licensed practitioners claimed an understanding of health and medicine that defined them as scientific and orthodox (see 'Trusting doctors' below). In making these claims, they asserted their superior skills and education. If science offered licensed practitioners a tool that reinforced their authority, they also used a range of rhetorical strategies to denounce quackery and alternative medicine as dangerous or fraudulent. New local and national grassroots associations and journals were formed in the late eighteenth and early nineteenth century to campaign for reforms to the licensing system. These organizations brought rank-and-file practitioners closer together, and in doing so strengthened professional ties. Tactics of exclusion were also adopted to marginalize alternative practitioners from medical institutions and from disseminating their ideas in the medical press. The emotional nature of these attacks suggests that there was more to professionalization that dispassionate claims to a body of knowledge or the nature of licensing.

In many accounts of professionalization, the role of the state in creating a standardized system of training and restricting entry into medicine in the nineteenth century has been identified as crucial in fashioning a monopoly for licensed practitioners and in dividing them into new categories. Broadly speaking the extension of state regulation over medical practice by nineteenth century governments brought a shift from corporate controls to bureaucratic regulation. Although entry requirements for medicine could be relaxed, as was the case in Soviet Russia during the Second World War (1939–45), or become subject to political manipulation, as in Nazi German (1933–45), common patterns emerged that were influenced by the reforms introduced in France following the 1789 revolution. Legislation in 1803 made France the model for the strict regulation of medical practise, stipulating educational requirements for different grades of practitioner and where they could work. The Napoleonic wars (1803–14) spread these reforms and new professional structures to other parts of Europe – notably to Italy, the Rhineland and the Low Countries – and equally inspired practitioners in other countries to press for reforms. Medical registers were established and controls were introduced that stipulated that only registered practitioners could legally practice medicine. Although in Prussia and then in unified-Germany regulation was relaxed after 1869, in most European states more rigorous qualifications were introduced. Periods of study were extended as training was standardized, with a university degree becoming the main route to qualification. New medical and university schools opened in response, reflecting a broader move in education that contributed to the rapid expansion of universities. However, statist concerns should not be overplayed at the expense of demand: practitioners placed a premium on medical training to improve their market position.

Greater regulatory controls might suggest that licensed practitioners were able to marginalize unlicensed healers, but they were only partially successful. The reluctance of bureaucrats and *laissez-faire* liberals to support outright controls limited the monopoly practitioners could secure. Regional inequalities in the distribution of practitioners and a concentration of medical services in towns ensured that in the countryside unlicensed healers prevailed. In Germany, where there were comparatively few academic doctors, medical care was often in the hands of unlicensed practitioners, a situation that continued to characterize medicine in interwar Germany. Even in France controls were ambiguous. The ongoing popularity of, and support for alternative medicine, particularly homeopathy, demonstrates how attempts to create a monopoly were not successful.

To see professionalization in terms of moves to limit competition reveals how concerns about status and income came to drive medical reform. Campaigns against quacks and alternative practitioners helped fashion professional identities and organizations by creating 'in' and 'out' groups, and by defining regular practitioners through whom they were not. That these efforts were not successful in creating a monopoly for licensed practitioners emphasizes how for many patients, access to, rather than the nature of care were often the determining factors. It was only with the growing therapeutic ability of conventional medicine after 1870 that unlicensed healers were gradually marginalized as greater confidence was placed in biomedicine.

A unified profession

The impression often given is that across Europe a modern medical profession had been created by the mid nineteenth century. Certainly, reform-minded doctors started to talk about medicine as a profession. Professional bodies and medical journals created a growing sense of unity and collective identity. In Germany, the *Deutscher Ärztevereinsverbund* (National Medical Association), founded in 1873, provided a national forum for issues of training and certification, while *Ärztekammern* (doctor's chambers) created self-regulating ethical bodies. Institutional training, associated with hospitals in Britain and France and universities in Germany, and greater state regulation, ensured both a more defined body of knowledge and clearer definitions of what constituted a regular practitioner. New hierarchies were established. Hospital consultants asserted their position as the new elite, even if it was the general practitioner who was the main local representative of mainstream medicine.

However, to equate the nineteenth century with a linear process of professionalization conceals elitism and intra-professional conflict as doctors struggled to fashion an identity. The mid nineteenth century was a period of upheaval and some practitioners gained status and authority at the expense of others. The divisions that emerged varied between countries in part because of the licensing systems established and qualifications demanded. In Belgium, for example, differences between university and non-university trained doctors created divisions along class lines, with the latter coming from the lower social orders. Nor was there a simple split between general practitioners and hospital consultants.

Distinctions were shaped by location, field of practice, institutional appointments, government positions (many of which were low status), and social or local standing. Those with hospital posts would undertake private practice, and those involved in general practice might hold institutional appointments, especially in rural areas. In France, this accumulation of posts – *le cumul* – was common. Many medical careers therefore fell somewhere between general and consulting practice.

The nineteenth century remained a volatile period for medicine notwithstanding the conventional image that medicine had emerged as a relatively homogenous profession. There are numerous examples of intra- and inter-professional conflict as individuals or groups of practitioners struggled to maintain their position in the medical marketplace. Tensions erupted between hospital consultants and general practitioners, and between general practitioners and public health officials, particularly over fees. Divisions existed between metropolitan and provincial practitioners, between urban and rural practitioners, with the latter often considered inferior. In France, for example, Parisian practitioners had very different ideas about medical welfare, professional qualifications and medical organizations to their country counterparts, whom they disdained. New or old treatments sparked controversy that could lead to splits, such as over the importance of bloodletting in the 1850s or the merits of antiseptics in the 1870s. Book reviews presented an opportunity for constructing and communicating knowledge, but also a mechanism for airing disputes and signalling allegiances.

One clear area of intra-professional conflict was specialization. Although historians have often described the growing split between specialists, consultants and generalists as an example of professionalization, specialization was also a source of tension. During the eighteenth century, low status practitioners had started to specialize to distinguish themselves in the medical marketplace. The development of obstetrics and the rise of the man-midwife is one such example [see 'Women and medicine']. In the nineteenth century, specialization took on a new momentum and meaning. Often the initial focus was at an academic and institutional level, only slowly did specialization come to influence practice. Scholars have tended to examine the development of major specialities to point to the factors that encouraged specialization. These have included changes within medicine with the shift to a localist pathology [see 'Anatomy'], growing patient demand, and the development of new instruments, such as the ophthalmoscope, but other forces were at work. In a comparative study of Paris and London, the historian George Weisz has shown how specialization was influenced by doctors' collective desire to expand medical knowledge and by institutional pressures and administrative reforms, processes that were most visible in Paris.[4] Yet, as Lindsay Granshaw has revealed through her research on London, professional concerns also had an important bearing.[5] Becoming a specialist was one way of gaining a position and status in an overcrowded medical marketplace.

However, whereas specialization offered professional advantages, it also encountered resistance. If this opposition was strongest in Britain, it existed elsewhere in Europe and broadly came from two sources: economic and intellectual. In Britain, general practitioners, fearing for their incomes, felt that specialists attracted patients away from them, starving them of work and income. At an intellectual level, opposition reflected a battle between different views of medicine. The main body of status-conscious practitioners believed that medicine was essentially holistic – that to understand disease it was necessary to understand the whole patient. This approach made sense for general practitioners as it emphasized the role of the doctor in treatment. Opponents of specialization characterized it as dangerous narrow-mindedness that put patients at risk. Specialization was therefore a threat to how many practitioners viewed medicine.

The development of a system of medical ethics provided a mechanism for policing these and similar conflicts between practitioners. In early modern Europe, medical practitioners responded to market-driven phenomena by creating ideas about what made a good doctor and what procedures characterized a bad doctor. Empirics were attacked and patients were criticized for not choosing licensed practitioners. Safeguarding the public became a repeated theme, but it was in the late eighteenth century that the ethical concept of the doctor-patient relationship was invented following pressure from rank-and-file practitioners as a response to overcrowding in medicine. Rather than regulating behaviour between doctor and patient, professional guidelines were designed to mediate between doctors and to prevent the poaching of patients. In Prussia, for example, state-sponsored *Ehrengerichte* (courts of honour) were established, not to minimize malpractice, but to protect practitioners by enforcing a code of ethics. Most of the cases brought before the *Ehrengerichte* therefore involved complaints brought by physicians for slander or excessive advertising.

Tensions between generalists and specialists did gradually ease, and specialization became a feature of practice in the twentieth century. By 1905, 30 per cent of medical practitioners in Berlin, slightly higher in Paris, identified themselves as specialists. Traditional arguments against specialization were redeployed to justify its inclusion. By the outbreak of war in 1914, specialists were among the leaders of the profession and the number of specialties rose dramatically, particularly after 1945. Cardiology, for example, emerged from general medicine; anaesthetics, which had been the province of the part-time generalist, developed as a sub-discipline with its own training and qualification. This move to specialization was reflected in hospitals as new specialist departments and clinics were established.

This did not mean that intra-professional conflict subsided in the twentieth century. Tensions remained between consultants and general practitioners, and between different fields of medicine, as reflected in the post-1945 debates between surgeons and radiotherapists over how to treat cancer. However, if doctors had not exhausted opportunities for infighting, during the early decades of the twentieth century more durable professional structures and identities had emerged. Licensed practitioners now formed a more cohesive group. Internal and external mechanisms – for example, state licensing – ensured that they shared similar education experiences, qualifications and professional codes of conduct. Practitioners increasingly saw themselves as belonging to a profession. It was this group identity, and the strategies that were used to define medicine as a profession, that were central to professionalization.

Women in medicine: 1800–1950

Many of the attributes and processes discussed in the previous sections can be associated with a masculinization of medicine and a marginalization of female healers. Women's efforts to gain access to medical education and to licensed practice have therefore often taken on a mythic quality. Invariably, the story is one of pioneering British women, such as Elizabeth Blackwell or Sophia Jex-Blake, and their struggle against a male-dominated profession. Accounts have stressed personal triumph over institutional obstacles; how male practitioners constructed theories that played on social prejudices to support claims that women were neither physically nor mentally suited to medicine. As the position of women in medicine attracted scholarly interest in the wake of the women's movement of the 1970s, different accounts emerged. Research into the strategies women adopted, and the links between these efforts and first-wave feminism, presented new views of patterns of professionalization, strategies of inclusion and exclusion, and fears of competition.

As discussed in an earlier section, women had an important role in medicine, both in the domestic sphere and as practitioners, but from the late eighteenth century, this role was eroded as medicine was increasingly defined as a masculine discipline. Traditional areas of female employment, such as midwifery, were redefined as women were pushed into more subordinate roles. This had the effect of marginalizing female practitioners but not excluding them from the medical marketplace as the continued attacks on the female practice demonstrate.

From the mid nineteenth century, a small number of educated women sought (re)entry to licensed practice. They were often liberal feminists and supported suffrage campaigns. Their efforts challenged the notion of separate spheres – which assigned men and women to distinct public (male) and private (female or domestic) spheres based on attributed natural character and perceived physical traits. Their attempts to enter licensed practice occurred against a background of campaigns for female enfranchisement and demands for greater access for women to secondary and university education. Several strategies were adopted. In those countries where women were excluded from licensed practice at a national level, as in Britain, they acquired qualifications that allowed them to practice from medical schools in Switzerland and France where there were fewer restrictions. Legalistic tactics – as exemplified by Elizabeth Garrett's efforts in Britain – and a move to establish all-female medical schools slowly replaced these approaches. The latter sought to provide opportunities for women to gain clinical training and experience and so enter licensed practice. In Britain, this strategy was necessary as attempts to challenge the male monopoly were resisted. Here medical schools and universities sought to exclude women, preventing them from securing qualifications that would allow them to practise. By establishing female medical schools, these exclusions were circumvented.

Although educational and legal restrictions were not uniform – for example, in Sweden, women could enter medical schools from 1870, while in the Netherlands all four universities granted medical diplomas to women by 1900 – many early female medical students faced opposition, as well as familial, economic and social restrictions. Inequalities in female education ensured that there were few opportunities for women to enter university, and this made it difficult for women to study medicine. Even where access to medical training was available, such as in Sweden, women often faced intense opposition from male students and staff. This was Jex-Blake's experience at Edinburgh. If opposition was never uniform, the presence of female doctors threatened the already insecure status of medicine and practitioners' incomes. In an overcrowded profession, female practitioners were seen as another threat. Opposition was informed by social and medical constructions of femininity, which drew on a biological determinism that associated women's roles with their reproductive functions [see 'Women and medicine']. This was used to support the belief that women were suited to maternity and the home. The implications of these ideas were considerable. They were used to justify socially-accepted norms of female behaviour to suggest that women were weak, physiologically prone to illness and should be subordinate to men. These social and medical constructions of femininity formed an important part of the licensed practitioners' exclusionary strategies of occupational closure as they sought to limit competition and raise the status of medicine. They were used to marginalize women, limit middle-class women's access to education and work, and confirm the masculine nature of medicine.

Yet, female campaigners manipulated these prejudices to their advantage: they re-deployed arguments about their domestic nature to support claims for a caring role, arguing that they were merely fulfilling their domestic duties by becoming doctors. Equally, female campaigners claimed a domestic understanding that they argued made them ideally suited to treating women and children and in dispensing advice on hygiene. Such arguments were employed as a way of generating support, and to counter existing prejudices to make the actions of early female doctors appear legitimate. However, rather than challenging the status quo, an emphasis on prevention and caring for women and children proved a double-edged sword: it was empowering but pushed women into certain medical roles.

Although opposition were most visible in Britain, at a European level the number of female practitioners remained small at the start of the twentieth century. In Germany, for example, there were only 138 women physicians by 1913. Whereas early female practitioners were able to secure high-profile posts, those who followed them frequently found themselves in low status areas of medicine that were broadly defined as suited to their talents and gender: public health, obstetrics and paediatrics. Few women were able to penetrate those areas of medical practice – internal medicine or surgery – where resistance remained strong, and they found it difficult to secure hospital posts. Most therefore built their practices around women and children and had to settle for low salaries.

The First World War (1914–18) has often been regarded as a watershed in securing women's entry to licensed practice, but the expansion of opportunities for women represented a temporary wartime expedient. Medical schools had admitted women to create durable sources of income and to fill vacant hospital posts as men went off to fight. After the war, many medical schools returned to their pre-war patterns. In Germany, women faced quotas and were used as scapegoats for the economic difficulties encountered by the country. Outside of Soviet Russia, where the growing importance of a technical and engineering education encouraged a feminization of medicine, female practitioners had to constantly prove their competence and were considered marginal to mainstream medicine. Many continued to be pushed into gendered career paths, such as obstetrics or paediatrics. Battles continued to be fought over low pay and access to hospital appointments. In the face of these difficulties, female practitioners used emerging disciplines, such as radiotherapy, to widen access to the medical profession in much the same way as marginal male practitioners had used specialization in the nineteenth century. Women's access to medical education and to the medical profession was therefore restricted or limited to particular areas. They encountered institutional obstacles and arguments that represented them as inferior or ill-suited to medicine. Even in the 1920s and 1930s, many of the obstacles that had restricted entry remained in place. If many of these barriers started to be lifted in the 1960s, by 1990 only a quarter of general practitioners in England – often seen as the area of medicine most open to female practitioners – were women.

Trusting doctors: status and authority

Medicine reached the height of its prestige in the 1950s, a prestige that allowed doctors to wield considerable cultural and expert authority and win public trust. The introduction of new drugs, such as antibiotics and steroids, the extension of immunization programmes, pioneering surgical techniques, as well as growing funding for medical research, encouraged a sense that medicine was contributing to an improving society. Modern medicine fitted well with the post-war 'Age of Affluence' with its promise of improved health. Television programmes, such as 'Dr Kildare', reinforced this perception. Yet, cracks began to appear in the 1960s and 1970s. Doubts were voiced about medical procedures, drugs and their side effects, and about professional values. The thalidomide tragedy, feminist and other critiques of medicine, and a new consumer perspective, all highlighted growing mistrust of medicine. The television series 'M*A*S*H', and films, such as 'One Flew over the Cuckoo's Nest' (1975), pointed to a darker side of medicine. Concerns about the nature of biomedicine and transplants were expressed, as reflected in the appearance of the Cybermen in the British television series Dr Who. Media coverage of medical malpractice stories further undermined confidence in doctors, if not in medicine.

Yet this distrust of medicine and medical practitioners was not new. Proverbial sayings, such as 'Physicians are worse than the disease', were current in sixteenth and seventeenth century Europe. Surgeons were accused of brutality and fraudulent treatments, physicians of only serving their own interests. Early modern poems and broadsheets offer numerous examples of the sexual indiscretions associated with physicians, accusations of manslaughter, incompetence and malpractice. Notions of credibility, honour and trustworthiness were central to social relationships and reputation, and such claims about physicians and surgeons pointed to the uncertain status of licensed practitioners in early modern Europe and the limited social trust in their abilities. These views were confirmed in the satirical outpouring against doctors and their therapeutic ability in the eighteenth century. The writers Voltaire and Moliere in France and the cartoonists Rowlandson and Cruikshank in Britain all satirized doctors. This anti-doctor satire revealed tensions in the customer–client relationship, and reflected how many patients were suspicious of licensed practitioners.

Accounts stress how during the nineteenth century contemporaries placed increasing trust in doctors' ability and authority. The advent of the medical expert and hospital medicine in the nineteenth century signalled a loss of patient control, a transformation that reflected doctors' growing ability to cure and the enhanced professional standing of medicine. The image of the doctor shifted as symbolized in the British artist Luke Fildes's image of the family doctor (see Figure 9.1) or in the celebrated French novelist Honoré de Balzac's *Medécin de Campagne*. Although this did not mean that licensed practitioners dominated medical encounters, it does illustrate how their status improved and how during the nineteenth century medicine was being recast as respectable and caring. Practitioners continued to modify their behaviour to take account of the wishes of private patients, but the growing status of medicine helped confirm their cultural authority as experts as medical discourses came to influence social and political debates. By the early decades of the twentieth century, medicine had secured a high status in popular culture, and licensed practitioners could feel more confident in their professional authority as reflected in their role in policymaking.

Although how much the public started trusting licensed practitioners, and

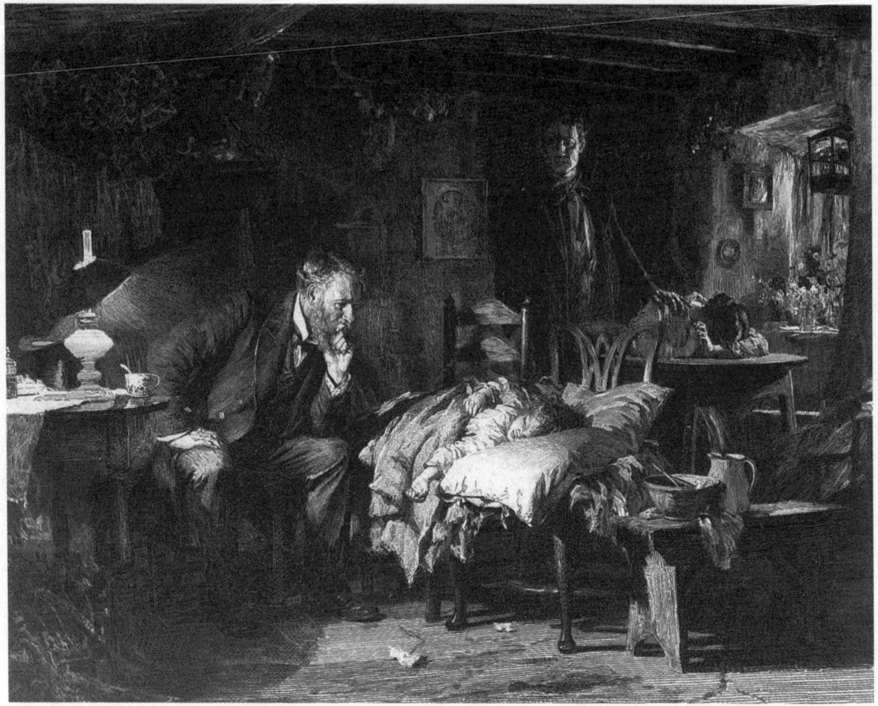

Figure 9.1 'The Doctor' by Salles (after Luke Fildes's painting of 1891).
Source: Wellcome Library, London.

whether this trust reflected an acceptance of medicine as a profession, are difficult questions to answer, a number of factors can be identified. Medical consumerism and rising demand for medicine in the eighteenth century created new opportunities to extend practices, but at the same time increased competition. This created an environment in which licensed practitioners asserted their expert credentials to defend their positions, while concerted attempts were made to reduce competition by marginalizing unlicensed healers through state regulation. Licensed practitioners introduced stricter self-policing measures, or campaigned for higher educational qualifications as in the case of Germany, to raise the status of medicine. A number of rhetorical strategies were also employed that co-opted an ideology of science to professional values and increasingly associated licensed practitioners with scientific knowledge [see 'Science and medicine']. These professional strategies of occupational closure, corporate controls, and an assertion of expert knowledge, elevated the status of licensed practitioners.

Further factors can be detected that had less to do with the professional strategies adopted by licensed practitioners. A growing idolization of science and the use of medical themes in European popular and literary culture strengthened licensed practitioners' claims to expert knowledge. These were supported by general improvements in health. Although rising life expectancy often had little initially to do with medicine, the growing perception that first surgery and then medicine – for example, through new vaccines – offered effective cures served to enhance doctors' reputations and contributed to their authority. The expansion of the state medical services improved access to doctors and enhanced their visibility and status [see 'Healthcare and the state']. In many ways, licensed practitioners were the obvious beneficiaries of the process of medicalization that many historians have associated with the nineteenth and twentieth centuries.

For sociologists, enhanced authority or social standing are evidence of professionalization, but where this was rising in the nineteenth century, securing public trust was not straightforward. Opposition to doctors did not disappear. Anti-vaccinators, for example, portrayed doctors as butchers, rapists and murders. Concerns about morphine addiction revealed unease about how doctors exacerbated existing ailments or caused new ones to generate trade, views that continued to be expressed in the twentieth century. Stories circulated about doctors mistreating or experimenting on their patients. These anxieties were embodied in contemporary literature. For the Irish playwright Oscar Wilde, Robert Louis Stevenson's *Dr Jekyll and Mr Hyde* (1886) read 'dangerously like an experiment out of the *Lancet*'.[6] This distrust was also gendered. Fears were expressed about male violence and sexual abuse. In Britain, women hence had a prominent role in mid-century campaigns against the Vaccination Acts and the Contagious Diseases Acts, as well as in the antivivisection movement. Concerns were repeatedly voiced in the twentieth century about the treatment women received at the hands of male doctors, and not just by feminist critics of male medical hegemony.

It would appear then that the public used different criteria from doctors to judge professional expertise. If medical practitioners were at the height of their authority in the 1950s, this should not blind us to the fact that it was only for a relatively short period that doctors' cultural and medical authority went unquestioned. This suggests that strategies of occupational closure, corporate control, and an assertion of expert knowledge by practitioners, should be balanced against the cultural authority they were able to wield and how this was shaped by socioeconomic, cultural and political factors. It was also informed by how practitioners were represented, both by themselves and by others. In the twentieth century, doctors could be both the comic figures of the British *Carry on* films of the 1960s, sinister characters in horror films, professional experts with claims to scientific knowledge guaranteed by licensing and professional codes of conduct, and individuals struggling with personal and professional dilemmas as seen in the television series *ER*. What this says about the nature of professionalization and the success of licensed practitioners in asserting their professional credentials requires further examination.

Further reading

On the importance of the concept of professionalization to the history of medicine see J.C. Burnham, 'How the Concept of Profession Evolved in the Work of Historians of Medicine', *Bulletin of the History of Medicine* 70 (1996), pp. 1–24. Most of the literature on early modern medicine relates to Britain, France and the Italian states. Margaret Pelling's chapter with Charles Webster, 'Medical Practitioners' in Charles Webster (ed.), *Healing, Medicine and Mortality in the Sixteenth Century* (Cambridge: Cambridge University Press, 1979), pp. 165–236, examines England, while David Gentilcore, *Healers and Healing in Early Modern Italy* (Manchester: Manchester University Press, 1998) and Laurence Brockliss and Colin Jones, *The Medical World of Early Modern France* (Oxford: Clarendon Press, 1997) examine Italy and France respectively. On the medical marketplace, see Mark Jenner and Patrick Wallis (eds), *Medicine and the Market in England and Its Colonies, c.1450–c.1850* (Basingstoke: Palgrave Macmillan, 2007) for information on how the concept has been used. Roy Porter, *Health for Sale: Quackery in England 1660–1850* (Manchester: Manchester University Press, 1989) is the standard account of quackery in Britain. Far less has been written on early modern female practitioners, although Mary Fissell, 'Introduction: Women, Health and Healing in Early Modern Europe', *Bulletin of the History of Medicine* 82 (2008), pp. 1–17, is a good starting point. The late eighteenth and nineteenth centuries have attracted more attention and there is a substantial literature on professionalization in Britain. Ann Digby's *Making a Medical Living: Doctors and their Patients in the English Market for Medicine, 1720–1911* (Cambridge: Cambridge University Press, 1994) and her *The Evolution of British General Practice, 1850–1948* (Oxford: Oxford University Press, 1999) are excellent accounts, while Irvine Loudon, *Medical Care and the General Practitioner, 1750–1850* (Oxford: Oxford University Press, 1986) remains a thorough assessment of medical reform. On the importance of France and the French Revolution, see Toby Gelfand, *Professionalizing Modern Medicine: Paris Surgeons and Medical Science and Institutions in the 18th Century* (Westport, CT: Greenwood Press, 1980) and Matthew Ramsey, *Professional and Popular Medicine in France, 1770–1830* (Cambridge: Cambridge University Press, 1988). Less has been written about German physicians, although Geoffrey Cocks and Konrad Jarausch (eds), *German Professions, 1800–1950* (New York and Oxford: Oxford University Press, 1982) and Charles McClelland, *The German Experience of Professionalization* (Cambridge: Cambridge University Press, 2002) are good introductions. Thomas N. Bonner, *Becoming a Physician: Medical Education in Britain, France, Germany and the United States, 1750–1945* (New York and Oxford: Oxford University Press, 1995) provides a comparative study of medical education, with Abraham Flexner's *Medical Education* (New York: Macmillan, 1925) giving a snapshot that has been used extensively by historians. There is a substantial literature of women's efforts to (re)enter the medical profession. Thomas N. Bonner's *To the Ends of the Earth: Women's Search for Education in Medicine* (Cambridge, MA: Harvard University Press, 1992) provides a good comparative account, while Ann Witz, *Professions and Patriarchy: The Gendered Politics of Occupational Closure* (London: Routledge, 1995) examines the idea of professionalization and the strategies used.

10

Science and the practice of medicine

The drive to science-based technocratic medicine became a key feature of most societies in the second half of the twentieth century, but the place and importance of science in medicine has a much longer history. Progress in medical science has traditionally been associated with key moments and discoveries, such as germ theory or penicillin, with great men – Isaac Newton, René Laennec, Joseph Lister, Robert Koch, Alexander Fleming – or with the emergence of a particular style of medical science in the nineteenth century associated with physiology, the laboratory and bacteriology. Such a view has reinforced ideas of inevitable progress, the cult of personality and a technological determinism in which hospitals, universities and laboratories provided the backdrop for advances is medical science. Although historians have come to reject such a positivist account of the history of medical science to examine instead how science was constructed and the values if reflected, many continue to take the rise of modern biomedicine for granted, while ideas that medicine before 1800 was somehow pre-scientific continues to find expression.

However, doctors in the past have never pretended that medicine was unscientific and over the last five hundred years, science has come to serve a number of functions in medicine. What this science has constituted and its roles in medicine have changed over time and this chapter moves beyond ideas of progress and technological determinism to explore the ways in which the role of science in medicine can be seen as meaning more than the application of laboratory methods or the triumph of biomedical science in the twentieth century. If it does not provide a chronological overview of how science influenced medicine, it does explore the contexts that shaped medical science and how practitioners used science.[1] The chapter also addresses ideas of revolutions in medical science to examine the nature of laboratory medicine, biomedicine and research in the nineteenth and twentieth centuries.

Science and medicine

Many historians agree that modern science has its origins in the Scientific Revolution of the seventeenth century, but that science in its modern sense is a nineteenth century phenomenon. They have argued that until then practitioners and patients were wary of science and saw medicine as an art or craft in which book learning, diagnostic skills and practical knowledge were crucial to what has been labelled bedside medicine. Although this assessment undervalues the importance of social criteria to practice [see 'Professionalization'], it suggests that before 1800 most doctors saw a limited role for science in medicine. In this account, often a distinction is being made between medicine – meaning clinical or hospital practice – and science – the experimentalism of the laboratory.

This distinction has marginalized other varieties of scientific medicine that existed prior to 1800 to favour an essentialist view of science that identifies it with one particular historical era. If we look beyond practice and employ different terms or categories – for example, mechanical philosophy which sought to explain physical properties and processes through the motion of the smallest parts that composed physical bodies – it becomes possible to construct longer histories of science in medicine. Many of these modes of inquiry were initially bound up with contemporary philosophical and theological questions. Although these often had little immediate impact on medical practice, they did contribute to new ways of understanding the body and influenced how medical practitioners were trained. Historians of science have therefore looked to the natural and human sciences of the Renaissance (roughly from 1300 to the mid seventeenth century), the Scientific Revolution (seventeenth century) and the Enlightenment (eighteenth century) for comparable structures of scientific practice and organization that predated the nineteenth century.

By thinking about the different forms science in medicine has taken, it becomes possible to see how natural philosophy (the science of nature) and moral philosophy (the science of action) offered early modern scholars and medical practitioners' ways of understanding the natural and physical world and the body. Although historians' views of the Scientific Revolution have undergone considerable revision, an array of cultural and scientific practices emerged in the seventeenth century as medical practitioners and natural philosophers endeavoured to understand and explain the natural world in new ways. A growing philosophical emphasis on empirical observation and experimentation encouraged investigations into how the body worked – for example, how blood circulated or how respiration functioned – rather than a reliance on the authority of Classical texts [see 'Anatomy']. These investigations contributed to the emergence of new models of the body, but they also reveal how the boundaries between the natural and the material sciences in early modern Europe were hardly airtight. For example, Newtonian mathematics and Descartes's Cartesianism (in which mind and body were separate) were incorporated into medicine. They informed iatromechanical and philosophical conceptions that represented the body as a machine (or watch) which stimulated interest in measuring physiological processes.

Nor were practices of observation and experimentation invented in the nineteenth century. The influence of medical humanism in the Renaissance and a questioning of Classical texts in the sixteenth century along with debates in natural philosophy in the seventeenth century encouraged a more experimental and observational approach in medicine [see 'Anatomy']. Philosophers and physicians, such as Thomas Sydenham in London or Herman Boerhaave in Leiden, emphasized the importance of observation to medicine. As practitioners sought to classify disease (or nosology) in the eighteenth century, they aimed to ground medicine in observation and experimentation. Efforts to explain the complexities of life and debate about whether or not it was purely mechanical or influenced by some vital phenomenon (known as Vitalism) encouraged physiological experimentation, as seen in the work of George Ernst Stahl in Germany or the experiments of the Bolognese physician Galvani with electricity. This experimental and observational approach equally influenced eighteenth century anatomists and hospital clinicians as they sought to identify and classify particular disease states [see 'Anatomy'].

Early modern medicine can therefore be represented as scientific on its own terms as natural philosophers, physicians, anatomists and other practitioners observed and experimented. Philosophical approaches and mathematical principles helped define inquiry. The result was often what the historian Susan Lawrence has referred to in *Charitable Knowledge* (1996) as 'safe science' in which innovation and experimentation was judiciously balanced against patient care. As Lawrence asks, how else could medicine advance?

If the use of different categories of science reveals a longer, more complex history of the relationship between science and medicine before 1800, this relationship was shaped by the cultural, political and socioeconomic context in which science and medicine was constructed and practised. This connection between science, medicine and their contexts is visible in early modern Europe. As the historian Charles Webster first revealed in *The Great Instauration* (1975), theological ideas in the sixteenth and seventeenth centuries were important in shaping how medical knowledge was generated and received. This interaction is evident in the ideas associated with the Renaissance physician and medical reformer Paracelsus and his influence on early modern medicine, but the religious censorship associated with the Counter-Reformation also created barriers to new forms of knowledge in Italy and Spain where new ideas came to be associated with heresy. Although the effects of the Counter-Reformation and Inquisition in southern Europe were not as stark as often suggested by historians, they did create a conservative intellectual culture that was to prove enduring in Spain. Nor did this relationship between medicine, science and theology disappear in the Enlightenment [see 'Religion'], while new social questions surrounding ideas of women's place in society and notions of race also influenced medicine and science and vice versa in the period [see 'Women and medicine'; 'Medicine and empire'].

Historians have used the social and political context of the German-speaking states in the nineteenth century to explain why Germany was at the forefront of medical science after 1850. In doing so, they have pointed to the crucial role played by the high value placed on the search for knowledge or *Wissenschaft*, and how this combined with middle-class and national aspirations to ensure that universities were well funded to promote a competitive culture favourable to research and experimentation. Conversely, in Spain the ruling conservative elite saw science within an explicitly Catholic framework, which restricted the practice of science and the questions pursued. Political contexts were important to medical science in other ways. Science was used to assert national agendas as seen in the work of the French chemist Louis Pasteur on rabies and anthrax. Popular sciences, such as phrenology, and medical sciences, such as physiology, offered flexible resources for those who sought political or social reforms.

In the twentieth century, medical research was harnessed to political and colonial agendas in new ways as industrialized states saw a connection between science, modernity and power and invested more heavily in particular styles of laboratory-based medicine. In Britain, anxiety about German competition saw state money injected into academic medicine and the laboratory sciences through the Medical Research Council (MRC), a policy that shaped interwar research and institutional provision, while in Spain the Francoist regime (1939–75) directed funding to those styles of science the regime deemed safe. If states employed medical science for political ends, the relationship was not one way. The German bacteriologists Robert Koch, for example, used rivalry between the new German state and France to argue for a research institute to match the Pasteur Institute in Paris. New funding opportunities in the twentieth century made it possible to develop research careers and develop a style of academic medicine that came to characterize how doctors were trained and how medical research was organized in universities.

Other sources of funding and institutional support equally fashioned medical research and the questions asked. In the nineteenth century, German chemical, dye and pharmaceutical companies started to invest in research, but in the twentieth century the connection between pharmaceutical companies, such as Burroughs Wellcome or Bayer, and research was to become essential to medical research. For example, Paul Ehrlich's work on Salvarsan for the treatment of venereal disease or Gerhard Domagk's research that led to the identification of sulphonamide as a means of treating streptococcal infection both relied on support from industry. New relationships were developed between the research laboratory, production plant and the clinic, while the association of medical researchers with commercial and pharmaceutical companies became commonplace after 1945. Philanthropy also shaped national and international scientific cultures. The best example of this is the activities of the Rockefeller Foundation. Incorporated in 1913, it launched an international scientific and medical programme in the 1920s and worked to export an American model of academic medicine to Europe. Although this brought an investment in capacity building, as could be seen in Czechoslovakia where the Rockefeller Foundation funded laboratory equipment, the Foundation had an inflexible approach that often lacked sensitivity to national sentiments. Funding from charities or industry often came with strings attached that influenced the type of medical science or research pursued.

Science was further made, negotiated and received in a range of sites. These multiplied from the seventeenth century onwards and were gradually institutionalized. Cities represented important locations and contexts for research, but, as studies in microbiology in the late nineteenth century demonstrate, the cities themselves, such as Paris and Hamburg, also influenced the form this research took. Cities were also home to a range of institutions from the hospital, laboratory and university to the meeting place of professional bodies, coffeehouses and public houses where medical science was formulated, observed and discussed. In the sixteenth and seventeenth centuries, anatomy theatres were central to the development of new knowledge about the body, while eighteenth century museums developed a range of functions for the production, discussion and display of new knowledge. In the nineteenth century, hospital patients as sources of information and the hospital as an experimental site grew in significance [see 'Hospitals'], while in the German-speaking states, universities were central to the growth of laboratory medicine (see below). By the start of the twentieth century, the hospital had become, along with the university, the premier site for medical research. Although it is a mistake to see hospital and university laboratories as the only spaces for medical science in the twentieth century, the emphasis placed on them as legitimate locations for research ensured that the place of medical science became more strictly defined. The result was that other forms of science, such as popular sciences like mesmerism, and the amateur, were marginalized.

These experimental sites or laboratory spaces were more than just passive locations. They were spaces where observations were made and new discoveries were displayed, but they equally affected the production and transmission of knowledge. As discussed in Chapter 8, hospitals were multifaceted institutions and not merely the backdrop for medical science. Science in them was shaped by competing professional and lay concerns, by internal tensions, by patient needs, and by finance. The impact of these institutions on medical science and discipline formation is evident in the different patterns of university expansion in Germany and Britain. Whereas in Germany an investment in universities facilitated the growth of a style of laboratory medicine that came to characterize late nineteenth century approaches to disease, in Britain only in those universities where medicine was peripheral, for example at Cambridge, or in medical schools with a strong university connection, such as Manchester, did medical research take root before 1890.

Nor were these experimental sites parochial in nature. Coffeehouses, museums and anatomy theatres were all part of what Jurgen Habermass referred to as the public sphere – an area in which people can get together and freely discuss and identify problems. These sites offered places of knowledge and cultural exchange. Practitioners did travel to observe others at work, a move initially encouraged by seventeenth century ideas about the importance of demonstrating knowledge as a means of asserting its validity. This was extended by the growth of published pamphlets and treatises that allowed those at a distance to observe. Scientific and medical societies, hospitals and universities, created new spaces in the eighteenth century where knowledge was displayed and ratified. Students, clinicians and researchers who travelled to foreign universities and laboratories to learn brought new practices back with them. For example, Russian physicians learnt about bacteriology in Paris having first travelled there with rabies sufferers to receive treatment from Louis Pasteur. International research networks became a feature of most institutional and commercial laboratories during the 1920s and by the second half of the twentieth century, few institutions or researchers could afford to be isolated.

Historians of science have argued that the shape and success of science has been further influenced by complex sets of social relations and by practitioners' abilities to make links with different communities (both within and outside science). The growth of universities not only fashioned new experimental spaces, but also professional researchers. The creation of full-time academic posts in the late nineteenth century provided opportunities for a range of practitioners to develop and consolidate their disciplines, as evident in the case of pathology in British provincial medical schools. These practitioners were helped by skilled technical workers, as well as by students, and this created environments that fostered the development of research schools. By the twentieth century, the existence of identifiable research disciplines was increasingly associated with such institutional and professional structures. At the same time, patronage and personal networks influenced how and what ideas were transmitted. Societies, journals and conferences not only communicated research, but also contributed to discipline formation. For example, publications in specialist journals, such as the German *Zeitschrift für Bakteriologie und Immunologie*, a dense network of personal contacts, and international meetings, helped shape bacteriology in the nineteenth century. The growth of an increasingly sophisticated publishing industry in the twentieth century offered a mechanism for communicating ideas, and for ensuring that busy or isolated doctors could keep up to date.

This is not to ignore the role of technology in framing medical science. In their groundbreaking work *Leviathan and the Air-Pump* (1985), Steven Shapin and Simon Schaffer drew attention to how seventeenth century debates about the nature of air depended on access to air pumps and the practical skill to operate them. Just like science, medicine is a practical activity and different technologies gave form to research and to new disciplines. Clinical thermometers aided studies of metabolism in the sixteenth century, while in the seventeenth century microscopes exposed new structures in human anatomy. In the nineteenth century, improvements in microscopes contributed to the growth of laboratory studies, while in the twentieth century the electron microscope aided advances in molecular biology, biochemistry, genetics and virology. By the 1960s, a number of medical disciplines were constructed around technological needs and their associated institutional spaces. However, the development of new technology should not be seen as sufficient in itself. For example, Julius Cohnheim's work on inflammation in the mid nineteenth century was not merely the result of new techniques or apparatus, but was also dependent on the institutional structures fostered by Rudolf Virchow at the Berlin Pathological Institute. New ways of seeing and new methods had to be institutionalized and taught, and this explains why medical schools and universities came to be central to medical science, research and discipline formation in the nineteenth and twentieth centuries.

In exploring these contexts, the pace of change should not be overstated nor routine work ignored. Continuities existed. Empirical and mechanical trends in seventeenth century natural philosophy did not immediately see older ways of conceiving the body displaced. Existing ideas were often reworked within new frameworks, as demonstrated by the endurance of the 'seed and soil' analogy in nineteenth century explanations of infectious disease. Nor did contemporary medical practitioners always view developments with the same enthusiasm as later historians. The proponents of scientific medicine, such as those who devoted themselves to physiological research in mid nineteenth century Britain, initially found themselves in a beleaguered clique. New discoveries, techniques, procedures or models were hotly debated and resisted. European universities in the sixteenth and seventeenth centuries, for example, resisted incorporating findings from anatomy or mathematics. Nor did a single or uniform chronology of medical science and research emerge. Whereas France and Germany are seen as countries that nurtured science – in France from the late eighteenth century to the 1830s and in Germany from the 1840s onwards – other countries did not embrace science in the same ways. In Spain, the socio-political structure limited the science undertaken and the questions asked, while in Britain the idea that science was a 'gentlemanly pursuit' was influential and the institutional support for medical science remained limited until the late nineteenth century. If simple chronologies do not work, the relationship between medicine and science was not a simple one. Not only did what this science represents change over time to produce a longer chronology of the role of science in medicine that does not over-privilege the nineteenth century, but, as we have examined in this section, it was influenced by a range of institutional settings and contexts. At the same time, it could serve political, economic or social roles. As we shall see in the next section, medical science was also employed to further professional ends.

Science and status

In medicine, science did not just have a practical value; it also had a rhetorical significance for practitioners in their claims to expertise. Although at times this often created the appearance of a distinction between basic and applied science that did not always exist in practice, science offered a flexible symbolic and cultural resource. Scholarship since the 1980s has pointed to how doctors used science in different ways. For the American historian Gerald Geison, late nineteenth century clinicians were sceptical of the practical contribution of science to medicine but embraced the laboratory for its ideological value and utilized science to assert their cultural authority, a view supported by Shortt who argued that physicians used the rhetoric of science to enhance their status (see Further Reading). Although counter-arguments have been presented, such as that of Christopher Lawrence in his compelling examination of the attitudes of elite British physicians to science, the idea that medical practitioners employed the language of science to confer authority was not limited to the nineteenth century. The networks of early modern science, linked to commercialization, print culture and a growing public sphere, offered opportunities for the middling sort and the gentry to define and assert their identity and authority. Learned and scientific societies, such as the Royal Society in London, were established which offered an arena for polite conversation among the emerging professions – clerics, lawyers and doctors – and also conferred identity and authority on their members. Such societies established networks that legitimated new knowledge and provided members with social capital [see 'Professionalization']. The salon served a similar function in France.

Science became a potent instrument of persuasion in the nineteenth century and assumed a key role in popular culture. In response, doctors increasingly emphasized their role as medical experts and scientific practitioners to exert their authority. One way they achieved this was by becoming involved in local and national scientific cultures and by using a range of rhetorical strategies to claim expertise, acquire cultural legitimacy, and insulate themselves from lay interference. Given that science was increasingly viewed as a force for modernity, medical practitioners readily incorporated a scientific culture and rhetoric into their professional identity [see 'Professionalization']. This rhetoric lent support to practitioners' claims that medicine was increasingly beyond lay comprehension, separating medicine from empiricism and defining legitimate medical knowledge. The credibility of the medical profession was further enhanced by the successes associated with laboratory medicine (see below).

However, what this science was had different meanings for different groups of medical practitioners at different times. Notions of science were used to support claims to identity and learning by different groups of medical practitioners as they vied for status: eighteenth century surgeons, for example, asserted the value of anatomy and a Hunterian tradition of surgery to distance themselves from craft associations and to present surgery as a learned profession [see 'Surgery']. But it was not just licensed practitioners who exploited science to enhance their status. Alternative medical practitioners equally used science to assert their rival claims to authority. The German physician Samuel Hahnemann, the founder of homeopathy, for example, equally drew on eighteenth century medical thought that emphasized observation and experimentation to justify his ideas. New forms of scientific knowledge affected systems of alternative medicine and contemporaries did not perceive them as antiscientific. French spas and hydrologists, for example, established a body of scientific literature through the creation of chairs of hydrology in medical faculties and new research institutes to convince other practitioners of their legitimacy. Developments in the physical sciences, such as the idea of radioactivity, were employed by naturopaths in the twentieth century to support ideas of human radiation.

Nor was this language of medical science restricted to practitioners. Nineteenth century radicals used phrenology in their critiques of the structure of society, while a language of germs and viruses quickly gained currency outside medicine. If the relationship between scientific developments and social views is not straightforward, as the example of eugenics reveals, by the late nineteenth century, science provided a powerful resource as enthusiasm grew that it offered a means to improve and manage society [see 'Public health']. Science was used to challenge older social models and was incorporated into a language of modernity and social reform. Lay groups equally used science to promote their own agendas. For example, in efforts to secure compensation claims, South Wales' miners used scientific evidence and expert witnesses in the twentieth century to make sophisticated appeals as they attempted to secure compensation for pneumoconiosis sufferers. By the late twentieth century, different groups were using the gene as the essence of identity and as an explanation for social difference.

There are problems with the above account. It presupposes that the public – however defined – uniformly accepted science and the authority it conferred. As already noted in Chapter 9, many contemporaries in the past remained uncertain of medical practitioners' authority. Although the popular effect of critiques of science are unclear, in the eighteenth and nineteenth centuries the public questioned medical science. Gothic representations, such as Mary Shelley's *Frankenstein* (1818) or H. G. Wells, *The Island of Dr Moreau* (1896), painted a darker picture of medical science that was influenced by concerns about anatomy, vivisection and experimentation. Such sensationalism and fears were not limited to the novel. Opposition to medical science was expressed in a number of movements, such as the protests against vaccination voiced in nineteenth century Britain. Physiological research and cases of human experimentation equally generated public and professional censure. This ethical dimension was clearly visible in nineteenth century debates about vivisection. The perceived torture inflicted on animals by physiologists drew on fears of immoral behaviour and cruelty; on support from a European movement for the protection of animals, and later on Charles Darwin's work on evolution, which emphasized the connections between the condition of people and animals. Antivivisectionists equated physiology and the laboratory with contested and questionable methods of experimentation. Laws were introduced to regulate animal experimentation, for example in Britain in 1876, while in other countries, such as Russia and France, antivivisectionists questioned scientific progress. If, as Shapin argues in *A Social History of Truth* (1996), there can be no science without a large degree of trust, notwithstanding the growing cultural authority of science this trust was by no means assured. The anti-vaccination and antivivisection movements reveal that just as medical practitioners were at times ambivalent about the merits and benefits of science (see below), so too were the public. Both hospital medicine and laboratory medicine were contested as doubts were voiced about the value of particular theories (anti-vaccination) or the practices associated with laboratory medicine (antivivisection).

Nor would it be wise to focus solely on the rhetorical value of medical science for practitioners. Accepting that the ideal of science was more important that the reality ignores the extent to which medical science informed clinical understanding or practices. As we shall see below, for science to flourish in medicine it often had to have a practical application. Anatomical investigations were institutionalized in the sixteenth and seventeenth centuries because they offered a way of understanding not only God's work but also morbid processes [see 'Anatomy']. Nineteenth century pathologists regarded their field of expertise as a bridge between the clinic and the laboratory and used their diagnostic work to assert their value and position. Biochemistry and haematology in the 1920s were equally framed in terms of their contribution to diagnosis and patient management, with their utility aided by the introduction of relatively simple tests. Diagnostic machines became emblems of scientific medicine that also had a practical value, while laboratory findings that had a practical clinical application were hailed as major breakthroughs.

Science could therefore serve a number of functions. It offered licensed practitioners both a means to assert their cultural or expert authority and a practical tool. By thinking about medical science in terms of its rhetorical value and how it aided diagnosis and clinical practice, it is possible to understand the multiple roles science has had in medicine and for the medical profession, but also how this science was contested. In the next section, we will explore some of these themes as we examine the 'Laboratory Revolution' and the development of laboratory medicine in the nineteenth and twentieth centuries.

A laboratory revolution

Just as the 'birth of the clinic' in Paris has been associated with the triumph of hospital medicine and the start of modern medicine [see 'Anatomy'], scientific medicine has been equated with the growing dominance of the laboratory and technology in the last years of the nineteenth century and the first two decades of the twentieth century. Historians have argued that this laboratory medicine represented both new knowledge and practical diagnostic work that contributed to rising life expectancy through the development of new cures and interventions and hence to the growing status of medicine. Whereas France had been the centre for hospital medicine, laboratory medicine was associated with the growth of universities and research schools in the German-speaking states. This laboratory medicine asserted a reductionist view that located disease at a cellular or biochemical level. It required new spaces, skills and methodologies, and changes in the ways that disease was interpreted, how research was conducted, and how doctors were trained.

Historians have suggested that the laboratory came to replace the hospital ward or clinic as the major site for research in late nineteenth century Europe and have pointed to an associated shift in the focus of medical authority. If studies have come to reveal how this was a contested process, historians have remained interested in laboratories as spaces in which scientific knowledge was produced and around which new disciplinary institutions and cultures emerged. There has been a tendency to assume that one consequence was a division between medical science and clinical practice that was only reversed after 1945 with the emergence of biomedicine. Yet, the laboratory was not a monolithic institution and significant links were fashioned between diagnostic and experimental sites and with hospitals and public health agencies. Laboratory medicine also covered a range of disciplines from physiology and bacteriology to biochemistry and genetics, which make generalizing difficult. Although historians are now more sanguine about the impact of laboratory medicine on clinical practice, how did the laboratory influence medicine?

Laboratories were being used in medicine in the sixteenth and seventeenth centuries. Under Philip II, distillation laboratories were created in Spain between 1564 and 1602 as part of Paracelsian practices, while in eighteenth century Germany apothecaries used laboratories in their research. Such laboratories had a practical purpose, but in the eighteenth century, medical science was firmly rooted in the bedside, the dissection room, and nosology. Although there was a link between the Paris Clinical School and the laboratory, it was clinical science and an interest in the structures of the body that dominated medicine in the early nineteenth century. However, with improvements in microscopes and developments in histology attention started to shift from organs to cells as exemplified by the work in the 1850s and 1860s on cellular pathology by the German pathologist Rudolf Virchow. Virchow uncovered new histological structures and encouraged research into histopathology and cellular pathology, promoting new analytical techniques that were more suited to the laboratory. Promise was also found in chemistry, especially in the work of the research school associated with Justus von Liebig's Institute of Chemistry in Giessen. Here Liebig's emphasis on laboratory-based experiments, accurate measurement and analysis provided a coherent approach to chemical and medical research. Following the work of the English physician Richard Bright on kidney disease in the 1820s, new chemical tests for analysing urine were introduced. If such work provided a practical focus for chemical analysis and research, it is around the development of physiology that historians have seen the emergence of a laboratory-based approach to medicine.

Notwithstanding the eighteenth century studies of the Swiss biologist von Haller and the French anatomist Xavier Bichat, it was in the mid nineteenth century that physiology moved beyond a focus on the functions of the body, such as digestion and respiration, and became a more experimental laboratory-based discipline. Although early physiological studies were initially dominated by clinicians (and in the case of France by veterinarians), they were influenced by the methods and advances in chemistry and physics and became coupled with experimentation, instrumentation and materialism. Ideas associated with the French chemist Antoine Lavoisier and Liebig's Giessen school were applied to examine how the body's functions were affected. The nervous system and metabolism attracted particular interest. Experimental methods were adopted as physiologists increasingly observed, measured and recorded the body's functions in a laboratory setting as evident in the work on nerves by the German physiologist Bois-Reymond and the German physician von Helmholtz. Encouraged by the methods adopted by Bichat and François Magendie in France, animal vivisection became the normal experimental process adopted. Most of the early experiments – chiefly on cats, dogs or rabbits – were basic in nature and concentrated on the functions of specific organs. After the basic functions were understood, physiologists turned to vivisection, chemistry and laboratory experimentation to determine the physical and chemical processes involved. In doing so, they elaborated a functional perspective on disease.

Initially these laboratories were primarily private spaces: for example, the German physiologist Bois-Reymond worked in his own apartment in the 1840s. As physiology rose in status, these laboratories were institutionalized and small-scale research was replaced by more cooperative experimentation. Even though few countries matched France or Germany in terms of investment in physiological laboratories, close links between physiological laboratories and clinical issues were forged everywhere in Europe, while laboratory teaching became a routine feature of medical training as physiologists eagerly showed how their experimental work delivered clinical benefits.

If physiology encouraged the growth and institutionalization of laboratories in the mid nineteenth century, it is the germ theory of disease, commonly associated with the work of the French chemist Louis Pasteur and his German rival Robert Koch, which has been cast as the new paradigm for the laboratory sciences. In the 1860s and 1870s, Pasteur isolated several disease-causing microbes, while in Germany Koch made advances in techniques to identify bacteria, establishing a procedure – Koch's postulates – to prove that a particular microorganism caused a disease. What was crucial was how their work gave new meanings to disease and its causes. Their research ushered in a period of rapid discoveries in which the organisms responsible for major infectious diseases were identified and new therapies were developed. New research institutes were established, with the Pasteur Institute in Paris becoming the model after it was opened in 1886. A decade later, municipal authorities, universities and medical schools could boast bacteriological laboratories for diagnosis and for the production of serums and vaccines.

Historians have spoken of these changes as a 'Bacteriological Revolution' (or in France 'Pasteurization'), and by the 1990s were associating this with a 'Laboratory Revolution'. This revolution was more than the development of bacteriology as a discipline. If bacteriology demonstrated the value of laboratory knowledge to medicine and public health, the Laboratory Revolution was an international movement that enabled widespread changes to medicine through the discovery of the microorganisms responsible for major infectious diseases, the development of new therapeutic agents, and a shift in authority from the ward to the laboratory. The formulation of germ theory became the icon of this revolution and has been represented as a watershed between traditional and modern scientific medicine. Examples of this process are seen in Joseph Lister's work on antiseptics [see 'Surgery'], Koch's postulates, and the new opportunities for vaccination and immunization. Just as with physiology, integration of germ theory and bacteriology was assisted by the promotion of the laboratory as a site for training doctors and for delivering clinical benefits. New diagnostic laboratories were opened in hospitals and by municipal authorities. By the 1890s, sputum, blood and urine from patients were being routinely tested. University and research institutes, such as the Institute for Infectious Disease in Berlin (1891), were established and research laboratories were opened by pharmaceutical companies. Research was framed as leading to new diagnostic and therapeutic techniques as demonstrated by the development of a diphtheria antitoxin (1894) and the production of Salvarsan for the treatment of venereal disease (1908), associating early laboratory studies with cures for dangerous infectious

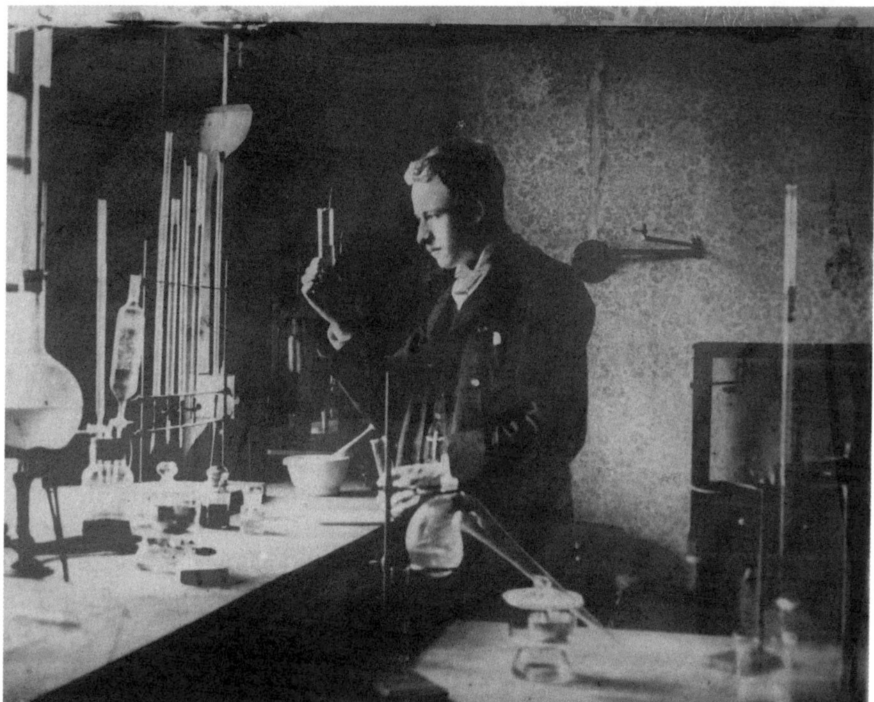

Figure 10.1 An experiment in a chemical laboratory.
Source: Wellcome Library, London.

diseases. Such was the power of the laboratory that emerging specialties sought to harness laboratory experimentation to acquire legitimacy.

The first three decades of the twentieth century witnessed large-scale efforts to introduce the laboratory into medical and commercial institutions, and an unprecedented rise in funding for medical research. Laboratory medicine and the search for further 'magic bullets' following the success with Salvarsan held out the promise of major advances. This was reflected in developments in vaccine therapy before the First World War (1914–18) and in the discovery of penicillin in 1928. Research into endocrinology and biochemistry in the 1920s and 1930s identified hormones, such as insulin, which could be used in the treatment (for example, in diabetes), while research on metabolism, digestion and deficiency diseases revealed the role of vitamins. If room remained for clinical experimentation, such as in cancer, new research institutes and university departments were established after 1919 that fostered an academic medical culture modelled on German universities and associated with Johns Hopkins University in Baltimore. Links with the pharmaceutical industry and with municipal authorities through public health work were consolidated. New techniques were introduced in the 1920s and 1930s that made serological, immunological and laboratory analysis easier. A growing emphasis on metabolic concepts saw blood-testing become key to the diagnosis and management of many disorders. As clinical biochemistry became important to patient management, specialized laboratory facilities were required. Subtle distinctions emerged between routine testing and research as a growing institutional investment was made in research and the appointment of full-time scientists.

This Laboratory Revolution in medicine was dependent on pragmatic local contexts and the perceived benefits. Where there were few direct clinical benefits – for example, in physiology – practitioners were more wary. Bacteriologists and pathologists were keen to show that their laboratory work had clinical relevance, reinforcing the role of clinical cases as the focus for investigation. For example, Koch's postulates were formulated to answer clinical questions. If in the 1890s bacteriology started to modify clinical and diagnostic practices, laboratory work frequently had a service role. Laboratories carried out routine testing on pathological or bacteriological samples for hospital clinicians, local practitioners, and public health agencies, and had a practical use in the production of antisera and vaccines. How they were used depended on local contexts and this ensured that the relationship between the laboratory and the clinic was seldom static. Different kinds of observation were combined: clinical and laboratory observations were both used to explain the particular case under investigation and to contribute to the development of new knowledge. There was often no clear demarcation between these different kinds of work. Clinical cases and routine testing were frequently the basis for research and for advancing scientific knowledge. At the forefront was the clinician-scientist who combined laboratory science with the clinical control of practice and research.

The above assessment would point to a triumph of laboratory medicine.

However, whereas historians are in broad agreement that by the 1930s medical and hospital practice and how doctors were trained were being structured around academic medicine and the laboratory, older ideas of a revolution and the nature of the relationship between clinic and laboratory have been challenged. Revisionists have encouraged historians to become more sensitive as to how 'the ascendancy of the germ theory in etiological explanations does not provide a straightforward indicator of the rising medical esteem for the laboratory'.[2] Received wisdom that germ theory was a defined entity has not held up to scrutiny. Its meanings changed over time and its acceptance did not mean the rapid triumph of laboratory medicine. New chronologies have therefore been put forward as historians have examined how national cultures led to different bacteriologies in France, Germany and Britain. Nor did the acceptance of germ theories see a simple or sudden switch from holism to reductionism. Existing ideas about disease that favoured metaphors of 'the seed and the soil' persisted. Rather than a bacteriological or laboratory revolution, change was uneven, shifts in medical or preventive practice were slow to materialize, older ideas persisted, and the authority of the laboratory was questioned.

Tensions also existed between the laboratory and clinic. This reflected intra-professional conflicts and unease about certain types of laboratory research or disciplines. Although attitudes to laboratory medicine were not straightforward, some doctors feared that bacteriology and the laboratory would turn medicine away from clinical practice. As Christopher Lawrence revealed in his article 'Incommunicable Knowledge', the view that medicine was an intuitive, clinical art remained a potent concept among elite British physicians in the 1920s and 1930s as some worried that laboratory methods were usurping traditional clinical skills and devaluing bedside investigations (see Further Reading). Nor was unease limited to Britain. A significant number of physicians in interwar Germany emphasized a holistic and intuitive approach to medicine that was at odds with laboratory medicine. Although resistance declined as more practitioners received training in laboratory methods, many remained cautious. Some sought to distance themselves from the ethical problems associated with the animal experimentation central to laboratory research. Attempts to introduce new medical practices and ideas about science into old institutions equally met with resistance. Universities and medical schools invariably recruited former graduates and suffered from inbreeding. This reinforced established practices and ensured that institutions were not always willing to invest in expensive laboratories or research activities. At its most extreme, opposition encouraged the development of alternative medical systems that emphasized the healing power of nature (naturopathy) or the individual (mesmerism).

As the above section illustrates, heroic narratives of laboratory medicine should be balanced against how the laboratory and laboratory knowledge were employed. New models for understanding and classifying disease were widely discussed and gradually used, and efforts were made to institutionalize the laboratory through medical education. However, changes in medicine were dependent on a wide range of factors and not just bacteriology or the laboratory. Values rooted in a clinical pathological approach and individualism remained strong, while new knowledge continued to be generated in a clinical setting that drew on practice. Given the dominant enduring usefulness of the pathological anatomical approach, the benefits of mastering new and difficult diagnostic tests or knowledge was not at first clear. New easier methods associated with analysing blood, urine or other bodily fluids had to be devised before they became clinically practicable. Clinical studies or innovations through practice, such as in surgery, remained important, as evident in the award of the Nobel Prize for Medicine in 1909 to the German surgeon Theodor Kocher for his work on the thyroid gland. Nor was laboratory medicine or knowledge uncritically accepted. Whereas some of the therapeutic agents associated with laboratory and pharmaceutical research, such as diphtheria antitoxin or insulin, were welcomed, others, such as organotherapy in the 1920s, which used extracts of animal glands and organs to treat disease, remained contentious. Developments in laboratory knowledge were slow to spread, especially to practitioners working away from medical schools or universities. Generation gaps existed and not all practitioners championed scientific or laboratory developments. By the 1920s, the laboratory had become a resource, but one that had an equivocal acceptance that was not always used in the ways that research papers or laboratory workers outlined. Rather than a laboratory revolution therefore, a process of accretion can be seen.

Biomedical science and research: 1945–2000

After 1945, medical research came to permeate every aspect of medical practice and laboratory research and clinical medicine became inseparable. As the previous section has illustrated, if this relationship between the laboratory and clinical medicine was being forged in the early twentieth century, biomedicine or the large-scale merger of laboratory-based and clinical activities became characteristic of the post-1945 period. The success of research programmes during the Second World War (1939–45) – for example, in the production of penicillin – encouraged a climate that favoured investment in biomedical research and academic medicine. Often labelled 'big science', large-scale programmes were developed as the number of researchers, university and medical school laboratories, and research institutes increased. Here the American biomedical model had a powerful influence. After 1945, medical research took on a transatlantic dimension as American biomedicine provided a resource and a reference point for European studies. Cancer and genetic research are ideal examples of not only big biomedicine and the development of transatlantic research programmes, but also of professional and public associations of disease with research, laboratory medicine and hopes for a cure.

In the post-war years, medicine in Europe was driven by a rapid expansion of biological and biomedical research and by the political and cultural climate of the Cold War. Modes of scientific practice based around institutional cooperation and collaboration increasingly came to define research. This promoted new research cultures. Institutes set up before 1939 experienced a period of growth and governments, charities and pharmaceutical companies established new research institutes. In France, support favoured government agencies, such as Centre National de la Recherche Scientifique, while in Britain the MRC undertook a programme of diversification and set up 109 research units, although support continued to build on a tradition of medical school-based research. Divisions between basic and clinical research areas gradually became more pronounced as established disciplinary hierarchies were perpetuated by how medical research was funded. New specialties were developed, while emerging health problems like cardiovascular diseases or AIDS attracted considerable research investment and effort.

Cancer research offers a case study of these processes. It received substantial investment not just from the state but also from charities, pharmaceutical companies and the tobacco industry. It provided the focus for the development of a number of disciplines and for biomedical science in general. Such was the scale of research investment that European collaborative partnerships were developed in the 1960s as the kind of work required was increasingly beyond the capacity of individual countries. However, despite the investment in research institutions and cancer research, Europe struggled to keep pace with the biomedical complex that developed around cancer research in the United States.

Although doubts were to emerge in the 1970s, in the two decades following the Second World War medical research contributed to a series of advances that fuelled faith in the ongoing ability of medicine to cure many diseases. This was matched by confidence in the application of science and technology to progress and make improvements. Notwithstanding attempts to distance legitimate research from Nazi science through the Nuremberg Code (1947), ethical concerns were not always an issue. Until regulations were strengthened in the 1960s following the thalidomide tragedy, controls on experimentation were lax and regulation minimal, leading to practices that would later come to be condemned. Dramatic successes with streptomycin in the treatment of tuberculosis and with penicillin not only helped generate optimism and change patterns of treatment – for example, by the 1950s many tuberculosis sanatoria had closed – but also stimulated considerable investment in developing chemotherapeutic agents. The need for a better understanding of disease mechanisms encouraged work on antibodies, enzymes, hormones and genes. Research into hormones, for example, saw the rapid introduction of fertility drugs and the contraceptive Pill in the 1960s. Virology, particularly in relation to work on live and inactivated vaccines, provided further examples of the clinical and preventive benefits medical and laboratory science offered. Following Watson and Crick's work at Cambridge in the early 1950s on the structure of DNA, research on genetic diseases and gene therapy promised further breakthroughs.

New tools and instruments fashioned not only knowledge but also new disciplines, such as molecular biology, genetics and virology, in the second half of the twentieth century. Although institutional and professional cultures should not be undervalued, the growing automation of the laboratory contributed to its increasing importance in the diagnosis and monitoring of disease. Many of the tests developed in the 1920s and 1930s were standardized and automated. New methods were introduced. The randomized controlled trial (RCT) – first developed in connection with a trial of streptomycin for the treatment of tuberculosis in 1946 – and the application of epidemiological methods to investigate clinical conditions extended clinical research. Although the use of RCTs was not without opposition as they ran counter to clinician autonomy, they became the gold standard and had a particular impact on cancer research. RCTs offered an efficient tool for organizing research and evaluating therapies as biomedical research and the development of new measurement techniques continued to extend the ability of clinicians to diagnose illness and examine the disease process. Sophisticated biochemical tests, such as for enzymes and hormones, became available. Radioimmunoassay, pioneered by Sol Berson and Rosalyn Yalow in New York in the 1970s, allowed very small amounts of hormones in the blood to be measured. Biochemical tests of blood and urine became essential to hospital work and to general practice.

Although European states invested increasing amounts in research in a Cold War climate that favoured scientific mobilization, the pharmaceutical industry assumed a major role in medical research. The wartime development of penicillin had relied on a combination of funding from governments and pharmaceutical companies in the United States and Britain and the same pattern was repeated after 1945 for other drugs, such as the anti-viral agent Interferon. Many academics initially viewed collaboration with pharmaceutical firms as an intrusion, but the realities of funding made such relationships increasingly important. Funding came at a price, however, as some researchers started to loose control of their work.

Some commentators have suggested that the pace of change had slowed by the 1980s and 1990s; that by the late twentieth century, there were no major medical breakthroughs that could rival, for example, developments in medical genetics in the 1950s. Older technologies, such as stethoscopes and X-rays, continued to be used. From the mid 1970s, funding for research decreased following the economic downturn precipitated by the oil crisis of 1973. Many older research institutes merged or were forced to seek external funding. Private and charitable income, for example from the Nuffield Foundation or Wellcome Trust in Britain, or from pharmaceutical companies, became increasingly important for universities and research institutes as countries began to re-evaluate their medical research programmes. Financial constraints stimulated debate on the value of medical research and its benefits, encouraging the growth of research programmes directed at applied work or major clinical problems, such as cancer or cardiovascular disease.

If new explanatory models and diagnostic tools directed therapeutic intervention, as exemplified in the post-war history of cancer, their direct impact was less tangible. For example, the substantial investment in cancer research did not result in the promised cures despite the advances made. Often the practical benefits of such medical research took longer to emerge, as seen in the case of Watson and Crick's work on DNA. By thinking about the above examples, it becomes possible to come to a more critical assessment of the relationship between science and medicine in the second half of the twentieth century and how notwithstanding the successes of biomedicine, this relationship did not necessarily imply progress.

Conclusions

As this chapter has shown, the role of science in medicine, and what this science has meant, has changed over time. Rather than an account that favours the nineteenth century and a laboratory revolution, this chapter has illustrated how it is possible to see a longer chronology and how different types of medical science existed in the past. It has shown how neither technological determinism nor inventions/discoveries adequately account for the relationships that were forged between science and medicine, and how the position and nature of medical science was often closely tied to political, theological, socioeconomic, institutional or professional contexts. In examining the nature and role of revolutions in medical science, the chapter has explored how change was uneven and how older ideas persisted, and, as the example of bacteriology and laboratory medicine reveals, how medical science was contested. For licensed practitioners, medical science had both a practical and a rhetorical value. If in a clinical or public health setting it was often the practical application of medical science that ensured its acceptance, science served other roles for practitioners as they used a language of science in their claims for expertise. Yet, as concerns about anti-vaccination and antivivisection reveal, it was not just Lawrence's elite British physicians who were ambivalent about medical science – contemporaries had their own ideas about progress.

Further reading

There is a substantial literature on science and the role of science in medicine from studies of individual disciplines to more thematic examinations. The further reading outlined here can hence only touch on the most important issues and studies. For readers interested in the history of science, Peter J. Bowler and Iwan R. Morus, *Making Modern Science* (Chicago, IL: University of Chicago Press, 2005) is an excellent introduction that also includes sections on biology and medicine, while Roy Porter, *The Greatest Benefit for Mankind: A Medical*

History of Humanity from Antiquity to the Present (London: HarperCollins, 1997) offers a detailed overview of medicine and science. There are few up-to-date examinations of the historiography, but John Harley Warner, 'The History of Science and the Sciences of Medicine', *Osiris* 10 (1995), pp. 164–93, remains a clear and concise assessment, while Ronald Doel and Thomas Söderqvist (eds), *The Historiography of Contemporary Science, Technology, and Medicine: Writing Recent Science* (London: Routledge, 2007) tackle approaches to the post-1945 period. There is a large literature on the Scientific Revolution, which is best approached through Steven Shapin, *The Scientific Revolution* (Chicago, IL: University of Chicago Press, 1996) and John Henry, *The Scientific Revolution and the Origins of Modern Science* (Basingstoke: Palgrave Macmillan, 2008). If there are few overviews of laboratory medicine, W.F. Bynum, *Science and the Practice of Medicine in the Nineteenth Century* (Cambridge: Cambridge University Press, 1994) is a clear introduction to the period. John Lesch, *Science and Medicine in France: The Emergence of Experimental Physiology, 1790–1855* (Cambridge, MA: Harvard University Press, 1984), Gerald Geison, *Michael Foster and the Cambridge School of Physiology* (Princeton, NJ: Princeton University Press, 1987) and Arleen M. Tuchman, *Science, Medicine and the State in Germany: The Case of Baden, 1815–1871* (Oxford: Oxford University Press, 1993) provide studies of physiology and experimentation in different national contexts. Robert Kohler, *From Medical Chemistry to Biochemistry: The Making of a Biomedical Discipline* (Cambridge: Cambridge University Press, 1982) does the same for biochemistry, and for pathology see Russell Maulitz, *Morbid Appearances: The Anatomy of Pathology in the Early Nineteenth Century* (Cambridge: Cambridge University Press, 1988). Although much has been written about germ theory, Bruno Latour, *The Pasteurization of France* tr. A. Sheridan and J. Law (Cambridge, MA: Harvard University Press, 1988) explores and questions the impact of Pasteur on France, while Michael Worboys, *Spreading Germs: Disease Theories and Medical Practice in Britain, 1865–1900* (Cambridge: Cambridge University Press, 2000) is a sophisticated study of how germ theories were used in practice. Stanley J. Reiser, *Medicine and the Reign of Technology* (Cambridge: Cambridge University Press, 1982) and Stuart Blume, *Insight and Industry: On the Dynamics of Technological Change in Medicine* (Cambridge, MA: MIT Press, 1992) present different perspectives on the role of technological change in medicine, with Joel Howell, *Technology in the Hospital: Transforming Patient Care in the Early Twentieth Century* (Baltimore, MD: Johns Hopkins University Press, 1995) offering a perceptive examination of the impact of technology on hospitals. On the role of the laboratory in medical education, readers should turn to Thomas N. Bonner, *Becoming a Physician: Medical Education in Britain, France, Germany, and the United States, 1750–1945* (New York and Oxford: Oxford University Press, 1995). For the twentieth century, the essays in Roger Cooter and John Pickstone (eds), *Medicine in the Twentieth Century* (London: Routledge, 2000) and the chapters by Chris Lawrence, Anne Hardy and Tilly Tansey in W.F. Bynum et al, *The Western Medical Tradition, 1800 to 2000* (Cambridge: Cambridge University Press, 2006) are excellent introductions, while Nikolas Rose, *The Politics of Life Itself* (Princeton, NJ: Princeton University Press, 2007) explores biomedicine, subjectivity and power. Harry Marks, *The Progress of Experiment* (Cambridge: Cambridge University Press, 1997) remains the best available account of clinical experimentation in the twentieth century, while the essays in A.H. Maehle and J. Geyer-Kordesch (eds), *Historical and Philosophical Perspectives on Biomedical Ethics* (Aldershot: Ashgate, 2002) address the ethical dimension. Readers interested in a sociology of science approach to twentieth century medicine should turn to Harry Collins and Trevor Pinch, *Dr Golem: How to Think About Medicine* (Chicago, IL: University of Chicago Press, 2005) with an introduction to this approach given by Sergio Sismondo, *An Introduction to Science and Technology Studies* (Oxford: Blackwell, 2004). On the pharmaceutical industry, see John Swann, *Academic Scientists and the Pharmaceutical Industry* (Baltimore, MD: Johns Hopkins University Press, 1988) or Miles Weatherall, *In Search of a Cure: A History of Pharmaceutical Discovery* (Oxford: Oxford University Press, 1990), while Robert Budd, *The Uses of Life: A History of Biotechnology* (Cambridge: Cambridge University Press, 1993) and Jean-Paul Gaudilliere and Ilana Löwy (eds), *The Invisible Industrialist: Manufacturers and the Construction of Scientific Knowledge* (Basingstoke: Palgrave Macmillan, 1999) examine biotechnology. On the importance of cancer research, see the special issue of the *Bulletin of the History of Medicine* in 2007. For those interested in the opposition medical science generated, a good starting point is Nicolaas Rupke (ed.), *Vivisection in Historical Perspective* (London: Routledge, 1987) and Nadja Durbach, *Bodily Matters: The Anti-Vaccination Movement in England, 1853–1907* (Durham, NC: Duke University Press, 2005). Christopher Lawrence, in 'Incommunicable Knowledge: Science, Technology and the Clinical Art in Britain, 1850–1914', *Journal of Contemporary* 20 (1985), pp. 503–20, provides a standard text on British physicians' attitudes to laboratory medicine, while Gerald Geison, '"Divided We Stand" Physiologists and Clinicians in the American Context', in Morris Vogel and Charles Rosenberg (eds), *The Therapeutic Revolution: Essays in the Social History of American Medicine* (Philadelphia, PA: University of Pennsylvania Press, 1979), pp. 67–90, and S.E.D. Shortt, 'Physicians, Science, and Status: Issues in the Professionalization of Anglo-American Medicine in the Nineteenth Century', *Medical History* 27 (1983), pp. 51–68, take a different approach to how science was. There is a large literature on popular science, but for science's impact on popular culture and vice versa see Colin Russell, *Science and Social Change, 1770–1900* (Basingstoke: Palgrave Macmillan, 1983) and Bernard Lightman, *Victorian Popularizers of Science: Designing Nature for New Audiences* (Chicago, IL: University of Chicago Press, 2007).

11
Nursing

Nursing history has often been described as the Cinderella of the history of medicine. Mostly written by nursing leaders, early nursing histories embraced an account that emphasized the importance of the nineteenth century to professionalization, tracing the perceived development from the ill-educated and drunken nurse epitomized by the comic figure of Sarah Gamp from Dickens's *Martin Chuzzlewit* (1843–44) to the trained, efficient nurses personified by Florence Nightingale. This triumphalist approach provided an unproblematic, moral tale of progress that reinforced both mid nineteenth century caricatures and the post-reform image of the professional nurse to foster a sense of identity and tradition. Although at first little influenced by the growth of women's history in the 1970s, in the 1980s work on nursing started to be shaped by feminist critiques, the social history of medicine, and by sociological studies that challenged ideas of professional authority. As historians began to re-examine the history of nursing they began to emphasize the difficulties of developing a new profession and in changing attitudes to nursing. Nightingale's contribution became the subject of considerable critical revision as attention turned to the work of nursing sisterhoods in the early nineteenth century as providing the foundations for nursing reforms. Studies revealed how reform was an intricate process that reflected wider socioeconomic trends, such as women's move into the public sphere, religious concerns, rising living standards, and developments in clinical medicine. Slowly the experience of ordinary nurses began to be examined and the realities of nurse training and the position of nursing in hospitals were re-evaluated as revisionists drew on feminist histories that demonstrated the inadequacies of a professional model when applied to women's work. Studies revealed how values of obedience and discipline were important to professionalization, and how reformers used socially constructed stereotypes of women for their own ends to create work identities and shape reform, although what nursing care meant and how to interpret this care remained problematic.

By the 1990s, historians of nursing were pointing to the revolution that had swept the discipline. Nurses were not a monolithic group as historians examined differences according to class, ethnicity, culture, religion and so forth nurses were no longer seen as a monolithic group. This chapter builds on this revisionist history to explore the parameters of nursing reform and Nightingale's contribution, alongside questions of class and gender to balance ideas of professionalization against nurses' experiences and the contexts that shaped reform.

Nursing, religion and charity: 1500–1800

Often the problem for historians looking at the period before 1800 has been separating out what was nursing from what was not as most nursing was an extension of the care provided by women on a relatively informal basis, either within families or in communities. These arrangements were shaped by the emphasis placed on women's role in the domestic sphere and the duties of women in caring for, and tending to the sick. Nursing care was further influenced by familial and community responsibilities and by an ingrained charitable imperative, which cast the care of the poor and the ill as a necessary part of Christian duty [see 'Religion'].

Although early modern women were expected to practise some form of medicine and nursing as a domestic art, during the sixteenth and seventeenth centuries, religious orders came to play a prominent role in the care of the sick poor and in allowing women to move beyond the domestic sphere and informal nursing arrangements. The San Giovanni di Dio nursing order, which originated in Spain in the late sixteenth century, not only established hospitals but also provided nursing care for other institutions, while the Ministers to the Sick (known as the Camillians) combined pastoral with nursing care, visiting the sick in their homes. In France, Catholic reforms stimulated changes to the structure of healthcare and emphasized the centrality of charity and spiritual motherhood. As hospital administrators sought to improve medical provision and rationalize care [see 'Hospitals'], they turned to nursing sisterhoods for a range of medical services. Nursing orders – the Daughters of Charity, the Sisters of St Thomas of Villeneuve, and the Brothers of Charity – were established and came to provide an important component in staffing hospitals.

Founded by Vincent de Paul and Louise de Marillac in 1633, the Daughters of Charity supplied a model for female pious activism and for later nursing organizations. Determined not to succumb to the pressures of the Counter-Reformation, de Paul saw the Daughters of Charity as not just spiritual workers but also as competent women who devoted their lives to the service of God through nursing, challenging ideas that women should lead a cloistered existence. As part of their routine training, a Daughter of Charity was taught to care for the sick in the community's infirmary (for sick sisters), shown how to grow and administer medicinal herbs, and how to perform minor surgery. Rather than being attached to a specific institution, they were contracted to municipal authorities, parishes or medical institutions. Evangelicalism proved a strong component of their work: a Daughter of Charity was to bring the sick poor back to God if they had strayed. However, they did take their professional duties seriously. This led to conflict with physicians and surgeons, and with powerful patrons, over how hospitals were administered, but at the same time, the Daughters of Charity had a significant impact on the nature of hospital services.

A different situation existed in England. The dissolution of the monasteries by Henry VIII had largely ended the care of the sick by religious orders, but public outcry ensured many existing hospitals (notably in London) were re-established as secular institutions. These institutions, such as St Bartholomew's Hospital, employed a number of nursing sisters. However, the bulk of nursing care was undertaken in a non-institutional setting and was left to domestic households and communities, a situation that remained a feature of English nursing care into the nineteenth century. Studies of female depositions to the London church courts in the late seventeenth and early eighteenth centuries suggest that nursing remained a relative small area of full-time employment for women. Most of those who assumed the duties of a nurse continued to be employed in domestic households as servants, cleaners or laundresses, or were themselves in receipt of poor relief who provided nursing as a form of outdoor relief. Those employed in the small number of hospitals in the period had functions similar to that of a domestic servant – administering food, changing linen, basic cleaning, etc. While some women gained a reputation for their nursing skill, most nursing arrangements remained informal, short-term or part-time and essentially involved often unskilled, manual labour.

One set of arguments would suggest that the professionalization of medicine and the exclusion of women by male-centred medical guilds in the eighteenth and nineteenth centuries forced women out of medical practice and into nursing. This influential view sees nursing only emerging as a separate female sphere as a consequence of men's increasing control of healing. The growth of hospitals in the eighteenth century did encourage a shift in nursing into an institutional context to create clearer divisions between caring and curing [see 'Hospitals']. However, many eighteenth century nurses remained little more than domestic servants. Nursing work had a poor and gendered image: most nurses had little formal education or training, and worked under poor conditions. These established patterns of nursing only began to be disrupted in the nineteenth century when nursing moved beyond informal domestic arrangements and limited institutional provision to take on new forms. Florence Nightingale has been seen as central to this reform of nursing.

Repositioning Florence Nightingale

The image of Florence Nightingale, the American poet Longfellow's 'Lady with a Lamp', has dominated popular perceptions of the history of nursing. Her contribution has been absorbed into a professional mythology as an icon of modern nursing. Born into a wealthy and cultured family, Nightingale sought to escape the claustrophobic nature of her background and trained as a nurse at Kaiserswerth in Prussia and in Paris. Nightingale achieved iconic status during the Crimean War (1853–56). Using her connections, she led a party of thirty-eight nurses to the English military base at Scutari. Her efforts there and her subsequent work in connection with the Nightingale Fund and St Thomas's School of Nursing were hailed as a revolution in nursing. Disseminating her ideas through a large body of writings, particularly her influential *Notes on Nursing – What It Is and What It Is Not* (1859), and through the Nightingale Fund and School, the charismatic Nightingale quickly became a central figure in nursing reform. Her work with the Nightingale Fund and St Thomas's came to symbolize the triumph of a modern system of nursing through the creation of a body of disciplined and institutionally trained carers who brought ideas of order and hygiene to the wards and to the care of the sick.

Just as historians of medicine have moved away from heroic narratives that stress the role of pioneers, so too has the myth surrounding Nightingale been questioned. The English writer Lytton Strachey in *Eminent Victorians* (1918) had already challenged the sentimental public image of the 'Lady with a Lamp', revealing another side to her as a woman with a harsh temper. The nursing

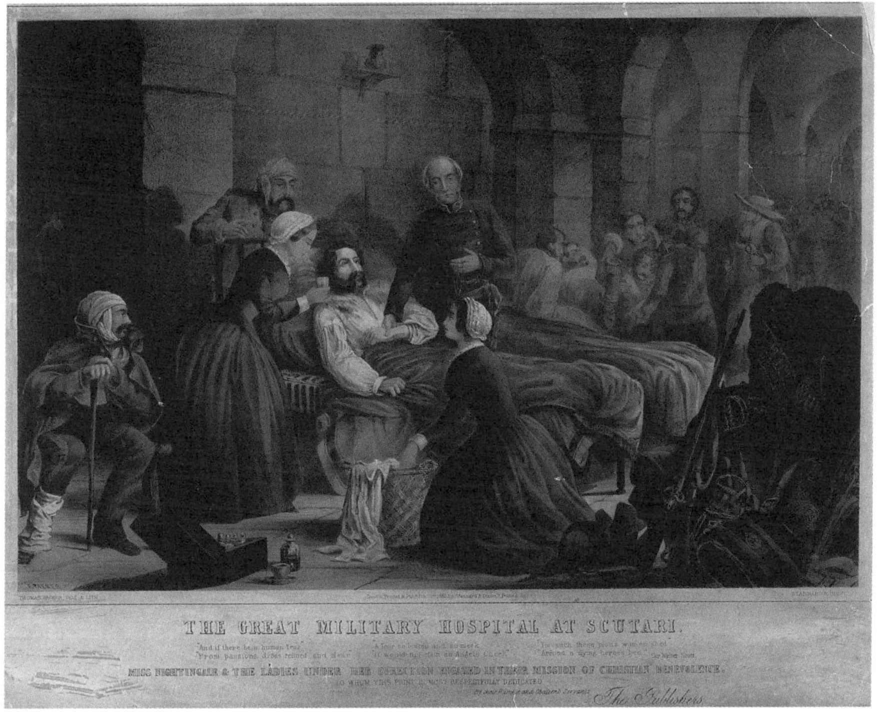

Figure 11.1 Florence Nightingale and her staff nursing a patient in the military hospital at Scutari, 1855. Lithography by Thomas Packer.

Source: Wellcome Library, London.

historian Monica Baly offered a less caustic but no less critical reassessment of Nightingale's contribution. In *Florence Nightingale and Nursing Legacy* (1986), Baly challenged the Nightingale myth, illustrating how the founding of nursing schools was tangential to Nightingale's interest in changing the way hospitals were constructed and to reforming the delivery of healthcare. Subsequent research revealed how Nightingale lacked any defined plans for nursing reform before she went to the Crimea; how the idea of the Nightingale Fund, its application to nursing reform, and the initial development of the St Thomas's scheme, relied on other peoples' initiatives. Far from being meek and selfless, Nightingale was increasingly presented as a complex and talented women; a tough-minded administrator who insisted on having her authority respected.

Studies have questioned not just the woman but also the nature of Nightingale's achievements. Although historians have continued to credit Nightingale with forging nursing into a respectable occupation – a crucial component in professionalization – her work in the Crimean has been placed in context. For example, a system of military nursing existed before Nightingale, with wards staffed by male orderlies, while her presence in Scutari met with a mixed reception. Nightingale was neither a lonely pioneer nor responsible for coming up with the idea of sending out a female nursing expedition to the Crimea. Rather, Nightingale was an excellent self-publicist and concentration on her work has obscured the contribution of other nurses in the Crimea. Perhaps most notable was the Jamaican-born 'doctress' Mary Seacole. Unlike Nightingale, who oversaw nursing activities from a distance, Seacole worked at the battlefront in Balaklava. Nightingale did not approve of Seacole, her aggressive medical tactics, or how she got round the Nurses Enlistment Centre, the institution controlling nursing activities in the Crimea. Although her efforts were appreciated at the front, Seacole remains a secondary figure to Nightingale in part because of her mixed racial background and low economic status. Nor was Seacole alone: most of the female nursing in the Crimean was outside of Nightingale's jurisdiction.

Rather than seeing Nightingale's activities in the Crimea as a defining moment, it is possible to push back the chronology to examine nursing reforms in the first half of the nineteenth century. Within this framework, nursing reforms can be seen in the context of changing patterns of hospital care, women's moves into the public sphere, and of the religious revivals of the early nineteenth century. The pioneering work of earlier nursing reformers and nursing sisterhoods were crucial to Nightingale's success.

Sisterhoods and nursing reform: 1800–1850

In the early nineteenth century, it was difficult to distinguish nursing from other areas of female employment. No specialized training or knowledge was required. Although hospital nurses were expected to be of good character, most were

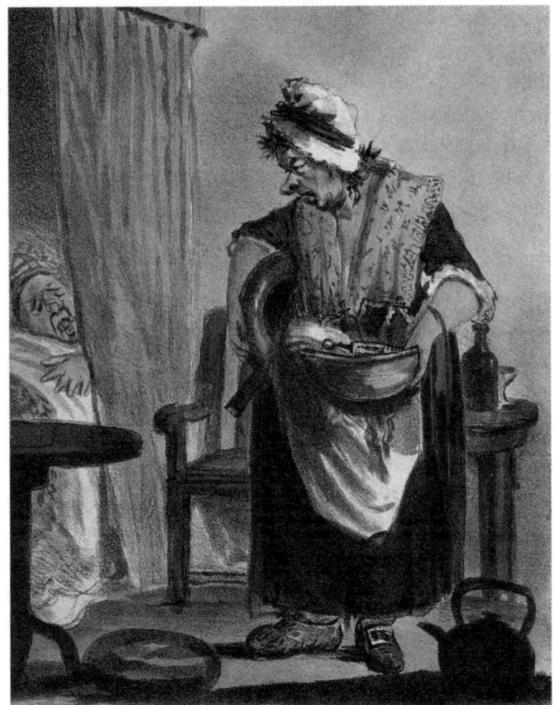

Figure 11.2 A dishevelled nurse with her disgruntled patient. This caricature illustrates early nineteenth century views of nursing and its negative associations.
Source: Wellcome Library, London.

casual, lacked training and performed mainly menial tasks. Even matrons were primarily housekeepers. Although nursing care remained essentially domestic in nature, it was in the hospital that attempts were made to improve nursing. This was achieved by raising wages, improving accommodation, and by the laying down of minimum standards as part of a drive to create a more ordered and respectable (or moral) environment. At Guy's Hospital in London, for example, insubordinate and drunken nurses were dismissed, salaries were raised, and scrubbing and other work associated with servants was prohibited in the hope that a better class of woman would be attracted. Without these provisions, it was not possible to attract and keep quiet orderly women.

Doctors had a crucial part in shaping these reforms, a role frequently overlooked in traditional accounts that favoured the heroic efforts of leading female reformers. In Germany, a six-month training course was established by physicians at the Berliner Charité hospital in 1832, while in London the medical staff of a number of general hospitals made similar moves to improve the quality of the nursing care. Conscientious doctors already offered some form of training for nurses and sisters on their wards, but changes to the nature of hospitals and clinical medicine required more far-reaching changes. A rapid growth in the number of hospitals, the influx of doctors into them with interests in research and teaching, and the changing nature of hospital medicine made the traditional system of hospital nursing no longer suitable. As hospitals became centres of medical education and prestige, and as shifts in medicine placed a heavier burden on those charged with caring for patients, unreformed nursing was seen as a hindrance to treatment [see 'Hospitals']. This required not only more nurses, but also nurses who were trained and subordinate to the needs of the medical staff.

To see medical and hospital concerns as the main drivers of nursing reform is to overlook the other factors at work. Moves to improve nursing were part of wider contemporary efforts to reform the workforce and instil character and discipline. At the same time, the early nineteenth century saw a series of religious revivals and the growth of evangelicalism. The latter provided a useful ethic for the emerging middle classes that emphasized hard work and charity to raise individuals out of their suffering and to reform morals. Whereas religion offered spiritual and practical benefits, philanthropy gave respectable women an important, socially acceptable public role that built on established traditions of caring. In nursing, this religious and philanthropic role was fused to create an ideal occupation for middle-class women to overcome their narrow social and economic roles. Early nursing reformers drew on these ideas. They saw in nursing a suitable occupation for honourable, single women who would not otherwise have work outside the home. This can be seen in the Dutch Society for Sick Nursing whose founders sought to engage decent – preferably middle-class – ladies as nurses.

In drawing on contemporary ideas of mortality, hard work, respectability and deference, reformers utilized constructions of femininity that stressed motherhood and nurturing as moral values for women [see 'Women and medicine']. Supporters of nursing reform argued that because middle-class women had these qualities and were used to dealing with servants they were ideally suitable for supervising nurses. They put forward a new concept of hospital nursing that involved vocation, training and a clear class hierarchy. This was a dramatic innovation: it recast the hospital as somewhere between a convent and an institutionalized version of a middle-class household.

Nursing sisterhoods were central in meeting this early demand for trained nurses and for respectable female employment. Although these nursing sisterhoods drew on established traditions of female religious orders, they introduced the concept of systematic hospital training for nurses. Here the Lutheran Order of the Deaconesses at Kaiserswerth (near Düsseldorf) in Prussia proved influential. The Deaconesses's Institute, established in 1836 by Pastor Theodor Fliedner for the order, not only revived a traditional church organization, but also created a hospital and nurse training school. The school aimed to create a sisterhood of hospital nurses who had received three years of training in order to produce a prototype professional nurse. Kaiserswerth served as a model for other nursing sisterhoods, including the French Établissement des Soeurs de Charité Protestantes and St John's House Sisterhood in Britain. Established to create a legitimate field of work for respectable women, these sisterhoods turned members of the order into trained head nurses or lady superintendents for hospitals and for domestic nursing. It was assumed that respectable women had the spiritual and social qualities necessary to provide proper nursing care and to instruct ordinary, often working-class nurses. However, it was not just a question of replacing drunken Sarah Gamps with more respectable women. The sisterhoods insisted on hospital training, a division between nursing and domestic duties, and ideas of morality that drew on contemporary notions of respectability. Concerned with the spiritual salvation of the sick poor, as well as their physical comfort and cure, they were successful in creating a new type of trained nurse who was efficient, respectable and moral. Hospitals bought in their services. The sisterhoods trained further women to be hospital nurses via a system of ward-based apprenticeship that was to remain a feature of nurse training throughout the nineteenth century.

The religious values associated with the work of the nursing sisterhoods played a vital role in re-constructing nursing as a respectable profession. By the 1840s and 1850s, the moral qualities attributed to philanthropic women and the vocation and training of the sisterhoods had combined in a model of nursing that gained widespread support. These ideas fitted neatly with wider middle-class notions of domestic femininity and respectability. Links were established between nursing and the ideal middle-class wife: both were expected to be good tempered, compassionate and sympathetic to the sick, quiet in their manners, neat, and have a love of order and cleanliness. Knowledge of medicine was not initially important. Nursing was shown to be naturally women's work. Combined these ideas became central to the feminization of nursing and to the entry of middle-class women into the field.

Although sisterhoods battled to improve patient care and ward management, they could not staff every hospital. Nor were they always welcomed. They posed a threat to medical authority while their religious credentials encouraged hostility. Most nurses continued to come untrained from the ranks of the working-class, and most hospital nursing remained menial in nature, similar to domestic service. However, to overstress the rough and lowly nature of nursing would be to accept the rhetoric of early nursing reformers at face value. Often the impression of early nineteenth century nursing depends on what sources are consulted. Research on English Poor Law nurses and other contemporary evidence suggests that not all nurses conformed to contemporary caricatures of them as drunken or incompetent. Many performed their duties in a competent and efficient manner though for most, nursing remained an informal occupation. They could easily move from post to post, ensuring that the turnover of nurses was high. It was only after 1850 that nursing started to be transformed from casual labour into a vocation.

Professionalizing nursing: 1850–1914

The changes that occurred in nursing in the second half of the nineteenth century were closely tied to socioeconomic and political change and to shifting patterns of hospital care. Industrialization and urbanization contributed to rising levels of ill health and disease and disrupted domestic and family care, encouraging the development of market and institutional solutions to meet a range of social needs. Religious revivals and changes in the pattern of philanthropy promoted ideas of active participation and reinforced the belief that social and nursing work was a Christian duty [see 'Religion']. The growth of hospitals and civic infirmaries created further demand for nurses as more patients needed to be cared for and supervised. Changes were also occurring with regard to the nature of hospital medicine with a shift to new supportive therapies and an extension of surgery, although it was not until the late nineteenth century that these had an obvious impact on nursing [see 'Hospitals']. New social structures were emerging. For middle-class women, nursing offered a way of entering the public sphere within socially acceptable gender norms. Because of these inter-locking forces, pressure grew for trained nurses and for nursing as a source of employment for respectable women. These two trends – the drive to separate nursing from domestic service and make it respectable, and the association of nursing with training and a recognized body of skills – marked what many nursing historians have seen as the start of professionalization.

As we have already seen, this drive to professionalize nursing is often associated with the work of Florence Nightingale. Revisionists have not only placed Nightingale within a broader reform movement that was gaining momentum independently of her, but also shown how professionalization was a longer and often contested process. In explaining these nursing reforms, sociological models of professionalization were found wanting and nursing emerged as a paradigm of the contradictions in the gendered nature of professions [see 'Professionalization']. Nursing reform drew on a conflicting set of ideals that emphasized traditional, socially constructed womanly values of caring and a rhetoric of training, morality, discipline and hygiene. If nursing reformers adopted a language of professionalization similar to other areas of medicine – for example, the need to protect the public through the exclusion of the untrained – and shared some of the same strategies – the creation of nursing organizations, professional journals and state regulation – the professionalization of nursing was equally shaped by gender, notions of respectability and domesticity, and by inter- and intra-professional tensions.

Whereas the appointment of a trained nurse in the early nineteenth century was seen as a way of promoting order and cleanliness in hospital wards, after 1850 the need for professional clinical nurses became the primary concern. Many nursing reformers shared a common view of the unsatisfactory nature of nursing standards. Combining the model embodied in the nursing sisterhoods with their values of vocation, training and class, reformers extended the idea that nursing needed to be transformed into a feminine profession for respectable women who, once trained, would impose morality, hygiene and efficiency on working-class nurses and patients. Reformers hence saw character and class as fundamental, and made ideas of order, discipline and obedience central to nursing reform. Moral and technical training were interlinked. These were important ideas in differentiating the trained nurses from other areas of female employment. They were also a practical response to a hospital environment in which discipline was necessary to cope with understaffing and poor educational standards.

Just as in the early nineteenth century, religious and charitable organizations and hospitals were central in promoting reform. Hospital administrators were keen to employ the cheapest, most efficient nursing force as pressure intensified for higher standards of patient care. Doctors continued to have a crucial role in influencing reform. In the Netherlands, for example, nursing reforms were spearheaded by doctors in Amsterdam who used training, textbooks, nursing organizations and journals to influence reform. As part of attempts to reform hospitals and patient care, doctors wanted trained nurses but ones that were subordinate to them. But it was not just doctors who pressed for reform. Nursing reform could also serve cultural and political ends. In France, during the Third Republic (1870–1940) nursing reform was linked to debates about the health of the nation, anticlericalism and the politics of gender. Pressure was brought to bear by the Republic on existing nursing organizations to initiate reforms which became closely tied to pressure for laicization.

By mid-century, the knowledge expected of an ordinary nurse required something more than picking up information by working on the wards for a few months: training was needed through hospital-based schools. These became central to the professionalizing process. Although many nursing schools were established to create both a cheap source of nursing labour and income for hospitals, they fashioned a particular type of nurse, style of training and conditions of work that strengthened professional identities. It was here that Nightingale had an important role. In her *Notes on Nursing* (1859) and through the St Thomas's School of Nursing, Nightingale outlined an influential model for the professional trained nurse. Influenced by the activities and ethos of the nursing sisterhoods, and by ideas of respectable female employment, hygiene and morality, she fashioned nursing as an appropriate occupation for lay women. Nightingale did this by claiming that nursing was part of the woman's sphere, by replicating existing class structures, and by making nursing subordinate to medicine. In doing so, Nightingale reinforced the close links between nursing, religious vocation and philanthropy. This was combined with values that stressed an unquestioning obedience to hierarchy. Nightingale's aim was to train sisters and matrons, using a two-tiered system of paying pupils, who trained for two years, and probationers, who came from humbler backgrounds and trained for one year. The Nightingale system hence recreated the middle-class household: paid, well-trained nurses worked under the supervision of ladies who acted as sisters and matrons who were in charge of the wards and the organization of nursing care. Nightingale further stressed the centrality of hygiene to separate nurses from domestic servants and created a strict division of labour between doctors and nurses. For Nightingale, the nurse was a competent assistant to the doctor; a woman who observed the patient, cared for their needs, and controlled the ward. Caring and morality were elevated over medical expertise. The system worked because it reflected expectations regarding the need for training and for a class-based hierarchy. It also worked because the responsibilities of Nightingale's nurses reproduced contemporary notions of the caring qualities associated with women.

The form the St Thomas's School of Nursing took from its creation in 1860 forced changes that shaped the nature of nursing reform. Officials at St. Thomas's had a different opinion of what student nurses should do from that held by Nightingale. Whereas she wanted them to become moral leaders, the hospital's governors wanted to staff the wards. Initially the system of nursing established differed little from the existing arrangements at St Thomas's in terms of the personnel and management. A system in which probationers were offered practical training in return for their work saw the hospital use the School as a cheap source of labour and work probationers into the ground. Nurses were hence at first little more than servants and received limited training: probationers spent most of their time on the wards unsupervised and the quality of the education was low. To cover up the cracks, Nightingale emphasized the Christian and philanthropic motivations of nursing along with ideas of obedience, sacrifice and calling. As Monica Baly explains, 'what we call the Nightingale system was a hotchpotch of what the Fund could wring out of St Thomas's – which was not much'.[1] The result reinforced the idea of nursing as a vocation, although the actual training offered reflected established patterns of ward-based training and the acquisition of practical experience. Nightingale's vision strengthened the idea that caring was more important than specialist knowledge or academic training.

Although the realities of training at St Thomas's did not match the image, the School quickly came to be regarded as an authoritative source of advice and guidance. The School and Nightingale's writings offered a language and vision of reform that provided a powerful model for the disciplined and professional nurse that was widely copied. The emphasis the School and Nightingale placed on the need for trained matrons in control of the nursing arrangements; that nurses should be reasonably paid; and that servants should do the manual domestic work was widely accepted as the desired model for hospital nursing that challenged older ward-based practices. Nurses trained at St Thomas's moved into other institutions, bringing with them Nightingale's conceptions of discipline and efficiency, although at an institutional level reform was more often shaped by the personalities involved, the situation in the wards, and the economic position of the hospital concerned. Other hospitals established similar schools, but St Thomas's retained its pre-eminent position. Women from other countries were sent to St Thomas's to train and reforms in other European countries drew on British experiences. For example, French nursing reforms borrowed heavily from British ideas and articulated the same programme of hospital nursing schools, vocation, hygiene, hierarchy and order. Training periods were gradually lengthened as nursing schools offered a source of cheap labour and income.

If the basic concept of the trained nurse did not materially differ from country to country, differences existed between countries over what constituted a trained nurse. For example, French practices were first shaped by traditional philanthropic ideas, which considered care of the sick poor a necessary part of Catholic practice, and then by the secularization policies of the Third Republic. In Germany, the emphasis was on the scientific rather than religious aspects of patient care. Differences can also be detected in how training was provided. Whereas emphasis in France was placed on the classroom, in England it was on practical experience in the wards.

Nor did all reformers share the same outlook. Nursing reformers often held contradictory views that reflected uncertainty about the role of the nurse. Those interested in reform did not always share the same values as rank-and-file nurses. Lady probationers sought to distance themselves from their working-class colleagues as existing class hierarchies were maintained. These tensions created conflict at an institutional and national level. For example, in Britain the leaders of new professional organizations and journals sought to exclude working-class women in their attempts to raise the status of nursing for lady probationers. Campaigns for state registration also saw lengthy infighting between nursing leaders, with tensions between the National Council of Nurses and the British Nursing Association over registration making it difficult for nursing organizations to work together. In Paris, proponents of lay nursing engaged in a fierce struggle with defenders of religious nursing orders. Between 1880 and 1908, struggles occurred over the desired qualities of the hospital nurse and who was most suited to that role, while the rank-and-file campaigned for improved working conditions.

The history of nursing is also more varied than the development of hospital training schools, institutional nursing, and the imposition of discipline. Home, rural and district nursing schemes followed a different trajectory. Domestic nursing, for example, either through private arrangements or within families and communities, remained an important component of care for all sections of society and most trained nurses entered private nursing. Where general hospitals took longer to emerge, as in the Netherlands, hospital-based training systems were slow to take shape. Home nursing often developed within the existing structures of local poor relief and philanthropy in those countries where household and community remained important. Domestic and public hospital nursing often existed side-by-side, creating two systems of care, but just as in other areas of nursing they gave the women involved opportunities for leadership, authority and power.

Notwithstanding these varied narratives, improvements to nursing undoubtedly occurred. By the end of the nineteenth century, the idea that all nurses should be trained was firmly accepted. Nursing reforms produced an inexpensive, disciplined and efficient workforce that emphasized moral training, order and hygiene, and saw patient care as their primary concern. By bringing nursing into closer association with the hospital, reformers promoted a particular type of nursing and a set of skills and discipline that was suited to hospital medicine. At the same time, nursing had achieved a degree of social acceptance as a respectable profession for women. The social background of late nineteenth century nurses suggests that nursing did provide employment opportunities and independence for middle-class, often downwardly mobile women. Most trained nurses appeared to be hardworking, if frequently exhausted and overworked. Those entering nursing did gain. In return for two (often three) years of arduous labour, they acquired training in an increasingly respectable skilled craft. For some, this promised opportunities for leadership and autonomy, for others economic security.

Limits of nursing reform: 1850–1914

Although the move to trained hospital nursing encouraged the feminization of patient care and witnessed the production of a cheap, disciplined and efficient nursing workforce, the process of reform was not the triumph of Nightingale-style changes. It often proved difficult to recruit, train and retain the kind of young women required by the Nightingale ideal. Reports in the 1860s and 1870s continued to point to hospital nurses who could not be relied upon to undertake orders swiftly, who drank, treated patients poorly, and who failed to conform to contemporary ideals of respectability. In some institutions, matrons remained nothing more than experienced housekeepers. In Paris, early moves to establish training schools filled an urgent need to provide basic education rather than trained nurses. European educational standards were generally poor. This ensured that professional training programmes were often slow to be established and were characterized by low enrolments and high dropout rates. Low salaries and poor working conditions as a result of hospital under-funding, as well as exposure to disease and limited training, discouraged many women from seeking a career in nursing when other areas of female employments were beginning to expand. Although widespread support for trained nurses was expressed across Europe, older associations of nursing with domestic service proved hard to dislodge, while the increasing financial demands on institutional medical services acted as a barrier to the appointment of trained nurses.

Whereas reformers prized order, punctuality and obedience, these very same values created obstacles to further reform. For example, Nightingale's efforts to model nursing on the middle-class household made nurses subordinate to doctors, limiting professionalization. A rigid hierarchy reinforced social divisions in nursing and prevented unity. Reformers' use of the idea that nursing was naturally women's work and an extension of motherhood was a double-edged sword that reinforced gender roles and nurses' subordinate status.

Nor were all attempts to create trained nurses initially successful. In Geneva, for example, a secular nursing school was opened in 1896, but opposition from political parties, doctors and religious-minded citizens saw the school close within a few years. Elsewhere nurse reformers encountered resistance, especially when they came up against entrenched masculine prerogatives or moved beyond safe feminine roles. Doctors wanted better-trained nurses to improve standards of care but were uneasy about the new style of nurses and matrons as they threatened to transgress established professional boundaries. The introduction of trained nurses, often with an independent income and a higher social status than the doctors themselves, was considered a challenge to traditional authority. Under the old system, the sister and the nurses were accountable to the doctor, under a reformed system their control was in doubt. For a matron to be successful a conflicting power base had to be established, challenging doctors' authority. These concerns did erupt into conflict as new style matrons clashed with doctors over issues of control. It would seem that despite the positive images of nursing hospitals exploited in their fundraising, not all welcomed the new style nurses.

In the face of these problems, nursing only slowly evolved into a feminine profession. If a professional ethos was strongest in England, elsewhere in Europe nursing held on to its religious origins. Familiar ideas of humility, deference and dedication associated with ideals of femininity and religious orders were repeated, even if they were increasingly articulated within a rhetoric that stressed professionalism. Although nursing was becoming a respectable livelihood for hard-up middle-class women, training programmes were not always successful at creating professional nurses. Many nurses in Britain and Germany continued to come from working-class backgrounds and much of the work remained menial in nature. Stereotypes proved hard to dislodge. In France, lay nurses were often characterized as ignorant, drunk or lazy. The same poor impression was reflected in James Joyce's coarse portrayal of Dublin hospital life in *Ulysses* (1922). Doctors were more likely to comment on nurses as attractive rather than professional.

Nor did the experiences of the rank-and-file always reflect professional concerns. The rank-and-file were often absorbed in daily work not professional struggles, and hospital administrators frequently treated them as little more than cheap labour. Underfunding of hospitals, especially in the public sector, limited what could be achieved and placed a considerable burden on nurses. Day-to-day work often had more to do with handling, managing and controlling patients, appearing neat and respectable, than it did with the values associated with the reformed nurse. It was this shared experience of the wards, rather than an ideal of professionalization, that shaped most nurses' aspirations and ideology. The professionalization of nursing in the nineteenth century was hence not without its limits.

Nursing in the twentieth century: 1900–39

The history of nursing in the twentieth century has been dominated by debates over professionalization, hospital nursing and the nature of training, and by an ongoing resistance to accepting women as professionals. Nursing remained a contested field in which various actors vied for influence. The moral authority of Anglo-American nursing reforms, aided by the missionary work of the International Council of Nursing, dominated, but away from debates about professionalization and training what happened at a practice level is less clear.

By the start of the twentieth century, the need for trained nurses was deemed essential to hospital medicine. Socio-political, economic and cultural changes, as well as ongoing specialization and the creation of new types of institution, such as the tuberculosis sanatorium, increased pressure for more trained nurses. Across Europe, government authorities, hospital administrators, doctors and reformers recognized that nurses had to offer more than physical and spiritual comfort. These new demands, along with changing views of the role of women in society and the growing women's movement, helped secularize nursing as a new generation of nurses sought autonomy. New supportive treatments and changes in surgery made nursing more demanding and time-consuming, and required the acquisition of new skills, as did the growth of specialist institutions, which necessitated the employment of specialist nurses, such as in paediatrics. New knowledge from biology, chemistry and pathology, along with new ideas about diet and cleanliness, also required changes. Emphasis was placed on formal training as nurses sought professional self-definition. Nursing gradually acquired what can be seen as classic professional qualities: restricted entry, an increasingly defined body of knowledge and expertise, and a distinct professional ethos linked to ideas of care, morality and order [see 'Professionalization']. However, reform was not unproblematic. During the first half of the twentieth century, nurses faced competing pressures as they struggled for professional autonomy.

The First World War (1914–18) is traditionally represented as an engine of change in gender roles as historians have asked was war 'good' or 'bad' for women. Nursing has been seen as an example of patriotic war work that helped re-shape women's economic, political and social position. The war did mark a turning point in the public image of nursing. The influx of middle- and upper-class volunteers into war hospitals helped recast nursing as a feminine patriotic service as volunteer nurses and the Red Cross drew comparisons with soldiering. Nursing acquired a new public status. As Katrin Schultheiss argues in *Bodies and Souls* (2001), the volunteer nurse was represented as a twentieth century cross between the Virgin Mary and Joan of Arc.

This pre-occupation with change has restricted the questions asked. Although the image of nursing improved, the dominant image was of womanhood and duty rather than a professional ethos, an image that undermined reformers' endeavours to establish nursing as a respectable career. Tensions also existed.

Volunteer nurses encountered hostility, often revolving around class and training. Trained nurses saw the more socially privileged volunteers as a threat and their shorter training as undermining professionalization. Experiences at the front were equally mixed. Whereas some volunteers demonstrated skill and understanding, the apparent incompetence of many lady nurses was criticized. Notwithstanding a shift in nurses' image, nursing under wartime conditions did not differ radically from established traditions.

Once war ended, many volunteer nurses quickly abandoned nursing, but the conflict did encourage a new wave of organization among nurses. Career nurses used the war to assert their professional capabilities and gain public acceptance. Pressure grew for regulation. Growing emphasis had been placed in the last decades of the nineteenth century on the need for state registration as the best way of regulating nursing. Registration, like medical licensing for doctors, was considered a means of ensuring common training and practice. Nursing reformers used wartime experiences to press for state recognition and regulation as demand for trained nurses increased as hospital facilities expanded. In Britain, a state Register of Nurses was created in 1919 and a General Nursing Council was formed to oversee registration. This guaranteed professional status to nurses who had completed three years training at an accredited training school and passed a nationally recognized examination. In France, regulation was slower to be granted, and was only partly recognized with the creation of a national diploma in 1922.

Although registration and regulation was considered a victory for professionalization, it was not without limitations. Existing hierarchies were maintained. Governments rather than nurses controlled the development of nursing programmes and nursing practices. Nowhere was this more visible than in Nazi Germany (1933–45). Training and practice were further shaped by the interests of hospitals, which relied on probationary nurses as cheap labour; by doctors who wanted to ensure nurses remained subordinate, and by entrenched cultural traditions that defined the role of women. Prevailing notions of femininity continued to be linked to professionalization. Just as in the nineteenth century, nursing leaders stressed that nursing belonged naturally to women, albeit women who were vigorously trained. In France, for example, reformers asserted that women had an innate aptitude for nursing that built on an inherent capacity for gentleness and sympathy. This image of the nurse as a self-denying angel remained a potent one: it anchored nursing to nineteenth century notions of womanhood and delayed the recognition of nursing as a legitimate profession.

Progress was also uneven. Whereas in Britain and France limited professional goals were secured along with state recognition, conditions in other countries, such as the newly formed Czechoslovakia, were poor. Nursing reformers across Europe encountered resistance, particularly from those who rejected the idea that nurses should be educated and have substantial authority in the wards. Nurses found it hard to assert their professional autonomy. In France, nursing

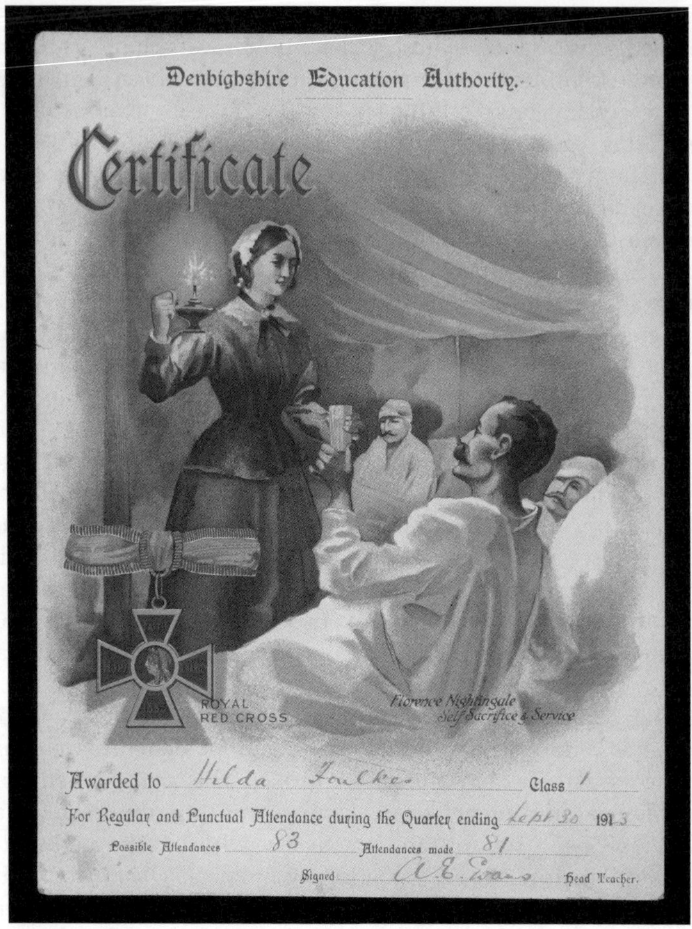

Figure 11.3 Certificate of attendance given to Hilda Foulkes for attending 81 out of 83 classes during 1923. In the certificate, Nightingale is represented giving a glass of water (comfort) to a patient, reinforcing the professional image and iconography of the trained nurse.

Source: Wellcome Library, London.

remained in an ambiguous position: it continued to be associated with domestic service, and charitable and religious duty. The position was not unique to France. Various attempts by the Swedish Nursing Association to modernize nursing appeared threatening to many nurses. Here nursing was dominated by its religious heritage which provided a barrier to reform. Conflict therefore remained a feature of interwar nursing in Europe. In France, disagreements emerged over the goal of reform, particularly between those who regarded nursing as a working-class occupation and others who asserted a model of nursing as a middle-class profession. These debates reflected wider uncertainty about the socioeconomic and political role of women.

In many respects, however, the 1920s and 1930s was most striking for the continuities in nursing. Control over training remained firmly in the hands of hospital schools, which had a stake in existing patterns of training. The life of ordinary nurses changed little. If successful nurses had greater career opportunities, nursing was subject to medical and lay controls. For many, day-to-day experiences remained restrictive and strictly disciplined. Nursing continued to be characterized by high levels of wastage and poor conditions, factors that contributed to a shortage of recruits as other career opportunities for women emerged and as demand for more nurses increased as hospital services expanded. By the outbreak of war in 1939, nursing remained in an ambiguous position, caught between professional values and the traditional problems that had faced early reformers.

Nursing in the twentieth century: 1945–2000

Although the Second World War (1939–1945) saw attempts to regulate and organize the nursing workforce, debates about the role, training and status of the nurse continued after 1945. Developments in medical technology and therapeutics altered the nature of hospital care and imposed one set of forces, while welfare reforms created new pressures on nursing and hospital management [see 'Healthcare and the state']. The traditional work of the nurse, their role and their responsibilities were challenged. Consequently, nursing became less patient-centred. At the same time, the emergence of lower-grade staff allowed a progressive dilution of nursing. Social changes, with greater educational and employment opportunities for women (not least in medicine), created further problems. These factors encouraged the continued decline of nursing as an attractive career for women. The result was a shortage of nurses. This was intensified by funding restrictions in many European health services. In Britain, for example, nursing services were the target of budgetary restraints in the National Health Service, with cuts heightening nurse militancy.

In response to these tensions, and to anxieties about the social standing of nursing and funding constraints in state healthcare, attention was directed at how nurses were trained and the tasks a qualified nurse should perform. Rather than tackling the problems of recruitment and status head on, Penny Starns has shown in *March of the Matrons* (2000) how wartime nostalgia and an obsession with uniforms, badges, rank, class and discipline among the old guard continued to shape attitudes. Nursing leaders initially sought to solve organizational problems by refining methods of selection and training. Professional status and questions of autonomy therefore remained central to debates about training as managerial and professional versions of nursing came into conflict. The nursing profession was constrained by traditionalism, ensuring that the gendered nature of nursing and ideas of good character, respectability and caring continued to be emphasized.

However, new ideas about nursing from the United States did encourage a gradual move from experience or ward-based training to theory-based training. In the 1960s and 1970s, the 'nursing process' became an important model for a style of training which rejected the traditional medical model of task-oriented nursing. The nursing process stressed an active response to the patient through an assessment of the patient's needs and the implementation of a nursing plan. Hospital-based training was slowly displaced by university-based nursing schools as nursing was recognized as a discipline. Ironically, these reforms restricted ward-based care, which had traditionally relied on student nurses. In the 1980s, a further shift occurred as attention came to focus on primary nursing and on the delivery of care by nurses to individual patients. These changes were reflected in the international guidelines adopted by the European Community in the 1970s and supported by the World Health Organization in the 1980s. In response to the changing market for medicine, these guidelines stressed minimal standards of education to harmonize qualifications between countries.

Just as the nature of how nurses were trained changed, so too did the nature of nursing. As in other areas of healthcare, nurses started to specialize. The spiralling cost of medicine in the 1970s saw some areas of nursing practice – represented by the nurse practitioner – move closer to medicine. By the 1990s, general practitioners in many European countries were delegating responsibility for screening and preventive treatments to practice nurses where they had previously sought to prevent nurses from undertaking medical procedures. In response to these changes, dissatisfaction with how nursing was organized intensified.

Conclusions

Attempts to reform and re-invent nursing in the twentieth century were only partially successful. If a view of nursing as patient-centred and problem solving came to dominate European models of nursing, by the start of the twenty first century, nursing continued to be a widely undervalued and underdeveloped profession. What does this say about the process of professionalization? If anything, it shows that the professionalization of nursing is full of contradictions. Although nurses were not passive victims, professionalization was as much shaped by the medical profession, the state, and by social and religious ideas of women's role and nature, as it was by nursing reformers and the values they espoused. Nor was professionalization an even process. It was characterized more by its limitations than its successes. Reformers continued to fight many of the problems that had plagued nursing: for example, making training independent from medical practitioners, conflicts between theoretical and practical concerns, and sexual harassment. Hospitals often favoured unquestioning obedience over innovation. Financial constraints ensured that hospitals provided too few nurses but expected tireless, efficient service. The problems inherent in nursing reform repeatedly resurface throughout the twentieth century. Debates over whether or not nursing was an occupation or a profession, and questions surrounding the need for nursing labour and better standards of education, were repeated.

Further reading

There have been a number of good historiographical surveys of nursing, but Patricia D'Antonio, 'Revisiting and Rethinking the Rewriting of Nursing History', *Bulletin of the History of Medicine* 73 (1999), pp. 268–90, and Barbara Mortimer, 'Introduction', in Susan McGann and Barbara Mortimer (eds), *New Directions in the History of Nursing: International Perspectives* (London: Routledge, 2005), pp. 1–21, are particularly good. On early modern France, see Colin Jones, *The Charitable Imperative: Hospitals and Nursing in the Ancien Regime and Revolutionary France* (London: Routledge, 1989), while Brian Pullan, 'The Counter-Reformation, Medical Care and Poor Relief', in Ole Peter Grell, Andrew Cunningham and Jon Arrizabalaga (eds), *Health Care and Poor Relief in Counter-Reformation Europe* (London: Routledge, 1999), pp. 18–39, covers the work of nursing orders. A good overview of nineteenth century nursing is outlined by Robert Dingwall, Anne Marie Rafferty and Charles Webster, *An Introduction to the Social History of Nursing* (London: Routledge, 1988). On Nightingale's contribution, Monica Baly, *Florence Nightingale and Nursing Legacy,* 1997 edn (Oxford: Blackwell, 1997) and Vern Bullough et al (eds), *Florence Nightingale and Her Era: A Collection of New Scholarship* (New York and London: Garland, 1990) provide excellent reassessments that examine the context of British nursing reform. Anne Summers's work on military nursing, *Angels and Citizens: British Women as Military Nurses 1854–1914* (London: Routledge, 1988) remains a key study, while Katrin Schultheiss, *Bodies and Souls: Politics and the Professionalization of Nursing in France, 1880–1922* (Cambridge, MA: Harvard University Press, 2001) is a compelling examination of nursing in France. Literature on European nursing is more limited, although the *Nursing History Review* contains a number of case studies that cover developments in Germany, the Netherlands and Finland along with a large number of articles on American nursing. More limited are studies of the twentieth century: Robert Dingwall et al, *An Introduction to the Social History of Nursing* (London: Routledge, 2002) and Anne Marie Rafferty, *The Politics of Nursing Knowledge* (London: Routledge, 1996) provide surveys of British nursing that cover the twentieth century, while J. Savage and S. Heijnen (eds), *Nursing in Europe* (World Health Organization, 1997) explores more contemporary issues.

12
Public health

The history of health in society has invariably concentrated on state initiatives or efforts to protect or promote the health of communities or populations. As historians have come to reject a view that characterizes sanitary reform as inevitable and beneficial or as a heroic response to epidemics and urbanization, the term public health has come to be used in a variety of ways – to refer to a movement, an administrative structure, a medical specialty, or a political idea. While historians have maintained a broad chronology of public health, which sees a move from the control of transmissible disease in the early modern period, to the control and improvement of the physical environment in the nineteenth century, and finally to the development of a 'therapeutic state' in the twentieth century, an examination of the wider national or local political and socioeconomic conditions and concerns that structured public health has revealed a more complex process. Often responses to epidemics enabled authorities to impose a range of civic regulations that were as much about preventing disease as they were about controlling the poor, pointing to the important political dimension to public health, albeit one that did not map neatly onto authoritarian or liberal political cultures. In thinking about the role of public health measures in mortality decline, either through an examination of responses to plague or more commonly by looking at nineteenth century sanitary reforms, historians have come to see how diversity, regionalism and local socioeconomic resources, policies and officials all influenced public health provision. By exploring these areas, and by thinking comparatively, ideas that public health reform was a natural or linear process have been rejected. This is not to overlook national cultures: these were important; for example, in how different European states responded to bacteriology in the nineteenth century. Nor does a more contextual or comparative focus downplay the emergence of a disciplinary culture associated with changing ideologies and practices in public health. These reflected the growth of a modern bureaucratic state as social relations were medicalized and the body placed under increased surveillance through a range of state agencies. Rather, such an approach encourages an examination of how public health was informed by ideas about how infectious diseases were spread, by shifts in thinking about the role of the state, by the cultural and intellectual contexts of reforms, by professional and philanthropic endeavours, and by local contexts. It is these areas that are explored in this chapter.

Plague and the early modern state

Responses to plague provide an excellent starting point for understanding the nature of early modern public health as the two were inextricably connected. This is hardly surprising. As explained in Chapter 2, plague killed a substantial proportion of the population in early modern Europe, but it also generated a range of regional and municipal responses that characterized early modern efforts to limit the spread and impact of epidemics.

The methods of plague prevention adopted depended on contemporary understanding of disease causation (or aetiology). At one level, plague was interpreted as a sign of divine disfavour or evidence of moral and physical uncleanness. This required prayer and penance, which served a symbolic and ritual function to bring communities together and discourage behaviours that were viewed as immoral, polluting and partly responsible for plague. Cities hence organized processions and religious services to curb the spread of the disease, and held prayers or built churches in gratitude when plague had passed. At another level, the re-emergence of the plague in the fourteenth century challenged existing ideas about causation, which were based on the works of the Greek doctor Hippocrates. The Hippocratic works had connected disease with environmental conditions and blamed epidemics on a combination of bad air (or miasma) produced by rotting vegetation, excrement, decaying corpses, etc., and individual humoral imbalances. Although these ideas were not abandoned, plague encouraged an emphasis on the role of person-to-person contagion. Such an understanding of how plague spread promoted a set of responses that favoured isolation. Tensions did exist between these approaches – for example, in 1630, Pope Urban VIII excommunicated Florentine health officials following complaints about secular interference with processions and liturgies – but it was within this broad framework that religious, regional and municipal authorities intervened.

Italian city-states were the first to introduce measures in the fifteenth century to limit contact between the sick and the healthy. Medicine was frequently marginal to these responses. When an outbreak occurred outside the city, the gates were closed and travellers were required to present testimonies of health. During a period when numerous small independent states existed, this policy of exclusion was relatively straightforward. When plague arrived, the sick (and often their households) were isolated in their homes or removed to lazarettos (a hospital or quarantine station); houses were fumigated and clothing was burned. Permanent boards of health were gradually established in most major Italian cities – Florence, for example, created one in 1527 – and represented the first systematic attempt to monitor and preserve public health. These boards not only imposed quarantines and isolated the sick, but also set about removing the insanitary conditions believed to generate disease. Although boards sought advice from physicians, they were essentially political bodies.

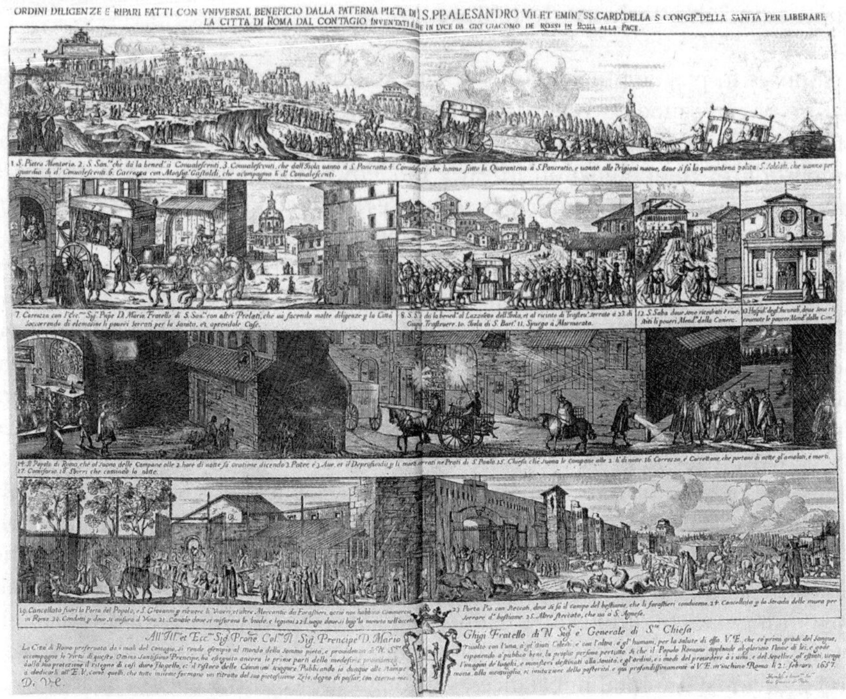

Figure 12.1 Responses to the plague in Rome, 1656. The etching by G. di Rossi depicts religious processions, transportation of the sick, removal of the dead, nightly prayers, quarantined sections, and the epidemic's impact on commerce.
Source: Wellcome Library, London.

European municipal and regional authorities developed routines for dealing with plague as epidemics waxed and waned. At a civic level, responses to epidemic emergencies allowed states to impose a range of regulations. As connections were made between poverty and disease, controls were introduced to clamp down on gambling and begging. Drawing on the Italian model, the afflicted were isolated and the dead certified. Burials were controlled and isolation hospitals were built. Normal activities, such as markets, were suspended and inter-regional trade was restricted. Printed bills of mortality or pamphlets allowed local communities to evaluate the threat and informed them of preventive measures. A range of officials were appointed from plague physicians and lay searchers to examine the sick to gravediggers to bury the dead.

Civic and medical authorities drew on ideas that the plague was contagious. In response to epidemics, they imposed precautionary measures until plague was reported and then established isolation hospitals, quarantines and *cordons sanitaires* to prevent infected ships or individuals from spreading the disease. Controls were not always rigorous, however. This was not a result of inadequate knowledge, but was often a feature of the severity of the situation and reflected concerns about how plague regulations would disrupt life in a city or region. The history of quarantine invariably alternated between success and failure, as can be seen in eighteenth century Malta. Over time, quarantines became more organized and harsher, aided by the international exchange of information and by stricter government regulation. When plague arrived in Marseille in 1720, for example, the Parlement de Provence established a *cordon sanitaire*, threatening anyone who left or entered the city with death. Quarantines and *cordons sanitaires* remained as mechanisms to check the spread of epidemic disease into the nineteenth century.

Rather than suggesting a uniform approach, precautions and regulations evolved over time and were invariably temporary measures put in place during periods of crisis. In France and Russia, ordinances against plague were introduced in the early sixteenth century, but in Naples and Switzerland management of epidemics remained haphazard until the mid seventeenth century. Controls were implemented on a trial and error basis at a local level. Only gradually did a practical set of policies emerge. Yet, plague controls were not always effective: the financial limitations of most poor parishes, where levels of plague were highest, hindered provision, while it was often difficult to recruit officials to treat or bury plague victims. Nor were these measures without criticism. Disputes in Britain emerged over the value of isolation, but more generally plague controls prompted conflict between residents and officials. As evidence from sixteenth century Spain and France reveals, it was not the plague itself but responses to epidemics that disrupted economic and social systems, and it was this that created opposition. Notwithstanding these problems, efforts to isolate and support the sick became permanent elements of local government.

Mortality from the plague began to fall from the mid seventeenth century onwards. Why this occurred has been a source of debate among historians [see 'Disease'], but scholarship has increasingly pointed to the role of public health programmes. Quarantines did limit the spread of rats and people and hence plague, and historians have argued that the *cordon sanitaire* established along the southern border of Austria-Hungary by the Habsburgs as a direct response to the 1708–13 epidemic, and then by Prussia in 1770, provided an effective barrier for Western Europe. This is not to suggest that the quarantine measures implemented were perfect. They were not. It was impossible to stop every ship or plague carrier, and by bending regulations where this would not endanger health, authorities sought to ensure cities and regions continued to function. However, given that plague spread haphazardly, even imperfect and porous quarantine measures reduced opportunities for infection.

Medical police and public health: 1600–1800

As noted in Chapter 2, whereas conventional accounts have connected sustained economic growth to a fall in mortality, industrialization in the eighteenth and early nineteenth centuries resulted in disruption, deprivation and disease. Rather than bringing progress, therefore, industrialization and urbanization initially saw sharp rises in mortality, particularly from infectious diseases. If patterns of socioeconomic change varied – France underwent gradual industrialization, while in Russia, industrialization was little in evidence until the late nineteenth century – many cities in the eighteenth century were inundated with people and filth as the urban infrastructure was overburdened, while the expansion of industry and trade both polluted the environment and contributed to the spread of disease. Many towns failed to adapt as they struggled to expand. City streets were often covered in filth and excrement, and rivers, such as the Tiber or the Seine, were little more than open sewers. Although mortality patterns owed much to local circumstances, endemic diseases, such as typhoid and typhus, as well as diarrhoeal diseases in the summer months, festered in these conditions and epidemics of smallpox, influenza, dysentery, diphtheria and other infectious diseases spread quickly and killed large numbers. These diseases and epidemics offset the decline in levels of plague. Faced with these conditions, contemporary commentators exhausted themselves in finding words to describe the sanitary horrors of the urban environment. If municipal authorities were often paralysed by the extent of the problems they faced, European states took an increasing interest in the health of the population.

Historians have turned to the idea of 'medical police' to explain the growing role of the state in the eighteenth century in responding to these conditions and meeting the health needs of the population through measures which centred on public health and controls on medical practice. The idea has been commonly associated with the work of the Austrian physician Johann Peter Frank whose first of six volumes, *System einer Vollständigen Medicinischen Polizey* (A Complete System of Medical Police) was published in 1779. Rather than referring to police in the modern sense, Frank's police represented administering a state. Frank's *System* outlined measures for regulating behaviour that might lead to disease and proposed hygiene measures to control and clean up the environment. His medical police blended paternalistic ideas with Cameralism – a German form of mercantilism – that viewed a healthy population as the source of national strength and the efficient management of the nation as a way of achieving this end.

Frank's ideas found a resonance in German-speaking countries, Eastern Europe and Sweden, but it is possible to move the idea of medical police back into the sixteenth and seventeenth centuries to trace continuities in public health between the sixteenth and eighteenth century. Early modern governments influenced by mercantilism began to collect information on mortality and introduced measures to promote health and productivity based on the sense that the wellbeing of society and state were connected. Although these measures often remained on a communal scale and were essentially defensive in nature, one way of understanding this growing interest in public health is to see these responses as shaped by a new interest in contagion encouraged by plague. However, rather than demonstrating a neat progression from anticontagionist theories, which emphasized the importance of the environment and miasmas, to a contagionist stance in the seventeenth and eighteenth centuries, these concepts were not mutually exclusive. The belief that certain diseases were spread by direct or indirect contact was supported by experience, but this did not rule out that other diseases were spread by miasmas. This mixed approach is found in early modern responses to epidemics. These combined measures that ranged from street cleaning and purification of the air – for example, by fumigating houses – to controls on public gatherings and brothels, restrictions on movement, and measures to isolate the sick as evident in the creation of lock hospitals in response to the rapid spread of venereal disease in the period. City councils initially favoured moves to clean up streets and houses when signs of an epidemic were reported, and when the epidemic appeared combined isolation and quarantine with environmental measures. Responses to epidemic disease therefore mixed precautions suggested by contagionist *and* anticontagionist theories.

As urban conditions deteriorated in the eighteenth century, more attention was directed at public health as part of a much broader contemporary interest in the social and physical environment. Socioeconomic change, population growth and urbanization required new approaches to epidemic and endemic disease. In Absolutist states, this merged with traditional paternalistic ideas, but in most European countries, the state of the nation became an increasing object of political concern in the eighteenth century. Efforts to determine patterns in nature and evaluate the strength of the nation – social mathematics in France or political arithmetic in England – contributed to this view and provided a language and means to inquire into health. Quantitative analysis and observation were used to establish connections between disease and environment. This interest in statistics had a powerful influence: it informed Frank's medical police and contributed to a belief that governments should intervene to prevent disease.

A revival of interest in the Hippocratic doctrine outlined in *On Airs, Waters and Places*, which linked diseased environments to miasmas, encouraged renewed attention in how epidemics were spread. A sense that disease was the result of poisons in the atmosphere generated by environmental conditions made sense given the conditions in many eighteenth century towns. What was new in the eighteenth century was that medical environmentalists began to suggest that these conditions could be remedied. The effort of the Société Royale de Médecine in France to collect empirical information from physicians and surgeons throughout France is symptomatic of this growing interest in medical environmentalism. Yet, although support for medical environmentalism grew, it continued to be combined with the belief that infectious diseases were transmitted between individuals and through the atmosphere. This fashioned a complex set of explanations that shaped eighteenth century approaches to public health.

Other forces were at work in the eighteenth century to promote public health. Enlightenment humanitarianism and political economy emphasized the idea that nature and humanity could be improved. Links between poverty and disease focused attention on the poor both as a source of contagion and as an object for reform as sanitation was subsumed as part of a civilizing process. New political and moral philosophies in the eighteenth century emphasized the utility of government intervention, a view that was to be embodied in Jeremy Bentham's Utilitarianism and in the belief that governments should strive for social welfare to increase national prosperity. Notions of democratic citizenship asserted in America following the revolution and Declaration of Independence (1776) linked despotism to disease and were given new form in Revolutionary France and the comprehensive health programme outlined between 1790 and 1794. Health was increasingly believed to be essential to political and economic strength. This interest in creating well-disciplined and healthy subjects can be read as evidence of a growing ideological shift to favour the extension of state control.

Although many of the methods adopted had been used by cities and states in the sixteenth and seventeenth century, European governments and municipal authorities targeted public medicine with a new aggressiveness after 1750. Port quarantines and measures to remove urban nuisances were enforced more rigorously. In Sweden, alarm about the population following the 1749 census saw strategies introduced to promote personal hygiene education, police socially transmitted diseases, and establish municipal hospitals. Elsewhere, cleansing and improving cities were increasingly seen as worthwhile precautions. When plague arrived in Moscow in 1771, for example, senators argued that noxious vapours from industrial waste and domestic filth were responsible and directed their efforts accordingly. Concerns about the injurious effects of pestilential exhalations saw moves to close and relocate urban cemeteries, first in France and then elsewhere in Europe, and similar efforts were directed at slaughterhouses and other noxious trades.

Not all the responses built on traditional methods as evident in the introduction of smallpox inoculation to Europe from the Ottoman Empire and then vaccination following the method developed by the English physician Edward Jenner. Both practices generated religious, popular and medical opposition, which was slow to dissipate, but they offered a solution to one of the most lethal epidemic diseases afflicting nations. If few states followed Denmark (1810) or Sweden (1815) in making vaccination compulsory, state-sponsored vaccination programmes were introduced in many European states. The gradual adoption of these methods represented an opportunity for the development of systematic policies to target disease.

By the end of the eighteenth century, officials were no longer just seeking to respond to epidemics, but were beginning to think in terms of prevention. A growing desire to regulate the urban environment and its rural hinterland did see a decline in such diseases as dysentery and fever. Yet too much stock should not be placed in these efforts. Although there was a more defined public health movement in the eighteenth century, action was frequently episodic and poorly organized. It was in the following century that clear programmes of sanitary reform took shape.

Victorian public health reform: the English case

In trying to understand why after 1870 mortality declined in Western Europe, historians have turned their attention to nineteenth century sanitary reforms. Whereas early modern initiatives were neither permanent nor extensive, nineteenth century public health focused on preventive solutions. Questions of water supply, sewage disposal, housing, factory conditions, food quality, etc., became integral to local and state sanitary programmes. The English's public health crusade has been represented as emblematic of this approach to sanitary reform. As the 'first industrial nation', England was at the forefront of tackling the problems associated with industrialization and the shift to a predominantly urban society. It pioneered mains drainage systems, clean water supplies and slum clearance programmes. Although a concentration on England marginalizes what was happening elsewhere – including Scotland and Wales – the English approach served to inspire public health programmes elsewhere in Europe.

The arrival of Asiatic cholera has frequently been cited as stimulating reform. Until the 1810s, the disease had been mainly limited to Asia, but from 1817 cholera spread across Europe, bringing with it mounting fear and throwing into question existing health measures (see 'Disease'). Cholera killed quickly and nastily and medical practitioners appeared helpless against its spread. In Britain, the 1831–32 cholera epidemic arrived at a time of political and social upheaval. In *Cholera and Nation* (2008), Pamela Gilbert shows how medical and sanitary authorities used the idea of the nation to both assert the threat of cholera and extend their power. In response, a short-lived Board of Health and some twelve hundred local boards were created and new restrictions were placed on the inhabitants of towns. Initially, contagionist policies were pursued, but with cholera able to bypass quarantine measures, and with isolation provoking social unrest, greater faith was placed in anticontagionism and miasmatic theory. The latter suggested that because certain diseases were the result of inanimate particles in the air produced by decaying organic matter they could be targeted through preventive strategies directed at the urban environment. Although the measures introduced in response to the cholera epidemic were temporary, reformers continued to use the threat of epidemic diseases to campaign for measures that favoured cleaning up the urban environment, and in doing so drew on interlocking narratives of sanitation, masculinity, professionalization, social and political reform, and empire.

This chronology should be challenged. Local boards of health had been established in response to yellow fever (1805–06) and in Irish towns during a typhus epidemic (1817–19). Questions about public responsibility for health had been raised in the 1810s and 1820s. As anxiety rose about the effects of urbanization, and as fears were expressed about the underclass and popular unrest, a range of social reforms were proposed that drew on investigations into the relationship between poverty and disease. How to deal with poverty, epidemics and the associated environmental conditions became a major preoccupation in the 1820s and 1830s, not only among politicians, but also among civil servants, clergymen, doctors, philanthropists, social reformers and industry (such as water companies). As the solutions were not cheap, those keen to promote public health turned to the government.

The work of the lawyer Edwin Chadwick is often cited as the starting point for a coherent English public health movement. An architect of the New Poor Law, Chadwick was a devotee of Bentham's Utilitarianism and the belief that society should be reorganized in a way that promoted wellbeing. He associated poverty with disease having observed that many of the poor were driven to the workhouse through illness. Chadwick believed that an assault on the 'filth diseases' that resulted from poverty and overcrowding would increase productivity and reduce expenditure on welfare. Following outbreaks of influenza and typhoid in 1837 and 1838, he conducted an investigation into urban conditions with the aid of several doctors. The resulting *Report on the Sanitary Condition of the Labouring Population* (1842) was an exhaustive statement on urban sanitary conditions, but it was not a sudden departure. Although the *Report* pioneered methods of social investigation, the 1830s had seen a series of statistical and aetiological studies into the geography of health as demonstrated in the epidemiological work of William Farr. Statistics were already being harnessed to moral and social reform and the *Report* reflected broader philanthropic and reformist goals.

Chadwick's *Report* emphasized the range of problems facing towns and asserted a statistical connection between the environment and disease. For some historians its findings represented a dogmatic adoption of anticontagionism, which provided a rationale that emphasized prevention and concentrated attention on the environmental and social causes of sickness. A broader understanding of the wider factors that caused disease was marginalized in the *Report* in favour of a concentration on places and infrastructures. As Chadwick had little faith in doctors, his programme involved systems of water supply and sewage disposal and proposals to remove the sources of urban and industrial pollution.

This Chadwickian ethos was embodied in the 1848 Public Health Act. A centralized General Board of Health and a system of local boards were established which rationalized existing *ad hoc* arrangements. The General Board could require the formation of local boards, although most of its powers were advisory. A system of local inspection was created through the appointment of medical officers of health (MOH) and municipal authorities were given more powers to intervene, with funding for improvements coming from the local rates. More than this, Chadwick actively promoted sanitation and gave public health a particular institutional structure. Action favoured small-bore sewers, sewage farms, and high-pressure water supplies, but the powers granted to local authorities also permitted wider reforms. However, measures were adoptive rather than compulsory and Chadwick's vision of centralization was resented. After the General Board's first five-year term it was dissolved and Chadwick pensioned off.

From Chadwickian sanitary reform, the adoption of an epidemiological approach, and a new concept of 'state medicine' has been detected as doctors gained greater control following Chadwick's replacement in 1855 by John Simon, surgeon and MOH to the City of London. Simon oversaw the development of a public health administration that was unparalleled in Europe. This chronology suggests that under Simon a broader conception of state medicine emerged that brought medical experts into public health. Whereas Chadwick favoured sanitary engineering, Simon supported research into the nature of infectious diseases and local outbreaks as reflected in the work of John Snow and William Budd. Alongside this shift, legislation became less permissive: Simon's medical department acquired greater powers to coerce individuals – as apparent in vaccination policy – and local authorities. The remit of state medicine was extended; for example, into measures against occupational diseases and food adulteration. New powers were given to local authorities to intervene in the provision of clean water, to regulate housing, and to provide isolation hospitals. The appointment of MOHs was made compulsory, so that their numbers rose from 50 in 1872 to 1,770 by 1900.

However, a straightforward view that locates reform within a framework that emphasizes a transition from contagionism to anticontagionism does not hold up to scrutiny. Although medical theory did influence public health reforms, ideas about disease causation were not straightforward. Sanitary reformers often drew on both contagionist and anticontagionist approaches, seeing some diseases in terms of miasmas and others, such as smallpox, as contagious. Nor were ideas of disease causation the only parts of the equation. Geography, trade, experiences of disease, politics and economics were among the factors influencing policies. Sanitary reform was shaped by legal and administrative complexities, by money and expertise, as well as by ideological factors. As the wretched living conditions in the early nineteenth century cities were believed to be a predisposing cause of immorality, early reforms drew on a strong current of humanitarian and evangelical ideas that aimed to address these problems. This contributed to a political and reforming agenda that combined paternalism with Utilitarian ideas in an effort to reform the urban poor. Concerns about the nature of the urban environment hence blended notions of civic improvement with a moral rhetoric and a vision of a reformed society.

Historians have equally questioned the role of central government in sanitary reform. Problems and solutions varied from town to town and reflected local physical and socioeconomic circumstances. Public health policy was often all about devising strategies to deal with local problems. Local acts shaped provision and national legislation emphasized the need for local action. The degree to which legislation was used also depended on local political, social and medical circumstances as sanitary projects from the building of reservoirs and sewers to controls on housing were essentially local in nature. Considerable responsibility therefore rested not with central governments but with individual towns, an approach reinforced by contemporary faith in local solutions and by a civic gospel of improvement.

The English pattern broadly mirrors what was happening elsewhere in Europe, although few European governments invested as heavily in administrative structures until the end of the century. Concerns about urbanization and industrialization and fears of popular unrest were European in scope. These prompted statistical and aetiological investigations into the relationship between social conditions and mortality as demonstrated in the work of French hygienists. Fears of social upheaval merged with medical theories of miasmas to produce a profound anxiety about urban conditions. Epidemics confirmed these fears to create a stimulus for reform. France, for example, established a permanent High Council of Health in 1822 following the appearance of yellow fever in Barcelona. Although the High Council was less concerned with the local context, the importance of local responses to public health was evident in France, Germany, Sweden and Russia. States worked with a range of local agencies, voluntary organizations and professional groups to promote reform. However, as we will see below, the growth of a sanitary state apparatus was contested.

Professionalizing public health

As the English case study demonstrates, the development of public health has been associated with the growing influence of medical experts both as promoters of new measures and as technical advisors. To explain this process, historians have turned to ideas of professionalization and medicalization to examine how doctors asserted their expertise [see 'Professionalization'].

Whereas early modern responses to plague had been largely implemented by lay officials, medical practitioners were able to gain greater influence in the eighteenth century because of the growing political importance assigned to hygiene. In the German-speaking territories, new regulations required administrative districts to appoint a *physicus* – an official with responsibility for public health – and in France and Hungary networks of medical officers were established. In France, this growing medical emphasis was embodied in the Société Royale de Médecine whose members used public health as a means to widen the medical domain and their influence. In Britain, the formation of medical associations and pressure groups in the 1840s and the appointment of MOHs were important in promoting reform. In Germany, Max Josef de Pettenkofer's appointment to the first chair of hygiene in 1865 created an environment that saw experts take an increasing lead in public health, and in 1900 an advisory health council of medical experts was created. This growing use of experts was part of a broader trend in government, but professionalization was also apparent in other ways in the nineteenth century. It was evident in the formation of professional bodies, which sought a greater role in public policy, in the establishment of academic posts, and in the creation of professional qualifications in hygiene. In this account, sanitary reform and then bacteriology (see below), and the links sanitary officials made between moral and physical conditions, allowed the medical community to assert their authority over the individual and social body and assert their voice in the public sphere. This authority was consolidated in the twentieth century as public health policies came to concentrate on risk populations and public health specialists extended their influence over a range of institutions, including schools, and social and political concerns, such as pronatalism or venereal disease.

The idea that doctors were quickly able to dominate policy needs to be qualified, however. In Sweden, low numbers of practitioners ensured that medical policy remained in the hands of lay officials until the late nineteenth century. The same pattern can be detected in France and Germany, while in England Chadwick limited medical influence on early legislation. Often middle-class perceptions of the need to reform the urban environment mattered more than medical views. Civil servants tended to dominate policy and lay authorities were reluctant to cede control to medical practitioners whose status remained uncertain [see 'Professionalization']. Outside Britain, full-time appointments were comparatively rare until the late nineteenth century and most were poorly paid. It was only with bacteriology that medical practitioners were able to gain greater influence over health policy.

An emphasis on medical experts and professionalization undervalues the importance of other agencies in influencing public health. New sanitary officials were appointed – water and food analysts, health visitors, surveyors, engineers and public vaccinators – that took responsibility for public health work. This created overlapping and competing spheres of influence, which resulted in tensions with doctors. Journalists and social commentators made regular forays into poor districts and published revelations of shocking conditions that helped stimulate reform. Governments frequently worked with voluntary agencies, many of whom provided a vehicle for women's involvement in the public sphere. This was in clear attempts to tackle tuberculosis and venereal disease after 1890 and in moves to promote infant and child welfare, but at the same time public protests against public health policies, for example, against vaccination in Britain or the regulation of prostitution and venereal disease, involved voluntary organizations in opposition to reforms. Although medical practitioners were involved with these agencies, and sought authority over a range of policymaking arenas, public health should not just be seen in terms of medicalization or professionalization.

Measuring progress: 1850–1914

Measuring the impact of public health in the nineteenth century has focused on mortality decline as an index of improvement. From the late nineteenth century, mortality fell across Europe. Although infant mortality remained high, life expectancy had risen, cholera had been largely eradicated from Western Europe, and levels of other infectious diseases had fallen. This decline in infectious disease can be seen in crude deaths rates for England and Wales (see Table 12.1), while in Paris crude death rates from all water- and food-borne diseases fell by approximately 75 per cent between 1854 and 1889.

Whereas Thomas McKeown in *The Rise of Modern Populations* (1976) dismissed the role of medicine, suggesting that improved nutrition was the key, this view was subsequently challenged. In an influential article published in the first issue of the *Social History of Medicine* (1988), Simon Szreter argued that McKeown underestimated the significance of sanitary improvements, a view that came to be supported by other revisionists [see 'Disease']. Although historians have recognized the role of improved living standards and increased social stability in health, the revisionist thesis has been widely adopted. Improvements in the quality of the water supply and sewerage reduced levels of infectious disease, since water- and food-borne diseases spread by faecal contamination were the diseases that fell most rapidly after 1870. In addition, better water supplies and sewerage allowed city dwellers to put ideas of personal hygiene into practice, resulting in behavioural changes that had an important bearing on morbidity and mortality. Other public health measures, such as the creation of isolation hospitals and disinfection, also limited the spread of infectious diseases like typhus or smallpox.

Table 12.1 Infectious diseases in England and Wales, 1848–1910: Change in mean annual death rates per million for men (all ages)

	1848–72	*1901–10*	*% change*
Infectious diseases (all)	7,517	3,282	–56
Tuberculosis	3,432	1,902	–46
Scarlet fever & diphtheria	1,341	289	–78
Typhus & typhoid	899	110	–88
Smallpox	299	16	–95
Measles	435	328	–25
Whopping cough	471	255	–46
Influenza	68	216	+318
Cholera	231	0	–100
Dysentery	81	9	–89
Diarrhoea & enteritis	1,102	874	–21

Note: the grouping of diseases reflects contemporary assessments.
Source: Registrar-General's Office.

Progress was far from smooth or even, however. Strong regional patterns emerged. Although all areas of Europe experienced a broad epidemiological transition after 1870, there was a split between Eastern and Western Europe. High levels of infectious disease remained a problem in Eastern Europe. For example, Russian experiences, where infant mortality remained high and the rural population continued to face regular epidemics, were different from the situation in Britain or Prussia. Nor were divisions limited to Eastern Europe. In Italy, living and working conditions in rural rice growing regions ensured that levels of malaria remained high throughout the 1920s and 1930s.

This diversity extended to the scale of reform. Intervention depended on a number of factors: the energy of officials, local pressures and resources, the scale of the problem, and ideologies of intervention. There was considerable diversity between states, regions and towns. Although Russian municipal councils had dramatically improved sanitary conditions by 1914, particularly with regard to isolation hospitals and disinfection, the tendency remained to prefer cheap to clean water. Germany was slow to embrace public health. The 1866 cholera epidemic did encourage more prosperous towns to clean up the urban environment, while national and international sanitary conferences stimulated a sanitary movement, but many German cities made little attempt to improve the urban environment until the 1890s. Nor was Germany unusual. It was not until the last decade of the nineteenth century that there was an upsurge in intervention in many countries as health services were reorganized and new sanitary measures were imposed.

A simple split between authoritarian states and liberal governments does not explain this diversity. A lack of political consensus or political divisions created obstacles that frustrated the kind of comprehensive sanitary facilities often required. This was evident in Britain in the first half of the nineteenth century where socio-political divisions created obstacles to reform, but it was also characteristic of France under the Third Republic (1870–1940) where inefficiency combined with pressure from competing groups to create instability in government that limited action on public health. Finance was also often a problem. In Russia, for example, a restricted municipal tax base acted as a barrier to public health programmes. Elsewhere, ratepayer resistance to expensive sanitary measures limited what was achieved. Although some towns were active in tackling sanitary problems, others were reluctant to spend money or intervene.

Even when intervention was seen as desirable, how to intervene was not straightforward. As Christopher Hamlin's important study of four British boroughs reveals, many local authorities were bewildered and frustrated by the technical and legal complexities, and were fearful of getting it wrong.[1] Nor were local powers always sufficient to solve local problems. As a report on the Welsh town of Merthyr Tydfil explained in 1901: 'The sanitary inspectors are continually coming across grave cases of overcrowding, and yet are unable to advise proceedings in most instances, as the person [who] would be evicted have nowhere else to go'.[2] Responses to sanitary problems further had a geographical and class dimension. Although the language of reform targeted the habits of the poor, and highlighted the dangers of overcrowded and insanitary areas, poor areas were not always given the same protection as prosperous districts. Responses were further constrained by an initial understanding of reform that only included structural works, such as building sewers or improving water supplies. Sanitary authorities adapted policies to meet local needs, but the burden of work was considerable, especially in those districts where sanitary officials were part-time.

At the same time, public health measures were contested. In Russia, divisions existed within the medical community over reform, limiting action. In France and Britain, general practitioners remained wary of sanitary policies, worried that public health initiatives would deprive them of fee-paying patients. These divisions combined with active resistance as fears were voiced about government coercion. Government intervention in matters of health and cleanliness were easily construed as a violation of individual rights. These concerns are visible in ballads and radical newspaper reactions to sanitary reform and in opposition to the British vaccination acts, which expressed a fundamental hostility to the principle of compulsion. Often such opposition reflected a liberal perception of the boundaries of state intervention in personal life and raised questions about the nature of citizenship. But hostility to reform or individual measures was not just ideological. Quarantine measures were opposed by businesses, while local inhabitants fearful of infection resisted the building of isolation hospitals. Sanitary reforms that sought to alter personal habits or business practices equally provoked resistance.

Questions should therefore be asked about the impact or extent of public health measures. Regional and local diversity ensured a wide variety of intervention and sanitary reforms were frequently limited to tackling the conditions associated with infectious disease. This ensured that other areas were often neglected while an investment was made in the appearance of cleanliness and order. When progress in public health is measured against the factors discussed in this section, a more halting process is revealed.

Bacteriology and public health: 1880–1914

Historians have claimed that in the last two decades of the nineteenth century science was harnessed to public health in new ways in a bacteriological era as influences on health came to be divided into social and environmental conditions and scientifically investigable causes. Bacteriology offered the hope that the causes of infectious disease would be discovered, that diagnosis would be improved, and that treatments would bring these diseases under control. This led to a heightened focus on risk populations and the social behaviour of individuals as carriers of infectious disease. In Germany, Robert Koch and his researchers' demonstration that tuberculosis was contagious and Louis Pasteur's work in France on the anthrax vaccine appeared to offer definitive moments that asserted the role of the individual in the spread of disease and the capacity for intervention [see 'Science and medicine']. The result was a broad shift in public health efforts from inclusive measures of preventive medicine to a more exclusive focus on disease agents to create new ideologies of intervention that increased the authority of medical experts just as European states were expanding their welfare agencies. This was apparent in the newly unified Germany and in France under the Third Republic where bacteriology provided a legitimation for the extension of public hygiene measures. People not environments became the main focus of action through a range of policies that emphasized notification, isolation and disinfection. This was aided by laboratory diagnosis and by the introduction of vaccines made possible by bacteriological research. Sanitary practices were consequently downgraded and a new bacteriological justification for action came to dominate public health.

Bacteriology offered both a rationale for existing sanitary measures and encouraged a renewed emphasis on the importance of isolating and disinfecting individuals. By providing a means to identify the microorganisms responsible for disease, it held out the promise of prevention and treatment through isolation. This presented less costly solutions that appealed to administrators and did not require intervention in socioeconomic conditions. For example, legislation to combat venereal disease and tuberculosis focused on person-to-person transmission and the isolation of infected individuals. Measures were introduced in Britain and France to make certain infectious diseases notifiable. Systems of medical inspection and home visiting were instituted and special sanitary facilities were established at ports and railways for migrants from Eastern Europe to target disease-carriers. New public health laboratories were opened to undertake testing and research. The best example of this process is France where Pasteurian ideas were institutionalized. From the 1880s, municipal laboratories were opened along with a series of Pasteur Institutes (the first in Paris in 1888), which provided centres for research and training. Bacteriology also offered new cures. For example, diphtheria antitoxin was introduced in 1894, and an antityphoid vaccine in 1896. New serums were developed and large-scale immunization programmes were initiated; for example, against tuberculosis in France in 1924 and in Sweden in 1927.

Notwithstanding the importance attached to innovations in diagnosis and the value of a few therapeutic agents like the diphtheria antitoxin, bacteriology did not suddenly transform public health. Whereas it offered new rationales for existing practices, an ongoing interest in non-specific causes, such as poverty, which could not be explained by bacteriological explanations of disease, persisted. Nor did all countries embrace the new science in the same way. If in France and Germany it received public support and investment, in Britain there was no medical consensus on the value of bacteriology before the 1890s and many MOHs remained committed to epidemiology and sanitary science. Even in France, reactions to Pasteur and bacteriology depended on whether or not practitioners deemed it useful: mixed responses existed, with general practitioners being generally distrustful, a pattern that was repeated elsewhere in Europe. The early promise of bacteriology was also slow to emerge. Anti-vaccination sentiments, as reflected in the Bernard Shaw's play *The Doctor's Dilemma* (1916), reveal popular and professional tensions. Difficulties were encountered in producing vaccines, while the failure of Tuberculin as a miracle drug to treat tuberculosis exposed the limitations of bacteriology.

Nor did an understanding of bacteriology mean that old ideas were rejected. A localist understanding of epidemics based around ideas of contaminated water and soil persisted because it offered plausible explanations and a framework for local action. In Britain, where sanitary measures had resulted in improvements, many MOHs merely added a bacteriological understanding to existing ideas about the spread of infectious diseases to create a blunderbuss approach. Pathogenic microorganisms existed in bodies and in places, which were tackled through hygiene and environmental controls. Although new languages of intervention were created, the object was frequently the same. Mixed measures were often adopted. For example, British responses to cholera focused on preventing carriers from entering the country and targeted the environmental conditions that allowed cholera to spread. Sanitarians and reformers therefore continued to think in terms of structural sanitary reform, personal responsibility, hygiene and morality. As responses to the 1918–19 influenza pandemic demonstrate, traditional methods often offered officials more effective means of action.

The contribution of bacteriology is therefore mixed. Although bacteriology encouraged a new understanding of how infectious diseases were caused and transmitted, the benefits were often less tangible, and traditional sanitary and epidemiological approaches remained important. Nor was bacteriology the only rationale for encouraging a growing emphasis on the individual. As we will see in the next section, other currents existed that encouraged an interest in the individual.

Degeneration and eugenics

The emergence of a morass of scientific and social theories linked to ideas of degeneration, national efficiency and eugenics have been seen as a twentieth century European phenomenon as societies grappled with ongoing industrialization, class differentiation and conflict, and a growing need for government intervention in an intellectual climate that favoured science. Whereas the ideas associated with eugenics had become a dirty word following the revelations of the racial hygiene policies adopted in Nazi Germany (1933–45), concerns about degeneration and eugenics branched out into other reform movements. In looking at degeneration and eugenics in this way, an uncomfortable picture emerges of the influence of scientific ideas and concerns about biological fitness on contemporary thinking and public health movements.

In debates about degeneration and eugenics, the idea that urbanization corrupted physical and moral health was paramount. As we have seen, these ideas were not novel. They were present in eighteenth century France and Russia, and emerged as a more general European phenomenon in the mid nineteenth century. They built on the rhetoric employed by early sanitary reformers who connected poverty to social conditions and on the growing belief that some diseases were hereditary. Charles Darwin's controversial ideas about evolution added a new dimension to these ideas that was manipulated by others. His selection theory, which he applied to civilization in *The Descent of Man* (1891), was developed by his first cousin Francis Galton. Galton claimed that in modern societies the unfit were no longer removed by natural selection and that as a consequence the level of poor heredity and hence disease increased in the population. As alarm about the negative consequences of urbanization intensified after 1870, these ideas gained widespread currency as confidence was expressed in the ability of science to manage society. Social Darwinists warned about the deleterious effects of urbanization on the future of the race, while social investigations pointed to the existence of a diseased underclass that many found threatening. Moral categories were added that combined ideas about behaviour with notions of heredity to scapegoat the diseased poor as a threat to the biological, social and moral order. Military humiliations – for example, Italy's campaigns in East Africa – and declining birth rates were used to justify these fears. Degenerationism served to provide a language that articulated a host of contemporary fears about heredity, health and the upheavals of urbanization and democratization, to focus alarm on the future health of the nation.

The emergence of eugenic movements in most European states in the twentieth century gave expression to these ideas. Eugenics was both a social movement and a science. Although national movements had their own particular composition, they shared common characteristics. Eugenics was loosely divided between 'negative' and 'positive' measures. The logical extension of hereditary notions was the need to prevent negative taints from being passed on to future generations – or negative eugenics. Environmental solutions could be rejected in favour of measures to protect the unborn using an argument where breeding mattered more than living conditions. 'Positive' eugenics favoured policies that encouraged a stronger, healthier society. Eugenics was hence concerned with improving the nation and the race through either controlling reproduction or the environment. However, such an assessment of eugenics pre-supposes a coherent ideology. Even at a national level, eugenics covered a wide range of conflicting aims, ideas and political perspectives. Distinctions were often blurred: eugenics was characterized by a complex set of scientific and political issues that were frequently in tension. This not only narrowed the grounds for agreement, but also ensured that clear policies often failed to emerge.

Notwithstanding the publicity that surrounded degenerationist and eugenic theories there was comparatively little eugenic legislation [see 'Healthcare and the state']. In Britain, leading medical officers opposed negative measures in

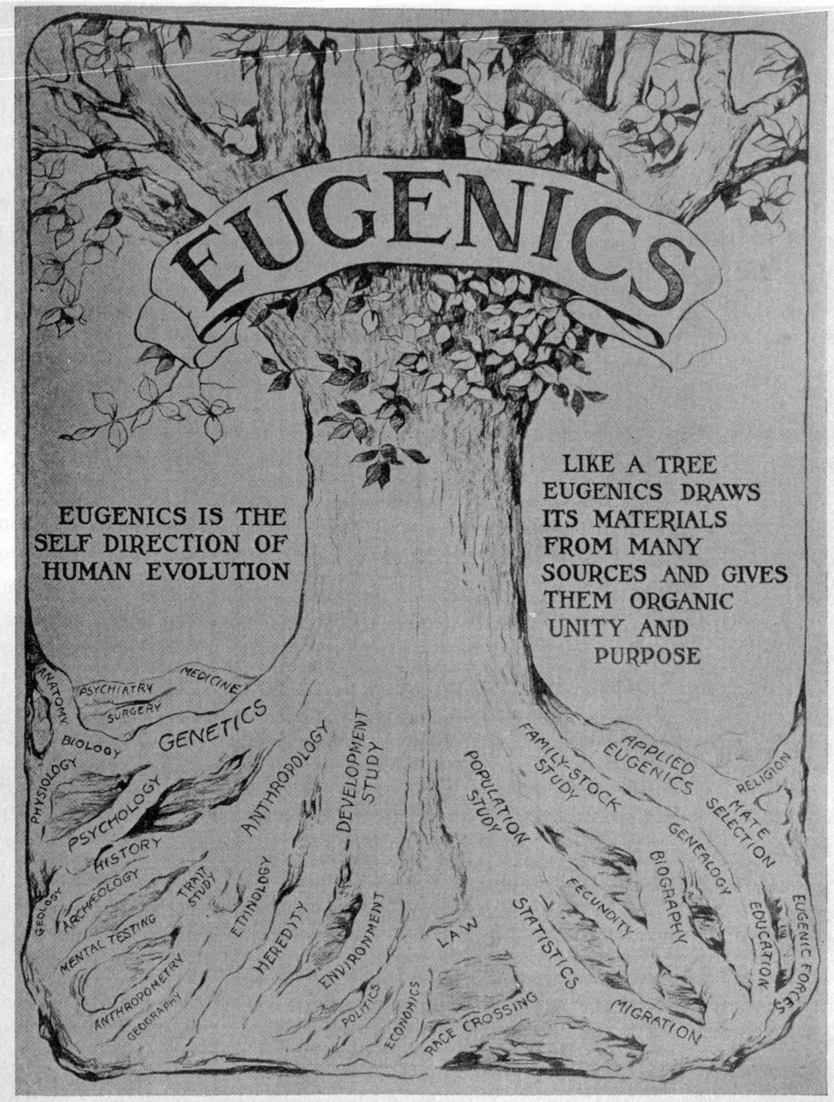

Figure 12.2 'The relation of eugenics to other sciences'. The illustration, used for the Third International Congress of Eugenics held at the American Museum of Natural History, New York, in August 1932, represents the 'tree' of eugenics and the range of ideas and disciplines that influenced its growth.

Source: Wellcome Library, London.

favour of comprehensive healthcare, while the 1904 *Report of the Inter-Departmental Committee on Physical Deterioration* – often seen as the highpoint of degenerationist thinking in Britain – favoured a range of social and environmental measures to promote general health. Yet fears of degeneration and a declining birth rate influenced the language of public health and health reform movements. Although it would be easy to suggest that these ideas reached their height in Nazi Germany, in most European countries they provided doctors with a powerful rhetoric that combined with existing concerns about urbanization and infant mortality to promote further public health measures. As the example of Sweden shows, doctors employed these arguments to acquire a key role in health policy. A degenerationist discourse and eugenics was harnessed to public health as evident in France, Italy and Spain. It informed child health and maternity provision [see 'Women and medicine']. It influenced measures to control the spread of venereal disease and tuberculosis, and informed the health reform movements of the 1920s and 1930s, which in advocating dietary restrictions, exercise, sunbathing and personal cleanliness, influenced health education and local initiatives to counter the dangers of urban lifestyles. However, as demonstrated in the next section, public health in the twentieth century covered more than these concerns.

Redefining public health: 1919–2000

The 1920s and 1930s have been characterized as marking a new era in state medicine [see 'Healthcare and the state']. If the state had played a minimal role in the 1880s, by the 1920s governments guided by medical experts and central health departments were becoming increasingly involved in the delivery of healthcare. Once confidence in preventing and controlling disease had recovered following the 1918–19 influenza pandemic, attention focused less on infectious diseases and more on the general health of the population and social diseases like venereal disease and tuberculosis as existing regulatory frameworks were adapted. This creates a problem. Much of the twentieth century history of public health is so caught-up with state welfare that often public health has been downplayed in favour of studies that have looked at, for example, pronatalism or the responses to tuberculosis. For scholars influenced by feminist and Foucaultian concepts of social control, these efforts have been subsumed into accounts that have examined the growth of surveillance and social disciplining as exemplified by responses to venereal disease.

In the 1920s, public health took on a stronger international dimension. Although internationalism was a feature of debates about the value of quarantine and disease controls in the late nineteenth century, after 1918 new international organizations were established and staffed by experts. The newly formed League of Nations (1919/20–46) directed part of its efforts to disease prevention, receiving considerable support from the United States-based Rockefeller

Foundation. An Epidemics Commission was established in 1920 to coordinate responses to outbreaks, and in 1925 further monitoring services were created in Geneva and Singapore. The League published monographs for public health workers, conducted investigations into cholera, rabies and tuberculosis vaccines, and organized national vaccination programmes. Malaria eradication was enthusiastically adopted in the 1920s, as well as investigations into tropical diseases. As a philanthropic body, the Rockefeller Foundation had its own programme. It favoured preventive measures on a country-by-country basis, evident in its support between 1916 and 1926 for the French campaign against tuberculosis. The Rockefeller Foundation equally invested heavily in Central Europe as it sought to transplant American models of public health to prevent rather than contain epidemics.

Whereas European states often resented the League or the Rockefeller Foundation's directives, at a national level, the extension of the franchise and movements for national self-determination and democratization after 1919 saw new agencies established to promote public health: for example, Poland created a Ministry of Public Health in 1918, and France created a Ministry of Hygiene, Assistance and National Insurance two years later. As governments stepped up their public health programmes, priorities came to favour the general health of the population, even if they remained constrained by existing infrastructures and an ongoing emphasis on preventing infection. A massive investment was made in public health in Soviet Russia (1922–91). Swamps were drained, land reclaimed and treatment programmes were introduced to combat malaria. Smallpox vaccination was made compulsory; tuberculosis and venereal disease were targeted through dispensaries. Although reforms were not as sustained in other European countries, the boundaries between public health and state medicine were increasingly blurred as ideas of positive health acquired a new political importance. This was clear in France under the Popular Front (1936–38).

For Dorothy Porter an important component of these new approaches to public health was social medicine. She argues that supporters of social medicine endeavoured to transform preventive practice as part of an international debate about the role of the state in social welfare.[3] As a concept, social medicine owed much to Soviet attempts to abolish the distinctions between curative and preventive medicine. It emphasized the social conditions within which disease occurred and stressed prophylaxis. Soviet ideas influenced a generation of public health intellectuals and various attempts were made to institutionalize social medicine in Belgium, Germany, France and Britain. In Nazi Germany, a different approach was adopted as racial hygiene came to dominate [see 'Healthcare and the state'].

However, public health infrastructures often remained unchanged. Just as before 1914, public health continued to be constructed around local or municipal services. Often capital expenditure was directed at those areas that municipal authorities had already invested in: for example, maternity, infant and child welfare, or tuberculosis dispensaries and sanatoriums. Less was done to expand other services. If public health programmes in the 1920s and 1930s were an extension of pre-1914 approaches, new rationales were developed around bacteriology and social hygiene. These provided a focus for a network of institutions and health professionals, as evident in the massive investment in tackling tuberculosis.

By the 1920s, the control of epidemic diseases had become routine and identification, isolation and vaccination were central to national health programmes. Large-scale immunization was started and vaccination against smallpox, diphtheria and tetanus became commonplace. In the workplace, there was a new enthusiasm to make factories efficient and healthy through medical screening, better sanitary facilities and canteens. A wide range of inspectorates and clinics were established to serve communities or particular groups. This was particularly manifest in the investment in clinics for infants and children [see 'Women and medicine']. Provision mixed concerns about socioeconomic deprivation with medical and educational policies, drawing on established ideas about environmental conditions and a rhetoric that blamed high infant mortality on maternal ignorance, particularly among the poor. Children also became targets through the provision of school medical services. Other services (both voluntary and municipal) were directed at promoting healthy bodies and habits through playing fields, social clubs and other physical activities.

New initiatives were launched and old ones were redefined. This can be seen in the substantial investment in anti-tuberculosis programmes in Britain, France and Germany. If the French pioneered tuberculosis dispensaries and German campaigns focused on the sanatorium, all three countries created networks of institutions backed up by inspectors, health education and nursing programmes. Prophylaxis was often central to these agencies' efforts, as can be seen in work of the French National Social Hygiene Office or in the anti-malarial campaigns in Italy. Contemporary interest in health as a personal responsibility and duty of citizenship encouraged investment in health education, much of which was directed at women. Radio programmes and films were produced, and hygiene, nutrition, domestic upkeep and work were all shown to be crucial as health education stressed the importance of physical culture and health [see 'Disease'].

The period following the Second World War (1939–45) witnessed a substantial investment in healthcare [see 'Healthcare and the state']. Although this favoured hospital medicine as social and political support for public health declined, traditional policies continued to be pursued, at least in the immediate post-war years. Wartime experiences had emphasized the value of vaccination. New programmes were initiated, aided by pharmaceutical companies' pursuit of vaccines for infectious diseases, such as whooping cough, polio and smallpox. Following the introduction of penicillin, the development of new antibiotics transformed the approach to tuberculosis and other infectious diseases. Other efforts were directed at preventing disease, as evident in the use of the pesticide DDT to combat malaria. Although continuities remained – for example, in slum clearance programmes or in measures to target environmental pollution as evident in British responses to smog – public health was gradually redefined. As chronic rather than infectious diseases came to dominate concerns, emphasis was placed on education as greater stress was given to social behaviour within a context that highlighted long-term risks and lifestyles [see 'Disease'].

By the late 1960s, public health was at a crossroads. A massive investment in biomedicine had seen a shift from preventive to curative medicine. The apparent success of biomedicine saw research and investigations into infectious diseases downplayed and the emergence of a different kind of population-based research more interested in chronic illnesses [see 'Science and medicine']. Public health had declined in importance and its officials had taken on an increasingly managerial role in coordinating non-institutional services. Welfare reforms, an ageing population, and epidemiological studies on the relationship between lifestyle and disease, necessitated a new role for public health that was more in tune with the contemporary emphasis on single issues, such as smoking, and ideas about personal responsibility. Partly in response to debates on smoking and the use of evidence-based medicine in policy, a new agenda that focused on risk and lifestyle choices came to dominate public health. Emphasis was placed on promoting healthy lifestyles just as the cost of healthcare was spiralling. In the process, the traditional role of public health specialists was eroded as new media techniques were employed, controls were introduced on advertising, and taxation (such as on cigarettes) was used to encourage healthy behaviour.

In the 1980s, fears of an AIDS pandemic and new international interest in environmental issues, as embodied in the World Health Organization's Healthy Cities initiative, revived debate about the nature of public health. Although there had been a growing emphasis on primary care in the previous decade, more funds were directed at health education and promotion, but tensions between values of liberty, privacy and compulsion became apparent in responses to AIDS. Reactions to Severe Acute Respiratory Syndrome (SARS) at the start of the twenty first century raised further questions about balancing individual rights with ideas of community health security. Concerns about the impact and cost of diseases associated with lifestyle, such as obesity, created new challenges and saw renewed educational efforts. The resurgence of tuberculosis and venereal disease alongside the emergence of new threats, such as BSE, required new responses, but it was the fears of a global pandemic that focused attention on ideas of containment and the role of public health.

By thinking about questions of compulsion, ideas of liberty and privacy, and health education it becomes possible to place twenty first century public health in a longer history. Although the sanitary engineering projects of the nineteenth century became less visible, public health continued to remain contested and influenced by international, national, regional, political, socioeconomic and professional concerns.

Further reading

The classic study of public health remains George Rosen's *From Medical Police to Social Medicine* (New York: Science History Publications, 1974). Dorothy Porter's *Health, Civilization and the State: History of Public Health from Ancient to Modern Times* (London: Routledge, 1999) presents a wide-ranging synthesis that examines the nature of public health and welfare. On plague, Paul Slack, *The Impact of the Plague in Tudor and Stuart England* (Oxford: Clarendon Press, 1990) provides a seminal study, while the work of Carlo Cipolla, *Fighting the Plague in Seventeenth-Century Italy* (Madison, WI: University of Wisconsin Press, 1981) and John Alexander, *Bubonic Plague in Early Modern Russia* (Oxford: Oxford University Press, 2003) explore Italian and Russian responses. All take in wider issues of public health, with Annemarie Kinzelbach, 'Infection, Contagion and Public Health in Late Medieval and Early Modern German Imperial Towns', *Journal of the History of Medicine and Allied Sciences* 61 (2006), pp. 369–89, offering insights into public health at a local level. A considerable literature exists on the impact of cholera, with Margaret Pelling, *Cholera, Fever and English Medicine 1825–1865* (Oxford: Clarendon Press, 1978) concentrating on the theoretical debates, while Richard Evans's *Death in Hamburg: Society and Politics in the Cholera Years 1830–1910* (Oxford: Clarendon Press, 1991) examines the social and political dimension. Peter Baldwin's *Contagion and the State in Europe 1830–1930* (Cambridge: Cambridge University Press, 2005) offers a comparative perspective on how contagious diseases affected public policy in Europe, while Ann La Berge, *Mission and Method* (Cambridge: Cambridge University Press, 1992) explores public health in early nineteenth century France. A good starting point for Victorian Britain is Anthony S. Wohl, *Endangered Lives: Public Health in Victorian Britain* (London: Methuen, 1983). For more detailed studies, Christopher Hamlin's *Public Health and Social Justice in the Age of Chadwick: Britain 1800–54* (Cambridge: Cambridge University Press, 2009) provides an unrivalled examination of the early public health movement, while Anne Hardy's *The Epidemic Streets: Infectious Disease and the Rise of Preventive Medicine 1856–1900* (Oxford: Clarendon Press, 1993) is an incisive analysis of the spread and demographic impact of the major killer-diseases in Britain. Less has been written about other European states. Accessible overviews are provided in Dorothy Porter (ed.), *The History of Public Health and the Modern State* (Amsterdam: Rodopi, 1994), with more detailed studies provided by Manfred Berg and Geoffrey Cocks (eds), *Medicine and Modernity: Public Health and Medical Care in Nineteenth- and Twentieth-Century Germany* (Cambridge: Cambridge University Press, 2002), N.E. Christiansen and K. Petersen, 'The Nordic Welfare States', *Scandinavian Journal of History* 26 (2001), pp. 153–56, and David Barnes, *The Great Stink of Paris and the Nineteenth-Century Struggle against Filth and Germs* (Baltimore, MD: Johns Hopkins University Press, 2006). On the impact of public health, the best starting point in Simon Szreter's article, 'The Importance of Social Intervention in Britain's Mortality Decline, c.1850–1914: A Reinterpretation of the Role of Public Health', *Social History of Medicine* 1 (1988), pp. 1–37. Although few studies have looked at gender, Alison Bashford's *Purity and Pollution: Gender, Embodiment and Victorian Medicine* (Basingstoke: Palgrave Macmillan, 1998) offers a provocative account. Less has been written about the twentieth century and for wider discussions of state welfare and eugenics readers should look at the Further Reading in Chapter 13, while the role of international organizations in public health is explored in Paul Weindling (ed.), *International Health Organizations and Movements, 1918–1939* (Cambridge: Cambridge University Press, 1995).

13
Healthcare and the state

Historians have often claimed that European states followed a similar evolutionary path and that patterns of welfare converged. One way of thinking about this expansion of state healthcare would suggest that rapid population growth from the sixteenth century onwards overburdened welfare institutions established in the medieval period and encouraged states to increasingly intervene. Whereas studies in the 1950s stressed benevolent progress, historians in the 1960s and 1970s explored how European governments pursued increasingly centralized welfare policies as pragmatic solutions to the problems generated by industrialization. Connections between welfare, the growth of government and the relative strength of Liberalism were detected and state intervention in healthcare became associated with welfare capitalism. By thinking in this way, the growth of social welfare in the nineteenth century became associated with what Derek Fraser has referred to in *The Evolution of the British Welfare State* (1973) as the 'logic of industrialization' and its resulting social dislocation and breakdown in familial and community ties. Such an approach suggests that progress was incremental as governments took an increasing interest in the welfare of their populations.

There are problems with this account. It does not explain why less industrialized societies like Sweden developed similar systems of welfare, while the notion of patterns of welfare converging and culminating in the welfare state reinforces the idea of inevitable modernity. It is also possible to put forward different national stories, but as Peter Baldwin makes clear in *Contagion and the State in Europe* (2005), the history of welfare is not reducible to interventionism versus *laissez-faire*, authoritarianism versus liberalism. As scholars have moved beyond national narratives and implicit assumptions about the unproblematic nature of welfare policy, they have emphasized the fragile relations that existed between central and local government and the considerable scope for local initiative. They have come to examine national cultures, changing class relations, the nature of state formation and the role of medical experts as ways of explaining the growing participation of the modern state in healthcare. As a consequence, more complex histories of social policy have emerged that analysed gender, eugenics and professionalization, and the connections between state welfare and modernity. For Foucauldians, welfare came to represent a means of disciplining first the deviant and the poor and then the social body. If the social-disciplining paradigm prominent in writing in the 1980s and 1990s at times overestimated the extent to which medical authority and the power of the state saturated society, it encouraged historians to examine the connections between the state and the growing authority of medicine.

Yet where to draw the limits of the state's influence remains problematic. It was not restricted to institutional provision or health insurance schemes. For example, European governments were actively involved in colonial and military medicine [see 'Medicine and empire' and 'Medicine and warfare']. Legislative control, for example of abortion and in licensing practitioners, involved the state both in medical debates and medical practices [see 'Professionalization']. It is equally hard to unpick the historiographies that surround poor relief and the involvement of the state in medical care. Historiographies of nursing and professionalization have emphasized the reluctant role of governments in shaping licensing requirements, drawing on notions of the market [see 'Nursing' and 'Professionalization']. Research on public health has attributed growing state intervention to epidemics, changes in medical knowledge, and growing professional authority [see 'Public health']. Often state or public medicine before 1939 has been seen to mean public health, but more broadly, social historians of medicine have pointed to a medicalization of society and the growing authority of medical experts and the state from the late nineteenth century onwards to define the normal and the pathological. This interest in biopolitics has come to associate medicine with the coercive aspects of twentieth century states to create new domains of power, an approach visible in research on state-sponsored social engineering in the Soviet Russia (1922–92) and Nazi Germany (1933–45) as public medicine was seen in a more authoritarian and controlling light.

Rather than dealing with how governments regulated medical practice [see 'Professionalization'] or tackled sanitary problems [see 'Public health'], this chapter concentrates on the eighteenth, nineteenth and twentieth centuries to examine the role of the state in the provision of healthcare. Although it is difficult to reduce national systems to a single pattern – there were similarities but also important differences in how European states defined and intervened in welfare – this chapter draws out broad trends. Rather than simply suggesting that important changes occurred at particular points in time, the chapter uses a chronological approach to examine a number of thematic questions: why did European governments become involved in healthcare? What was the extent of doctors' influence? How much was state involvement influenced by political ideas, ideologies of intervention, or by social and class pressures?

State, medicine and welfare: 1600–1870

Closely tied to systems of poor relief, the dynamics of the state's responsibility for healthcare in sixteenth and seventeenth century Europe reflected the small, decentralized and fragmented nature of early modern states. Medical services were structured around poor relief and were essentially local in nature, dependent on local resources, and directed at the poor or transient as other social groups were expected to pay for care or medicines. Provision drew on an intricate network of agencies and authorities that included the Church, parishes, municipal authorities, charities and individual benefactors. The devastating effects of plague and other epidemics forced local as well as central states to act and establish isolation hospitals and introduce quarantine and other measures [see 'Public health']. For example, Verona responded to regular epidemics by creating an almshouse and introduced further taxes to aid the poor. By the early seventeenth century, many city authorities had developed a complex, if informal system of medical relief for the poor. This was dispensed either through institutional care or in the form of outdoor relief by providing medicines, food or medical assistance to the poor in their homes. As the examples of Italy and Spain demonstrate, civic authorities also managed common poor funds and hospital foundations [see 'Hospitals']. Elsewhere, civic authorities appointed surgeons, physicians and other healers to treat the poor. Parish records demonstrate that the sick poor generally received sympathetic and humane treatment and had access to a range of medical services.

Historians have argued that the expansion of systems of poor relief was necessitated by the considerable socioeconomic changes that affected sixteenth and seventeenth century Europe. Population growth and economic expansion required new forms of relief, but provision was also shaped by fears of vagrancy and social disorder. As suggested in Chapter 3, the Reformation and Counter-Reformation created new rationales for poor relief, which were used to uphold religious identities and reinforce community values. Systems of relief were therefore more than just anxious reactions to an increase in the numbers of the poor. They mixed economic, moral and religious concerns as distinctions were made between the 'deserving' poor, who were victims of their condition or who had fallen on hard times, and the 'undeserving' poor, a group that included beggars and prostitutes.

From these early modern origins, the expansion of social welfare in the eighteenth century has been associated with the emergence of a capitalist and market economy, the growth of towns, and the resulting breakdown of social and familial networks of support. Certainly, population growth, increased social mobility, and industrialization stretched systems designed for pre-industrial economies, but as discussed in the previous chapter, concern for social welfare also reflected a growing interest in mercantilism and the population as a source of national prosperity. If the idea of 'medical police' – which outlined the need for hygiene and other welfare measures as a means to strengthen the nation – offered a rationale for regulation, Enlightenment humanitarianism and new political and moral philosophies also emphasized the utility of government intervention. Whereas in some states, such as Russia, this took the form of Enlightened Absolutism, many European states increasingly perceived health as essential to political and economic strength.

Governments responded differently to the same problems but broad patterns can be detected. Measures focused on tackling epidemics [see 'Public health'] and in providing aid to the sick poor through the growth of specialized institutions, such as isolation hospitals, limited institutional support, and outdoor relief. In Germany, a network of municipal hospitals, dispensaries and convalescent homes were created, while in France an institutional framework was established under Louis XIV that responded first to epidemics by dispatching boxes of remedies and medical personnel and then in the nineteenth century saw public support for hospitals and public assistance programmes introduced. Although in Britain the New Poor Law (1834) was designed to deter people from applying for relief, a system of institutional relief evolved around the workhouse. Following scandals in the 1860s, greater attention was directed at offering the sick poor medical care as contemporaries started to talk about workhouse sick wards as public hospitals. Legislation allowed for the creation of separate Poor Law infirmaries and efforts were made to improve services. If these institutions often offered only basic provision, they became important providers of medical care for anyone who could not obtain care by other means. Beyond these institutions, many European states appointed or paid for doctors to oversee measures to prevent disease or to provide medical assistance to the poor. Outdoor relief was often valued over institutional care. In France, for example, a generous public assistance programme was adopted in 1794. *Bureaux de Bienfaisance* (welfare bureaus) were gradually established in each administrative district to supply medicines and to pay physicians to treat the sick poor. Gradually, European states acquired new obligations, including vaccination programmes or the care of the insane [see 'Asylums'], and exerted a supervisory role over medical provision.

To explain this process the historian Peter Laslett advanced the idea of 'nuclear hardship' whereby the shift to nuclear families in the late eighteenth and nineteenth centuries encouraged individuals to become progressively more dependent on formal systems of relief. Whereas Laslett's hypothesis draws attention to how a lack of local or familial resources shaped poor relief and individual decisions, it does not work for all European countries. Nor does it tell the entire story. Public funding for, and involvement in medical care was not simply demand driven or the result of industrialization. Changing attitudes to poor relief also played their part as after 1750 European states became alarmed about pauperism. These concerns merged with desires to improve national efficiency and a need to reduce the cost of poor relief to create systems of relief that were designed to impose social and moral controls. For Foucauldians, such attempts to create well-disciplined and healthy subjects were part of a growing ideological shift to support the extension of state control. One commonly used example of this process is how the system of poor relief in Britain was reformed through the 1834 Poor Law Amendment Act around the principle of 'less eligibility' and the workhouse test to discourage pauperism and reduce the welfare bill. Similar debates surrounded the introduction of the Elberfeld System in Germany, which aimed to cut relief expenditure by providing care based on need to encourage the poor to return to work. These ideas have been used to explain why conditions of indoor (or institutional) poor relief were often deemed demeaning or inadequate.

Renewed concerns about the strength of the nation equally had a role in promoting new programmes of poor relief and state-funded institutions. In Sweden, these fears saw a raft of measures introduced that favoured acute care. In France, similar anxieties stimulated debate about public welfare, but it was the Revolution (1789–99) that provided a mechanism for change as legislators attempted to establish a state-directed *bienfaisance*. French reforms reveal the tensions between different political approaches and values that informed welfare programmes. Ideals of equality and fraternity encouraged a sense that welfare was a right or civic responsibility, but the hopes of the revolutionaries were countered by those who resisted state intervention. They were further constrained by ideas of economic freedom, the sanctity of property, and a strong sense of local autonomy. In France and elsewhere, powerful *laissez-faire* ideas and faith in the role of charity served to limit state intervention.

In thinking about the changes to poor relief and the nature of public welfare in the nineteenth century, historians have come to emphasize how tensions existed between national legislation and local implementation, with the later crucial to how services developed. In Prussia, the state initially kept a distance from intervening in local welfare systems, believing that local solutions were best. In Sweden, the idea that parishes were responsible for their poor parishioners was enshrined in legislation in 1847. Cities and municipal authorities were often central in introducing health services. This is evident in Russia where the creation of new local administrations or *zemstvos* in 1864 saw a community-based system of free medical care established in many rural communities. Elsewhere in Europe, demand for services at a local level often forced the pace of change, ensuring that urban and rural patterns of care emerged that reflected local ideologies of welfare, population densities, geography and accessibility.

Nor does state provision fit with a simple model of progress. Although in Paris and Berlin public welfare institutions offered high standards of care for all sections of society, this was not replicated elsewhere in France or Germany. Some cities or regions were reluctant or unable to invest money: by 1871, over 40 per cent of communes in France lacked a welfare bureau. Financial support for welfare was often limited and the medical care offered by municipal authorities was generally considered to be of poor quality. For example, if municipal medical services did expand in Britain, they were constrained by opposition to adding to the burden on local rates. Hence, in many areas, the organizations responsible for local welfare continued to follow traditional, localized patterns of relief.

Rather than the nineteenth century witnessing an inevitable shift to public relief, voluntary organizations remained crucial to the provision of medical care. They were supported by Catholic and Protestant faith in the value of benevolence, by civic pride, and by the range of selfless and self-interested factors that influenced charity. Medical self-help and mutualism created networks of mutual aid societies that provided support during times of sickness. Yet, notwithstanding the strength of the voluntary sector, distinctions between private, charitable and public provision were not rigid. In France, *bureaux de bienfaisance* were financed by a combination of public and private charity, while in Spain, civic governments worked with the Catholic Church to create institutions for socially marginal groups. Such services limited the burden on the public purse and created what has been described as a 'mixed economy of welfare', the boundaries of which were gradually redefined during the nineteenth century.

The perceived stigma surrounding public medicine has encouraged historians to believe that poor relief was shunned and that its provision was a middle-class attempt at control. This idea owes much to work in the social sciences on the stigma of poverty and creates a simplistic picture – one that emphasizes opposition and obscures the fact that the medical relief available from state agencies was an important source of assistance for many. Although indoor or outdoor poor relief was often inadequate or demeaning, recipients were far from helpless or hopeless. In Britain, the poor had a right to relief under the New Poor Law, which, notwithstanding initial intense opposition, they did use. Scholars have increasingly come to recognize that relief was frequently negotiated; that the poor had agency, with the need to use public-funded services shaped by household structure and access to familial or community resources. Individuals or heads of households frequently made decisions to use municipal services to avoid hardship or because the services dispensed were desired.

As this section has illustrated, efforts to extend poor relief remained fragmented and shaped by a range of factors that had as much to do with political ideas, conceptions of relief and local resources, as they did with industrialization and demand. Although the boundaries of state intervention in medical care and welfare grew, a localized and flexible framework dominated relief. Rather than recipients being simple victims of surveillance, they employed a range of strategies to secure what they believed was their entitlement. The result was a mixed economy of care in which the state had a limited if growing role. As the next section demonstrates, the boundaries of this mixed economy of welfare changed in the late nineteenth and early twentieth century.

Health and the state: 1870–1914

Historians have commonly described the years 1870 to 1914 as a period in which access to medicine and medical care expanded. They have attributed this expansion to the state as across Europe governments established new welfare services and insurance schemes. The process of nation-building encouraged new views of the state and nation to emerge as existing welfare arrangements became unable to meet the problems facing modern industrialized societies. New rationales for intervention were put forward that challenged *laissez-faire* ideas. For example, republicans in France espoused Solidarism that asserted the need for mutual dependence and justified a broad welfare programme that balanced the rights of the individual with ideas of social responsibility. These changing attitudes to welfare were aided by the rediscovery of poverty by social investigators, and by mounting anxiety about degeneration and social upheaval. Existing concerns about the dangers of urbanization and fears of a breakdown in social and familial institutions were reworked as health and welfare became political issues.

European governments responded to these concerns and extended or established systems of relief, insurance schemes and medical services as it became clear that voluntary organizations – such as charities and churches – could no longer meet demand for welfare and that more collectivist solutions were needed. By the outbreak of war in 1914, the dimensions and coverage of public medicine had grown considerably. At the same time, medical practitioners had become more closely involved with nation-states and policymaking. New health priorities encouraged a shift in policy as social reforms and insurance schemes were enlarged to cover larger sections of the population. This was evident in Britain: Poor Law medical services were extended to the non-destitute as many towns after 1870 followed London's lead and built public infirmaries and dispensaries. Although facilities were limited when compared to those available in charitable hospitals, demand for municipal health services rose. Often healthcare could not be separated from other social questions – such as unemployment or pronatalism – but the growing involvement of governments in health provision encouraged changes in the relationship between the state and the individual.

Although the acceptance of statist solutions varied as governments struggled with the medical profession, developed new systems of funding, and tried to persuade the public that state-sponsored programmes benefited all segments of society, a large body of historical literature argues that only minor differences existed in terms of chronology and emphasis. European governments did copy each other, adapting welfare programmes to suit their needs, finances and political systems, and to reflect prevailing attitudes to state intervention. Limited insurance schemes for accident, sickness and unemployment were created. Specific diseases believed to be undermining the nation were tackled through clinics and institutional solutions [see 'Public health']. Women and children became prime targets for assistance as governments embraced pronatalist policies within a framework that utilized structures and practices that reflected contemporary gender ideologies [see 'Women and medicine']. School medical services were established in Germany, France and Britain; public-funded midwifery care was extended, milk supplies were regulated, and emphasis was placed on improving infant and childcare. Many of these measures were not just about curing the diseased but also about promoting healthy lifestyles.

Historians have traditionally argued that Germany embodied a move to progressive social legislation that was copied by other European states. Prussia took the lead and following unification in 1871 social policy was extended. Compulsory health, accident and old age insurance was introduced under the 'iron chancellor' Bismarck in the 1880s, mixing contributions from employers and employees. Initially insurance was only compulsory for low-paid manual workers, but by 1919, the majority of the German population were covered. This created a substantial fund not only for the treatment of individuals through hospital and doctors' services but also for the modernization of these services. Other European states followed, although as the example of Sweden demonstrates some sickness insurance schemes were voluntary in nature.

A different pattern is believed to have existed in France. Scholars have argued that France under the Third Republic (1870–1940) was slow to introduce effective welfare and medical programmes. This has been attributed to economic and social backwardness, resistance to state intervention, and the strength of narrow-minded business interests. There is some truth to these claims. During the early years of the Third Republic, welfare was not a priority as the future of the republic was debated. Attempts to establish public assistance programmes were discussed but were resisted in favour of local and charitable provision and state support for self-help institutions.

However, this view of France as backward is one of perspective. By thinking about the history of welfare in France differently, it becomes possible to show how neat chronologies of welfare do not always work. Although from its inception the Third Republic made an ideological commitment to health, it was only during the two decades before the First World War (1914–18) that a substantial investment was made in medical care. In 1893, the public healthcare system was overhauled. Workmen's compensation was introduced in 1898 and gradually extended to provide general medical coverage to a substantial proportion of the population. Four years later, municipalities were required to establish bureaus of hygiene. Nearly a third of French doctors were involved in public programmes by 1914 and the state was spending over 204 million francs on hospitals and hospices and 28 million on free medical services or just under half the total expenditure on welfare. This more positive assessment of welfare under the Third Republic is further supported when pronatalist measures are considered. Infant welfare clinics (*gouttes de lait*) were established which encouraged mothers to breastfeed and provided regular health checks. In 1904, every department was required to create a *maison maternelle*, which offered a full range of prenatal and obstetric services. Welfare under the Third Republic hence moved from earlier conceptions of social aid for the poor to favour more universal measures.

This expansion of state medicine has been interpreted as part of a process of modernization and medicalization as attempts were made to target specific groups, such as the tubercular or venereal, and establish systems of surveillance that aimed to define and control the deviant. Social reforms have also been shown to reflect a collectivization process and the growth of nation-states as part of a drive to modernity that included democratization, economic development and the growth of state education provision. Encouraged by a Marxist approach, scholars have attributed the development of state welfare to the efforts of working-class leaders to translate growing political power into state programmes designed to aid them. In Britain, for example, the extension of municipal and national suffrage to men has been shown to have had a profound effect on welfare, creating a more assertive working-class (and parliamentary Labour Party) that demanded better provision. However, welfare could serve other functions. For neo-Marxists, it was a form of control, an ameliorative measure to reduce social tension and protest. For example, the social insurance programme introduced in Germany by Bismarck has been characterized as an anti-socialist measure and a means of political pacification and social integration. Whereas these arguments draw attention to the political and electoral advantages of healthcare reforms, bourgeois parties equally played their part, as did peasant organizations and commercial interests. Often the middle classes had an important role. Their need to protect themselves from risk influenced moves to extend state welfare, while the rising cost of care and the desirability and expense of hospital admission added further incentives. The medical programmes introduced were hence often the result of a multi-class coalition of interests that required delicate political balancing acts.

Feminist scholarship in the 1980s and 1990s began to stress the importance of gender ideologies and women's agency to these welfare reforms. As interest shifted from critiquing the discriminatory nature of welfare programmes and how they reinforced gender ideologies to examining questions of agency, attention was directed at women's political activism and influence. Middle-class women had an important role in stimulating welfare reforms, particularly in connection with child and maternal welfare. An interest in maternalist ideologies and policies in various national settings emphasizes common patterns to reveal how as women entered into new relations with the state they challenged existing social and political institutions. Hence, welfare reform was one component of what many contemporary European writers labelled the women's question.

Historians have equally highlighted the role of doctors in the development of state medical services as they have made links to a growing faith in scientific solutions to social problems and the influence of medical experts. In the Third Republic, physicians exerted a marked influence on new social laws, while significant numbers of doctors also served in the Italian, Spanish, Russian and Turkish governments and promoted social reform. State appointments offered some doctors not only financial advantages but also increased their political influence and their authority as medical experts. Yet, it was not just medical experts who endorsed biological ideas that favoured state intervention. As demonstrated in Chapter 12, medical and popular models of degeneration were widespread in *fin de siècle* Europe and exerted a strong rhetorical influence on the provision of medical services, particularly in relation to tuberculosis, venereal disease, and infant and child welfare. Historians have been fascinated by the impact of fears of national decline and degeneration on social policy and have connected them to the emergence of pronatalist, eugenicist and racial hygiene movements and the expansion of medical welfare programmes [see 'Public health'].

The importance of degenerationist ideas has become central to how historians have approached French welfare provision under the Third Republic. Concerns about depopulation – which affected France more than any other European nation in the late nineteenth century – and degeneration were encouraged by the defeat in the Franco-Prussian War (1870–71), falling birth rates, and by colonial fears. The apparent population crisis provided a potent language that redefined the social question and raised the spectre that France was loosing its vigour in the face of venereal disease, tuberculosis, alcoholism and high infant mortality. These fears were intimately tied up with arguments about the role of women in society and found expression in cross-party support for pronatalism that often reduced women to breeders of healthy offspring. As in other European countries, a range of solutions was suggested from physical exercise and immigration policies to an investment in human capital. Although the pronatalist movement failed to convince French couples to have more children, public assistance programmes became crucial components of attempts to improve the nation's health.

At a European level, ideas of degeneration and eugenics were highly flexible, but where fears of racial decline influenced some health strategies directly, others indirectly, it is surprising how few explicitly eugenicist measures were implemented before 1914. The complex set of scientific and political issues that made up eugenics movements were frequently in tension, producing a narrow ground for agreement from which it was difficult for clear policies to emerge. The lack of unanimity and contradictions in the movement, as demonstrated by the British Eugenics Society, and divisions between those who supported positive methods – for example, school medical services to promote a stronger, healthier society – and those who favoured negative solutions – such as sterilization of those deemed unfit – frustrated action. Even in France, where concerns about degeneration and pronatalism were highly visible, eugenics as a movement had limited success as the emphasis was not on the survival of the fittest but on strengthening an ill-defined French nation.

Although governments did move into areas previously held to be private, important political, social and ideological barriers limited the nature of this intervention. Traditional welfare institutions continued to dispense relief, and a mixed economy of welfare between state, mutual aid and charity remained essential to provision. For example, in France charitable efforts overshadowed the relief provided by public institutions. Although medical services were provided at a municipal level – such as through Poor Law infirmaries or isolation hospitals in Britain – many hospitals remained primarily voluntary institutions. Private and philanthropic initiatives were important in developing new services; for example, in the sanatorium and the treatment of tuberculosis, and in stimulating debate, as seen in organizations founded in Belgium (1899), France (1901) and Germany (1902) to tackle venereal disease. At the same time, many state schemes were outgrowths of mutual or charitable schemes. In Belgium, a system of social insurance developed from a network of voluntary sickness insurance programmes, while in Britain health insurance was based around approved societies funded through a combination of individual, employer and state contributions. As the example of health insurance illustrates, public and private medical agencies frequently worked alongside each other, creating mixed systems that were financially practical and socially acceptable.

Whereas charity and mutualism remained important in structuring care, few welfare programmes in this period were comprehensive or universally welcomed. Important differences between urban and rural services remained and considerable disparities existed in terms of spending between cities. Although services were extended to new groups, the main emphasis remained on the poor and working classes and services were limited. Specific programmes reinforced gender assumptions of the male breadwinner and notions of female dependency, and that motherhood was a woman's primary duty. Doctors may have sought to extend their authority through public medicine, but this did not mean that they uncritically accepted a new role for the state. Many felt their therapeutic autonomy was threatened by state medical services. They often viewed public medicine as a second-class service and those with local government positions argued that they were underpaid and overworked. These complaints and fears about autonomy were fought out at a national and local level. German doctors, for example, resented being dependent on health insurance organizations. When their complaints went unheeded, German doctors went on strike, forcing an agreement with insurance organizations that gave them greater autonomy and control. Similar resistance from rank-and-file doctors was expressed in Holland and Spain, while in France a strong and organized medical profession was successful in shaping welfare legislation. Nor was opposition limited to medical practitioners. New measures threatened working-class budgets and traditions of self-help, while health visitors and other inspectors were unwelcomed intruders in working-class homes. Different social groups and parties expressed very different ideas about the nature of state responsibility. Local elites often used voluntary networks to enhance their political careers and social standing, and hence resisted central or municipal initiatives. As the example of Switzerland suggests, this could result in national welfare programmes being derailed.

As the above discussion reveals there is more to late nineteenth and early twentieth century medical welfare than a simple narrative of expanding state services. Not only was the role of the state contested, but it was also shaped by a range of actors and ideas. The extent to which fears of degeneration influenced the extension of state welfare programmes needs to be balanced against support for pronatalism and the emergence of working-class movements and the women's question. Although the boundaries between the state and traditional welfare institutions changed as new services and insurance schemes were established, the expansion of access to medical services was not simply a state-driven phenomenon, nor one of medicalization and control.

State medicine: 1914–39

The idea that the British welfare state was born out of the experiences of the Second World War has ensured that the 1920s and 1930s have invariably been represented as a backdrop to post-1945 reforms. However, the First World War caused both a disruption to existing welfare services as countries were placed on a war footing and stimulated reform in areas deemed essential to the war effort. In response to the war, European states adopted measures to promote the health of the nation as civilian health became militarily important [see 'Medicine and warfare']. Governments impinged more directly on their populations: controls were introduced over daily and working life and public health services were extended. Existing provision for the treatment of venereal diseases and tuberculosis, and for infant and maternal welfare were extended. Measures were established to improve health conditions (and hence efficiency) at work. Rather than representing a watershed, the war accelerated existing trends.

Although the expansion of the state during the First World War had occurred without an ideological change, post-war ideas of reconstruction and the desire to rebuild nations after the losses in the trenches favoured intervention and created a new set of health priorities that facilitated reform. In the Weimar Republic (1919–33), for example, the expansion of sickness insurance provision was shaped by ideas of rebuilding the German nation following the defeat of 1918. Across Europe, hope was expressed that social and medical welfare programmes would remove the causes of poverty, reduce social conflicts and build healthy nations as existing concerns about eugenics and pronatalism acquired a new currency against a backdrop of concerns about the health of the nation following the losses sustained during the war. In this sense, war encouraged the growth of strong social reform movements in Europe.

In the 1920s and 1930s, national governments guided by medical experts and newly formed central health departments became more involved in the delivery of healthcare. As interest extended beyond a traditional public health focus, new relationships were forged between the state, the voluntary sector, families and businesses. The nature of these relationships varied between nations, but attention focused less on infectious diseases and more on the general health of the population. Services were either free or paid for through health insurance schemes, with the former directed at the poor or at social diseases like tuberculosis and venereal disease. The result was that access to public-funded medical services and expertise expanded, a transition bolstered by rising expectations of curative and hospital medicine. Social policy in Europe further converged as states investigated and compared provision and established similar welfare programmes. Country after country implemented pensions, unemployment insurance and family allowances, established health and welfare clinics, funded clinics for venereal disease and dispensaries and sanatoriums for tuberculosis, and invested in infant and child welfare and maternity services. Faith was placed in the value of preventive medicine: vaccination and immunization programmes were extended, notably for tuberculosis, and health education programmes were developed [see 'Public health']. Wider conceptions of welfare were put forward that encouraged efforts to coordinate and extend public provision as demand for public services increased. In France, for example, the Republic stepped-up its involvement in healthcare through subsidies and a programme of modernization, providing over 43 million francs in grants to hospital projects by 1933. By 1939, over 20 million Frenchmen and women had medical insurance. Elsewhere in Europe, attempts were made to systematize healthcare through the work of central health departments and through government funding. The result was a creeping nationalization of local welfare and medical initiatives in many European states.

Eugenics and pronatalism continued to enjoy widespread popularity. Eugenics ideas spread from England to North America, Latin America, Scandinavia, continental Europe and Asia, while ongoing fears of degeneration encouraged governments to launch campaigns against tuberculosis and venereal disease, but nowhere in Europe was there sufficient support for eugenics to bring in extensive legislation. More persuasive and pervasive was pronatalism. The demographic losses of the trenches gave pronatalist groups national audiences and a sense of urgency permeated efforts to tackle infant and childhood mortality and morbidity. In France, where these concerns were most visible, the creation of local *Conseil supérieur de la natalité* and legislation throughout the 1920s aimed to limit population decline (including prohibitions on abortion), increase the birth rate, and develop childcare resources. Elsewhere in Europe, pronatalism was equally manifest in policies to promote large families (as in Sweden) in efforts to extend ante- and postnatal care and reform midwifery, and in the extension of state benefits to pregnant women. Only in the 1930s was greater attention directed at maternal health [see 'Women and medicine'].

The national nature of healthcare provision should not be overestimated: one characteristic of the 1920s and 1930s was that welfare remained fragmented. Government initiatives suffered from economic restrictions and were often resisted by both left and right. Although central financial control was extended, there remained marked regional variations in welfare provision and municipal authorities retained considerable scope for initiative. This was not a simple case of central innovators versus local conservatives. In France, local experiments and debates were important in determining national policy, while municipal authorities took the lead in funding hospital services. A similar situation existed in Denmark and Norway where municipalities were central in initiating social policies. In Britain, the interwar years marked the height of local government responsibility in healthcare as they both resisted and exploited national initiatives. In the 1920s, there was a rapid expansion of clinics and dispensaries, with infant and child welfare and tuberculosis services dominating local initiatives. The permissive 1929 Local Government Act stimulated local boroughs to extend their commitment and investment in health provision. Poor Law hospitals were transferred to municipal authorities and were developed as general hospitals. In most European states, the expansion of health services reflected growing support for municipal control and increased state responsibility for healthcare.

Notwithstanding the striking involvement of medical practitioners with public-funded services, this expansion was not without opposition from doctors who sought to defend their professional or financial autonomy. Active resistance and distrust on the part of doctors reveals how there was more to public medicine than a simple model of medicalization. A similar picture is produced when attention is turned to those who used these services. Although those accessing public medical care often received a lower quality service, many were not passive recipients of care. They negotiated relief, campaigned for better conditions, and resisted medical authority as the idea grew that access to medical services was a right of citizenship.

Nor should a focus on central or local government obscure the relationships that evolved between state agencies and charities. Although complex and uneasy partnerships were established, shaped by ideology and pragmatism on both sides, voluntary organizations worked with public bodies, the result of which was a flourishing of a range of welfare agencies during the 1920s and 1930s. In Denmark, for example, public and private agencies combined to create a joint system of pensions and health insurance that reflected conservative notions of self-help and government assistance. By 1934, voluntary organizations in Britain were receiving 37 per cent of their funds from the state, while at a local level attempts were made to promote greater cooperation. This represented a practical arrangement for governments, which were often reluctant to overspend, and allowed voluntary bodies to keep pace with rising costs. Not all charities or local authorities welcomed the relationship although wariness existed on both sides. However, notwithstanding this wariness, European governments relied upon private charity to fill the gaps in their welfare programmes.

The global depression of the 1930s had an important bearing on welfare provision. High levels of unemployment saw issues of health, nutrition and unemployment become crucial, but at the same time assistance policies started to blur the boundaries between different forms of relief. This is apparent in the work of School Medical Officers in Wales where health inspection and free school meals were as much to deal with poverty, as they were to tackle health. The depression not only helped to politicize recipients of welfare but also meant that longstanding divisions between the deserving and undeserving started to breakdown. Although at a local level, high unemployment acted as a catalyst for changing attitudes to welfare, governments wanted to control spending. Social welfare budgets were cut. In Norway, for example, state support for tuberculosis sanatoriums was reduced and welfare legislation was dropped. Elsewhere, central control was exerted over healthcare spending. Local bodies tried to subvert these central policies, revealing different attitudes at a local and national level to welfare provision.

By the late 1930s an intricate network of provision had emerged that reflected the haphazard, often piecemeal nature of healthcare provision. The 1920s and

1930s had seen creeping collectivism as states' responsibility for healthcare expanded. Although one result was a wide range of anomalies, as the example of France suggests, mini-welfare states were created at a municipal level. Localism continued to be valued, but a growing body of opinion favoured more national approaches, a view reinforced by investigations that revealed that the existing provision available from charities and local authorities were inefficient and uncoordinated. If discussions about the future of state welfare had a limited impact on policy in the 1930s, they stimulated growing debate that influenced wartime discussions.

Nazi welfare: 1933–45

Historians have argued that Germany followed a special path or *Sonderweg* in the twentieth century. Although National Socialism and Fascism should not be considered aberrations, the view that German welfare reforms were somehow different has drawn on the example of Nazi racial policies as historians have explored questions of modernity. However, rather than seeing Nazi policies as marking a break with earlier welfare policies, it is possible to detect continuities with the social welfare programmes of the Wilhelmine (1871–1919) and Weimar (1919–33) periods. From the 1890s, for example, like many European states, initiatives to improve infant and child health and broadly eugenic policies were adopted in Germany along with efforts to tackle the perceived racial poisons of alcoholism, venereal disease and tuberculosis. Under the Weimar Republic, social hygiene offered an ideology for welfare intervention that was used by both left and right and mirrored what was happening elsewhere in Europe. Rather than a German *Sonderweg*, therefore, the policies pursued under Hitler can be represented as a radical and violent expression of racial hygiene thinking present elsewhere in Europe.

Under Hitler, welfare programmes focused on creating a racial national community or *volksgemeinschaft*. Health and fertility were identified with German nationalism and social problems were medicalized. Although the Nazis drew on a range of other social and political sciences – such as urban planning and economics – racial hygiene was elevated into central policy. This did not mean that the existing system of welfare was radically changed. As noted above, welfare under the Weimar Republic already contained a stress on social hygiene, but under Hitler greater emphasis was placed on racial hygiene, marriage and the family as the active responsibility of the state as ideas about *Erbgesundheitspflege* (protection of hereditary health) and *Rassenpflege* (protection of the race) were enshrined in welfare policy. New welfare agencies were established. Laws were passed that emphasized individual responsibility and racial hygiene to improve the race and to limit or eradicate those racial groups perceived to be inferior and/or alien. Access to birth control was limited and natural childbirth was promoted. A sterilization programme was started in 1934 and quickly became big business. Genetic health courts and appeals tribunals were established. The systematic mass murder of the mentally ill and physically impaired, often euphemistically known as the euthanasia programme, started in 1939–40 with the systematic extermination of Jews following. Nazi policies and structures were exported to occupied countries where, as in the case of Czechoslovakia, new healthcare policies were imposed.

Many German doctors took an active part in Nazi welfare programmes, while elite physicians readily participated in the forcible sterilization and euthanasia programmes. Historians have been fascinated as to why so many doctors participated. There are three main schools of thought. Early research emphasized how medical thought and training contributed to an objectification of the patient that made Nazi policies easier to accept. This explanation has been replaced by a model that points to a combination of the growth of narrowly deterministic explanations of mental illness, the perceived inability to help incurable cases, and the growing cost of institutionalizing them to encourage a belief that the elimination of the hopeless would permit resources to be concentrated on the curable. Professional agreement on the need to reduce the burden of those defined as less valuable certainly existed in the 1920s and made it possible for the Nazis to radicalize these ideas. However, for other historians, the answer rests with the authority the Nazis conferred on doctors, although it should be acknowledged that careerism, greed and in some cases brutality, were factors. Nazism not only encouraged doctors to think of themselves as custodians of the health of the German race, but also increased their earnings and opportunities.

It is easy to look at the euthanasia programme and the Holocaust and argue that Nazi policies were brutally efficient in pursuing racial hygiene. Yet, progressive social policies were implemented. Physical fitness and diet was promoted. Smoking was denounced. Holistic medicine and the idea of the general practitioner as a family doctor were supported. Welfare policies equally shared similarities with pronatalist policies and support for families and child health found elsewhere in Europe. This is not to diminish the brutality of the Nazi regime, but to show how there was more to Nazi welfare policies than just sterilization or extermination. Nor were Nazi welfare policies universally successful. Whereas they worked in some parts of the healthcare system, they failed in others. Hence, a view of Nazi welfare is needed that sees continuities, recognizes the similarities with what was happening elsewhere in Europe, and shows how racial hygiene dominated German approaches to welfare.

Medicine and welfarism: 1939–2000

In the years immediately after the Second World War (1939–45) renewed effort went into extending public welfare programmes, but it is not simply a question of expansion. The policies adopted, the chronology of reform, and the nature of services varied between nations and the post-1945 history of welfare falls into a number of phases. Whereas before 1939, planning had been piecemeal, as nations pursued plans for reconstruction in the years immediately after the war public expenditure on healthcare rose. The period to the mid 1970s has consequently been identified as the era of the classic welfare state, characterized first by early legislative activity and then by expansion. Although the percentage spent on healthcare as a proportion of GDP broadly rose with the cost of delivering state healthcare (see Table 13.1), expansion slowed in the 1970s and 1980s as economic instability ushered in a period of anxiety and reform, while in the 1990s questions about the boundaries of welfare coloured debates about the future of state welfare. While this might suggest consensus, the participation of the state in healthcare often proved controversial, and the nature of the programmes established were invariably the result of compromise. For different reasons, Sweden and Britain have come to exemplify this process.

Although some welfare systems were more generous than others, there was a degree of convergence. Even in Soviet Russia, the ideologically driven health policies of the interwar years were overshadowed in the 1950s and 1960s by approaches that favoured clinical medicine. Historians have debated the reasons for this expansion. Interpretations of twentieth century social policy have moved away from favouring wartime experiences as creating a sense of solidarity or a welfare consensus. Instead, historians have come to point to the necessity of political parties to gain electoral support, the growing influence of welfare professionals, population growth, a sense that existing provision was failing, and the need to adapt welfare policies as part of a programme of modernity to explain growth. Strong ideological currents have been also detected that

Table 13.1 State expenditure on health (per cent of GDP)

Country	*1980*	*1985*	*1990*	*1995*	*2000*
France	5.6	6.3	6.2	7.4	7.1
Germany	6.6	6.8	6.3	8.2	8.1
Italy	5.5	5.3	6.1	5.1	5.8
Netherlands	5.1	5.2	5.4	5.9	5.0
Norway	4.9	4.5	4.3	4.3	4.0
Spain	4.2	4.3	5.1	5.4	5.2
Sweden	8.3	7.6	7.4	6.2	6.3
Switzerland	3.6	3.9	3.9	4.6	5.0
UK	4.9	4.9	4.9	5.6	5.5
US	3.7	4.1	4.8	6.2	5.9
OECD (Total)	4.5	4.6	4.7	5.1	5.3

Source: OECD Health Data: *OECD Health Statistics* (database).
Based on data from OECD (2010), OECD Health Data 2010: Statistics and Indicators, www.oecd.org/health/healthdata.

favoured state intervention. For example, Keynesian ideas, Richard Titmuss's influential work on social policy and social integration, and ideas of citizenship and universalism, contributed to a climate in which state intervention in welfare was seen to promote economic growth and individual liberty.

Traditionally, historians of social policy have considered the Beveridge Report – published in Britain in 1942 – as the blueprint for the classic welfare state and presented the Second World War as fostering conditions in Britain that favoured the construction of a solidaristic and universal welfare system. The demands of the war economy, the Emergency Medical Service (EMS), and the slow modernization of public hospitals have been identified as facilitating and legitimizing a more direct role for government in healthcare, which came to fruition in the National Health Service (NHS). In these accounts, the EMS has been credited with establishing an embryonic health service that exposed deficiencies and promoted the case for a nationalized hospital service. Although such a system was implicit in the Beveridge Report, it is necessary to question ideas of wartime solidarity and point to continuities with the 1930s. The question becomes how to balance the creation of the NHS with longer-term trends.

The volume of social legislation in the 1940s and the move from welfare as a concession to a right was significant, but antecedents existed. Although municipal authorities in the 1930s had taken on greater responsibility for healthcare, central funding had underwritten expansion. Ideas of administrative efficiency, seen in the 1929 Local Government Act, reinforced this trend towards centralization. Even Beveridge drew on interwar surveys to devise his blueprint for social welfare. However, opposition to municipal control and the compromises negotiated with the British Medical Association and hospital consultants were crucial to the process of nationalization as earlier plans for municipal control was rejected. In this respect, the medical profession exerted a strong influence on the new service, a position of strength it exploited until the 1980s. Rather than being a product of consensus therefore, the NHS grew out of opposition from doctors and compromises between politicians and professionals.

The NHS was designed as a comprehensive service, funded by central taxation and free at the point of delivery. The new health service was an enormous improvement on the ramshackle system that had previously existed. A tripartite system was created – hospital, general practice and community medicine – that reflected professional hierarchies and reinforced existing power relationships among medical practitioners. Access to general practitioners, dentists, ophthalmic care and prescription medicines was extended to all, but the main emphasis was on a nationalized hospital service. Public health and primary healthcare were relegated as a substantial investment – ideological, professional and material – was made in hospital medicine [see 'Public health']. The NHS proved immediately popular, resulting in a rapid uptake of services.

However, the NHS did not represent the only system of post-war healthcare. Although Beveridge offered a blueprint for universalism, three basic models evolved. In Britain, Sweden and Spain a public system was implemented whereby medical services were nationalized, with Italy, Portugal and Greece moving towards a universalization of access in the 1970s and 1980s. This did not mean that the state crowded out the voluntary or private sector – welfare pluralism remained, as did private healthcare – but that universalism became integral to social policy. More widespread in Europe was a model that mixed public and private provision based on the insurance principle in which social insurance guaranteed access to medical services provided by private agencies. This approach characterized France and Germany. In West Germany, aspects of Nazi welfare policies survived and there was a continuing reliance on family care and compulsory institutionalization, while in France, a decentralized system was created in which contributions from employers and employees provided the mainstay of funding. A third system, characteristic of the United States, was an essentially private insurance system with subsidized care for special groups, such as the elderly or poor. In the 1990s, this private insurance model came to attract increasing attention in Europe as the cost of welfare rose.

The nature of welfare programmes, and the pace at which public-funded services were extended, varied between countries. In Denmark, the Social Democrats and others on the left quickly expanded state healthcare and moved towards universalism, while in Soviet Russia poor economic performance undermined optimistic healthcare programmes. This variety and the delays in implementing welfare programmes in part reflected the complex pattern of interactions between vested interest groups, legislators and finance. If women had a less central role in policymaking, the Catholic Church, trade unions, insurance companies, pharmaceutical companies and later self-help groups all influenced policy. This is apparent in post-Franco Spain and in Sweden where the labour movement pressed for the expansion of state welfare, while the development of AIDS policies and services in the late twentieth century drew attention to the role of self-help groups. The resulting negotiations not only caused delays, but also influenced the structure of the services established.

It would be easy to assume that doctors were the main beneficiaries of welfare programmes, but their relationship with the state was seldom straightforward. Doctors, who had been used to self-regulation and autonomy, frequently resisted reforms. In France, the Confédération des Syndicats Médicaux effectively vetoed health service reform until after the collapse of the Fourth Republic (1946–58). However, as the example of the NHS shows, welfare systems often reinforced established medical hierarchies. Health professionals were able to exercise power, not only over policymaking but also in dispensing care and in defining priorities. Unsurprisingly, unease was quickly voiced about the limits of medical authority.

Just as concerns were voiced about professional dominance, initial optimism began to wane in the 1950s and 1960s as evidence pointed to ongoing health inequalities. Comprehensive systems of healthcare proved difficult to manage and fund. Rising patient demand and expectations, new and more expensive medical technologies and procedures, and demand from doctors, all contributed to rising costs, as did inflation. Demographic change, with the post-war baby boom, and shifts in morbidity patterns to favour chronic and degenerative diseases, added further pressures. The result was that short-term welfare crises became characteristic of the 1960s. Managerial solutions were developed that tried to fuse central planning with health needs and funding. European states reorganized services, introduced patient charges, or extended their control over care providers. Constant reforms in the NHS in Britain are an ideal example of this repeated reorganization.

The economic downturn that followed the oil crisis of 1973 had an effect on welfare programmes as costs started to exceed the ability of nations to afford services, especially expensive hospital services. In Denmark, rising unemployment and an aging population forced a retrenchment in public welfare. Similar restrictions were imposed on social spending in West Germany as health insurance benefits were cut. A common pattern emerged: the rising cost of medicine, an ageing population and an increase in the number of longer-living chronic sick combined with higher expectations and demand to increase healthcare spending.

Criticisms and the economic downturn did not lead to radical reforms, however. The pace of expansion slowed and efforts were made to bring spending into line with economic growth. In the 1980s, governments continued to look not to drastic reforms but to reducing expenditure, maximizing efficiency and transferring some of the cost onto patients. Attention was directed at health education, which focused on promoting healthy lifestyles and against the risks associated with particular behaviours – for example, smoking, drinking, and unprotected sex – in an attempt to reduce costs [see 'Public health']. Governments became increasingly concerned with monitoring the effectiveness and quality of care to evaluate value for money and encourage accountability. Budgetary constraints saw rationing of healthcare. In France, charges for hospital beds were introduced in 1983 and stricter financial controls were implemented in the following year as efforts were made to curb spending. Policymakers and healthcare providers came to place more emphasis on the selection and prioritization of patients.

However, economic factors were only part of the equation. Other explanations can be found for why welfare reforms were implemented. These included political necessity, generational changes in policymakers, and new views on the nature of welfare and citizenship. The need for a new welfare contract between citizen and state was expressed as support for universalism came under attack for failing to help those who needed free care most. Although studies in the 1980s questioned conventional assumptions that the less well-off had benefited, anxiety was expressed that universalism was creating a dependency culture. Following work by American theorists, greater weight was given to the notion that welfare should be distributed selectively as the structure of families, patterns of employment, growing inequalities and an ageing population placed growing demands on public-funded services. If little was actually new in these ideas – in many ways they repeated concerns first expressed in the 1950s – the United States model of a public-private welfare state proved increasingly influential in Europe. Italy, for example, moved closer to the US model following reforms in the 1990s that aimed to create a decentralized system of managed competition. These ideas equally found expression in Margaret Thatcher's Britain (1979–90) with its support for NHS reform, quasi-markets, competition and consumer choice, and private medicine, which not only saw reorganization, but also made managers key figures in the delivery of healthcare. Individual over collective solutions came to be valued as the culture of welfarism was challenged.

Conclusions

If the renewed emphasis on community, individual and local responsibility resulted in complex networks of interactions between the state, insurance companies and professionals, viewing these changes in the long-term suggests parallels with earlier approaches. The conflict between local and centralizing forces, especially between municipal authorities and the state, and a mixed economy of care have been a feature of welfare since the eighteenth century. The provision of state medical welfare in the eighteenth, nineteenth and twentieth centuries can therefore be placed in the context of how new relationships have evolved over the last three-hundred years between the state, voluntary and private care, and how these relationships were influenced by socioeconomic, political and ideological change and by expediency. States' responsibility for medical care should not therefore be read in terms of modernization, nor just as a result of demand or medicalization, but as a complex and halting process informed as much by negotiation as it was by conflict and consensus.

Further reading

Although it is hard to recommend a single overview, good starting points are George Rosen, *From Medical Police to Social Medicine* (New York: Science History Publications, 1974) and Dorothy Porter, *Health, Civilization and the State: History of Public Health from Ancient to Modern Times* (London: Routledge, 1999). On early modern poor relief, see Brian Pullan, *Rich and Poor in Renaissance Venice: The Social Institutions of a Catholic State to 1620* (ACLS History E-Book Project, 2008) and Paul Slack, *Poverty and Policy in Tudor and Stuart England* (London: Longman, 1990), with Ole Peter Grell and Andrew Cunningham (eds), *Health Care Provision and Poor Relief in Northern Europe 1500–1700* (London: Routledge, 1996) providing a comparative perspective. A larger literature exists on the nineteenth century. Studies of the British Poor Law abound and a good starting place is Anthony Brundage, *The English Poor Laws 1700–1930* (Basingstoke: Palgrave Macmillan, 2001). For France, see Jack Ellis, *The Physician-Legislators of France: Medicine and Politics in the Early Third Republic* (Cambridge: Cambridge University Press, 1990) and Timothy Smith, *Creating the Welfare State in France 1880–1940* (Montreal and Kingston: McGill-Queen's University Press, 2003), while Young-sun Hong, 'Neither Singular Nor

Alternative: Narratives of Modernity and Welfare in Germany, 1870–1945', *Social History* 30 (2005), pp. 133–53, examines how German welfare has been approached. On the influence of eugenics, Robert Nye, 'The Rise and Fall of the Eugenics Empire: Recent Perspectives on the Impact of Biomedical Thought in Modern Society', *Historical Journal* 36 (1993), pp. 687–700, offers an excellent examination along with M.B. Adams (ed.), *The Wellborn Science: Eugenics in Germany, France, Brazil and Russia* (New York and Oxford: Oxford University Press, 1990) and Gunnar Broberg and Nils Roll-Hansen (eds), *Eugenics and the Welfare State: Sterilization Policy in Denmark, Sweden, Norway and Finland* (East Lansing, MI: Michigan State University Press, 2005), with Daniel Pick's *Faces of Degeneration: A European Disorder c.1848–1918,* 1993 edn (Cambridge: Cambridge University Press, 1993) providing a seminal study of the influence of degenerationist ideas. The best survey of women and healthcare policy is provided by Seth Koven and Sonya Michel, 'Womanly Duties', *American Historical Review* 95 (1990), pp. 1076–1108. The dimensions of public medicine in the twentieth century are such that the range of literature is extensive. Here Helen Jones, *Health and Society in Twentieth-Century Britain* (London: Longman, 1994) and Anne Hardy, *Health and Medicine in Britain since 1860* (Basingstoke: Palgrave Macmillan, 2001) provide excellent introductions, while Peter Baldwin, *The Politics of Social Solidarity: Class Bases of the European Welfare State 1875–1975* (Cambridge: Cambridge University Press, 1992) gives a comparative dimension. On interwar municipal medicine, Becky Taylor, John Stewart and Martin Powell, 'Central and Local Government and the Provision of Municipal Medicine, 1919–39', *English Historical Review* 122 (2007), pp. 397–426, illustrates the varied nature of provision and the importance of local services. On responses to venereal disease, see the collection edited by Roger Davidson and Lesley Hall (eds), *Sex, Sin and Suffering: Venereal Disease and European Society since 1870* (London: Routledge, 2001). A considerable body of literature exists on tuberculosis, with Linda Bryder's *Below the Magic Mountain: A Social History of Tuberculosis in Twentieth-Century Britain* (Oxford: Clarendon Press, 1988) remaining a seminal study. On pronatalism and maternity, see Deborah Dwork, *War is Good for Babies and Other Young Children: A History of the Infant and Child Welfare Movement in England 1898–1918* (London: Tavistock, 1987) or Susan Pedersen, *Family, Dependence, and the Origins of the Welfare State: Britain and France 1914–1945* (Cambridge: Cambridge University Press, 1995). Paul Weindling, *Health, Race and German Politics between National Unification and Nazism 1879–1945* (Cambridge: Cambridge University Press, 1993) and Michael Burleigh, *Death and Deliverance* (London: Pan, 2002) are insightful examinations of Nazi welfare policies, while Susan Gross Solomon and John F. Hutchinson (eds), *Health and Society in Revolutionary Russia* (Bloomington, IN: Indiana University Press, 1990) and M.G. Field, 'Soviet Medicine', in Roger Cooter and John Pickstone (eds), *Medicine in the Twentieth Century* (London: Routledge, 2000), pp. 51–66, are good English-language studies of Soviet healthcare. For reading on public health, see the Further Reading in the previous chapter. On the impact of the Second World War, see the Further Reading in Chapter 15 along with the monumental *The Health Services since the War. Volume I: Problems of Health Care. The National Health Service before 1957* (London: HMSO, 1988) by Charles Webster. Although there is a wealth of literature on the NHS, Charles Webster's *The National Health Service: A Political History* (Oxford: Oxford University Press, 2002) and Geoffrey Rivett's *From Cradle to Grave: Fifty years of the NHS* (London: King's Fund, 1998) are accessible introductions. For a comparative approach, see Ellen Immergut, *Health Politics: Interests and Institutions in Western Europe* (Cambridge: Cambridge University Press, 1992) or Anna Dixon and Elias Mossialos, *Health Care Systems in Eight Countries* (European Observatory on Health Care Systems, 2002). For readers interested in twentieth century health policy, see James Morone and Janice

Goggin, 'Health Policies in Europe', *Journal of Health Politics, Policy and Law* 20 (1995), pp. 557–69, and David Wilsford, 'States Facing Interests', pp. 571–613, in the same volume, while Christopher Pierson, *Beyond the Welfare State?* (Cambridge: Polity Press, 2007) explores the political economy of welfare.

14

Medicine and empire

Imperialism has come in many forms – formal and informal, cultural, political or economic – and these forms have shifted over time. The early modern period saw the establishment of colonial possessions, first in the Americas and then in the Pacific, as long-distance trade stimulated an awareness of the wider world. By the seventeenth century, European powers, including France, the Netherlands and Britain, had found strategic and commercial advantages in colonization. Conquest, trade or settlement drove expansion, aided by unequal treaties, armed intervention and an interventionist ideology that linked together commercial, missionary, military and medical interests. The nineteenth century was an 'Age of Empire'. European nations became involved in aggressive and competitive campaigns to acquire new colonies, particularly in Africa, and extended their informal empires in South America, China and Japan. Although not all colonies were the same, or were established for the same reasons, empire exerted a strong fascination as faith was placed in the belief that European nations were bringing civilization to the world. Developments in medicine, especially towards the end of the nineteenth century, fuelled this self-confidence.

With the beginning of decolonization in the 1960s, historians began to examine the history of medicine in a colonial context. By the 1990s, interest in empire had become fashionable and had moved beyond the diplomatic histories of the past to show how empire was multifaceted, and how it had a profound effect on the making of the modern world. This shift across a variety of sub-disciplines reflected the adoption of postcolonial theories and contemporary concerns about the global political order. In writing on medicine and empire, a number of broad trends emerged. One approach focused on how Western medicine – essentially clinical practice, sanitation, immunization, health education and personal hygiene – shaped the development of non-Western countries. Initially, scholars argued that Western medicine spread – or was diffused – from the centre or metropolis (London or Paris) to the periphery (Bombay or Cape Town); that the adoption of Western medical knowledge and practices in colonized territories aided modernization, which resulted in improvements in health. Later studies began to suggest that medicine should be viewed as 'a tool of empire'. Within this framework, the conflict between Western and indigenous medicine was exaggerated, reducing colonial medicine to problems of hegemony and resistance.

Although the concept of centre and periphery has continued to be used by historians, a more critical approach emerged in the 1980s, which rejected the idea of a rigid dichotomy between centre and periphery to emphasize the traffic in ideas, practices and careers. Influenced by new imperial history and subaltern studies, scholars from the late 1980s began to explore the extent to which colonial contexts not only promoted the development of new disciplines, such as tropical medicine, but also influenced European practices and ideas to suggest how reciprocity was more common than diffusion and empire exerted a considerable influence on the metropole. Whereas in some areas, European and colonial physicians dismissed local healing practices (for example, in southern Africa), in others they displayed a more grudging admiration (for example, in China). Historians came to accept that there was no single model of colonial medicine; that different ways of healing coexisted and overlapped. Scholarship further revealed how medical practitioners were never simple tools of empire and how colonial medicine was not merely medicine in the colonies but was often negotiated, adapted and assimilated. The result, as evident in Arnold or Harrison's work on India, was a more nuanced understanding of the ways in which medical ideas and practices were negotiated and accommodated to indigenous environments (see Further Reading). This did not mean that the idea that colonial medicine served to uphold ideas of European control or the values of the white ruling groups was rejected, but that control was often an unexpected result rather than a goal in itself. Rather than medicine being diffused as a colonizing force, colonial medical policies, such as in South Africa or India, were shown to be enclavist, primarily serving colonial armies and administrators.

This chapter builds on these historiographical trends to explore the nature of colonial medical encounters and their impact on medical practices and institutions. Rather than examining indigenous systems of medicine – for example, Unani or Ayurveda in India – it concentrates on the relationship between Western medicine and colonialism. However, before thinking about this relationship, it is important to stress that not only has the period of colonialism covered nearly five hundred years, but also that colonial encounters have occurred in a variety of different regions, geographies, climates, and socioeconomic and political contexts. Marked differences existed between those regions and contexts: between white settler colonies like Australia or New Spain (Mexico), where self-sufficiency was sought, and Africa and South Asia. In the so-called informal empires, such as in Argentina or China, economic, cultural and medical influence went hand-in-hand. Different imperial powers adopted different approaches. Spain, for example, followed a more centralizing approach to colonial government than Britain. These differences shaped the form of colonial medicine and in part accounts for its complexities.

Race and medicine

Historians of medicine often assumed, as Warwick Anderson has explained, that 'the body of biomedicine was [a] generic one' and was above all white.[1] For contemporaries such an idea carried with it an implicit faith in European superiority as reflected in the writing of Rudyard Kipling and other authors. Notions of racial difference came to permeate colonial encounters and ideas of empire and influenced colonial administration and practices. Influenced by the work of Edward Said, scholars in the 1980s began to explore notions of racial difference to uncover the extent to which medicine was not only a potent agent of cultural imperialism, but also how colonial expansion contributed to the emergence of racial categories and scientific racism. Historians, anthropologists and literary scholars interested in questions of power pointed to the ways in which race started to acquire a solid intellectual currency in eighteenth century scientific and intellectual circles and highlighted a shift from scientific-based racism in the nineteenth century to racial hygiene in the twentieth century. Although a consensus on how and why this transition occurred has proved elusive, agreement exists that scientific racism and colonial rule were mutually reinforcing and how framing racial hierarchies reinforced faith in European superiority. Racial ideas therefore offer a useful starting point for thinking about European notions of colonialism.

European colonial expansion in the seventeenth century encouraged an interest in racial difference. Although ideas about race drew on long-established views about religious and social differences, existing division between racial groups were given new meanings, which were often conceptualized in terms of blood or anatomical differences. In this framework, Africans were explicitly related to apes and defined by their perceived unruly sexuality, lack of reason, violence and ugliness. These ideas contributed to a sense of European superiority that justified colonial power, but it was in the eighteenth century that race started to take on new configurations. Although as Daniel Defoe's *Robinson Crusoe* (1719) shows, popular views continue to be informed by fanciful accounts that dwelled on cannibalism, new views of race offered a means of understanding the perceived differences that were felt to exist between Europeans and non-Europeans. These views were shaped as much by culture, religion, politics and heritage, as they were by biological concerns and anatomical investigations. Colonialism was crucial to this formation of new ideas about race and provided a testing ground for racial theories.

In the eighteenth century, the voyages of discovery saw Europe flooded with new specimens of plants, animals and humans. Anatomists used these specimens to construct hierarchies of racial variation that had a strong geographical component and drew on contemporary thinking about gender and sexual difference [see 'Women and medicine']. Adopting the model of the 'Great Chain of Being', in which nature progressed in one smooth process from the simplest forms to the most complex, anatomists and naturalists, such as the Swedish botanist Carl Linnaeus and the German physician Johann Blumenbach, developed comprehensive categories to classify man along with other animal groups. Scientific racism grew out of these studies, but cultural concerns, personal beliefs and assumptions embedded in the institutional and social contexts of the anatomists and naturalists concerned were as important as the biological or anatomical ideas they advanced. In their investigations, anatomists constructed the European male as the standard of excellence: Africans were seen as a distinct, lower race, while Aboriginals were deemed organically incapable of civilization and were hence doomed, views that were supported by apologists for slavery.

Numerous theories of racial variation were asserted to explain these perceived differences, theories that increasingly acquired scientific justification. Drawing on Biblical ideas, environmentalists argued that because humanity had a common ancestry with Adam and Eve, racial characteristics were shaped by environmental factors, such as climate, diet, culture and disease, which produced modifications to the body and behaviour. This belief derived from popular and Hippocratic notions of environmental determinism. The extreme climate found in India and the natural fertility of the soil, for example, was felt to produce a lethargic race, while French writers stressed how tropical climates made women over-sexed, views that found visible expression in discussion surrounding the Khoikhoi women (known as 'Hottentots'). Although the anti-slavery movement adopted these ideas in their efforts to emphasize how all men were naturally equal, environmental explanations continued to favour a belief that racial difference was a process of degeneration from a white European origin. These ideas allowed early nineteenth century writers to express unease about foreign exposure (see below).

Between 1780 and the 1830s, this environmental approach was challenged as the boundaries between races became more fixed. This shift in thinking about race owed much to a more pessimistic assessment of the fixity of human characteristics and drew on comparative anatomy, reports of colonial encounters with indigenous peoples, ideas of racial immunity, and on investigations in physical anthropology, phrenology and craniometry (the measurement of cranial capacity). The result was a view of race that upheld an understanding of racial hierarchy that was used to support social and political divides. Scientific ideas about racial difference were developed and were widely diffused so that by mid-century race had acquired a clear biological meaning in which established ideas about the influence of climate (especially in French medical writing) and the centrality of innate racial characteristics were stressed. The growing colonial dominance of the European powers and their own sense of superiority further served to reinforce the belief that they represented an ideal physical and racial type. New ideas of nation and nationhood sustained these views, with race used to strengthen nationalist claims. Industrialization and technological development further emphasized differences and was used as evidence of European superiority. In addition, the disease experiences of European settlers made it easier to accept the idea that European bodies were different from their colonial subjects.

at Last I have met with a True Broad Bottom
real flesh no Deception in I wonder if Broad Bottoms
would breed in this Country
me hear of your Bottom me Long to See
it me write to you about it
oh sure a Pair were never Seen
so justly formed to meet by Nature
Charming Indeed. oh I am so happy
the Family is not Extinct
LOVE at FIRST SIGHT: or A PAIR of HOTTENTOTS,
with an Addition to the Broad Bottom Family

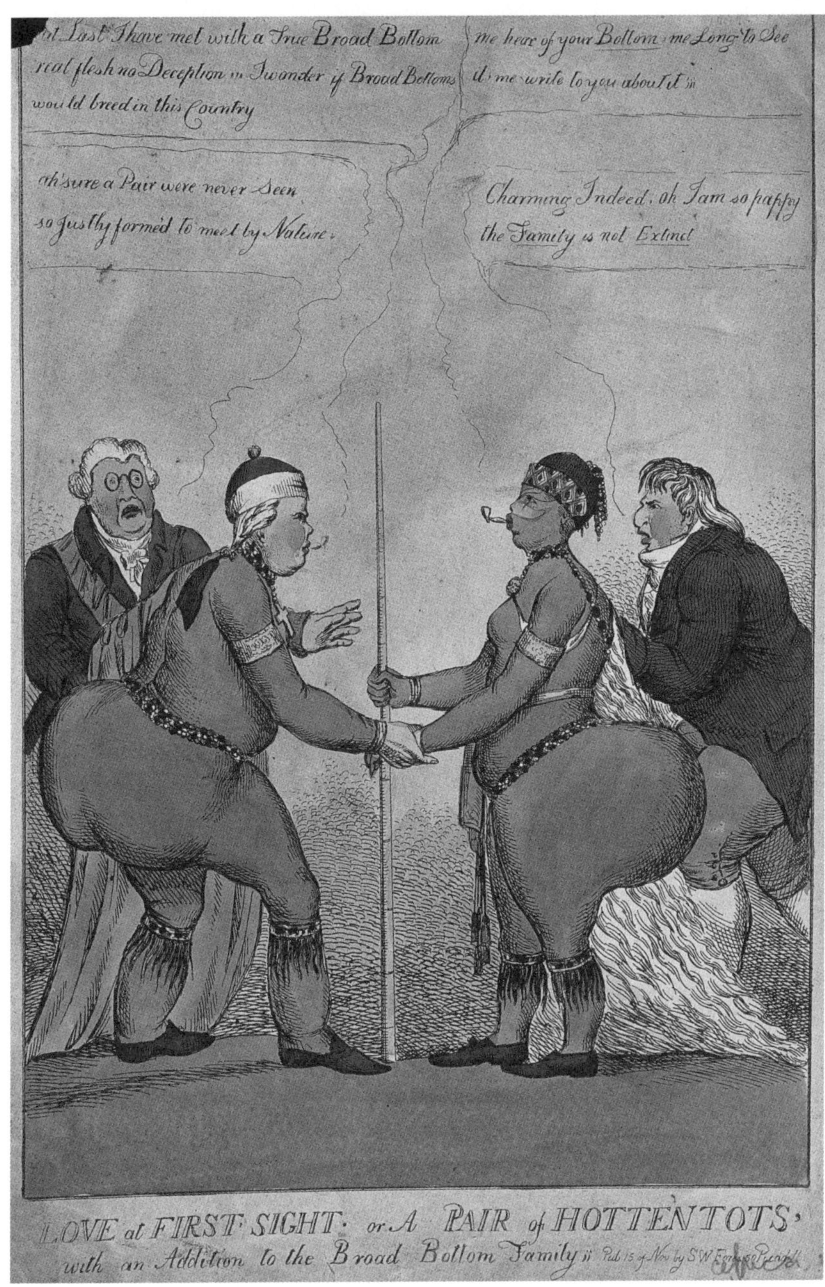

Figure 14.1 The 'Hottentot venus'. The etching represents two large women, one of whom is the 'Hottentot venus'.

Source: Wellcome Library, London.

Phrenological investigations and skull measurements in Britain, Austria and Germany reinforced this belief by advancing the idea that the skulls of diverse races reflected their intellectual powers and that some races, notably Africans and Aboriginals, were inferior. These views appeared to be confirmed by the emerging social sciences of ethnography and anthropology and the work of geographers. They added what was seen as quantitative evidence to support ideas of racial hierarchy.

These views were not all encompassing. Ideas of racial difference and racial inferiority were not entirely straightforward, as can be seen in Jean-Jacques Rousseau's concept of the noble savage. Imperial notions were often limited by distance, by low levels of education, and by a concentration on European or local affairs. The same might be true about racial thinking. Notwithstanding these caveats, ideas of racial hierarchy were eagerly used to support claims that those nations or peoples deemed less advanced deserved subjection and that even more developed peoples required European tutelage. Scientific racism was not a pre-requisite for empire, but concepts of racial hierarchy and colonialism were mutually reinforcing. Imperialists seized on these theories of racial hierarchy because they offered neat justifications for colonialism.

The idea of biological racial difference became central to the high imperial era (c. 1880–1910). Whereas early settlers may have intermarried with indigenous populations, as was the case in India and the Cape, as white families became more established, traditional relationships were redefined. Greater stress was placed on biological differences, the limitations of human adaptation, and an evolutionary hierarchy. Although a racial hierarchy was taken for granted by the mid nineteenth century, the publication of Charles Darwin's *Origins of Species* (1859) and *Descent of Man* (1871) encouraged others to apply his evolutionary concepts and selection theory to human society and construct racial hierarchies. Darwin did not emphasize the physical and intellectual differences between races, but others did to create a malleable social Darwinism. Ernst Haeckel in Germany, for example, identified twelve species that he saw derived from Darwin's ape-man and argued that Mediterraneans were the most evolved. The result was a belief that non-Europeans were primitive, lazy, lascivious and untrustworthy, a mindset that produced a view of non-European races that was generalized and negative. Although it was acknowledged that Europeans were vulnerable to tropical disease, it was argued that those lower down the racial scale, such as the Australian aborigines, were predestined to social failure. That such racial stereotyping was used more widely in contemporary debates demonstrates how ideas developed in a colonial context were applied back home. This is evident in how a language of race and racial metaphors were employed in debates about the nature of urbanization and the urban poor. There was often a slippage between categories of race, class and poverty, with social commentators regularly talking about 'primitives' or 'savages', invoking images of Africa, as can be seen in William Booth's *In Darkest England and the Way Out* (1890). Fears of bad blood, immigrant groups and the

Negro came to form a staple of Victorian gothic literature and late nineteenth century adventure stories.

The physical anthropology and a race-oriented ethnography of the 1890s and 1900s reinforced these views by providing apparent mathematic precision for existing racial arguments. Ideas of 'racial progress', 'racial decline' and 'racial hygiene' became part of wider organic metaphors that influenced the social sciences and debates on the condition of the nation. The eugenics movement strengthened belief in white superiority [see 'Public health']. It merged with fears about the declining fitness of the imperial race and the ability of European nations to defend their colonial possessions. For eugenicists, race was a convenient and malleable concept. It fitted well with their concern for national biological standards and fears of the polluting effects of the unfit on the national stock. In the 1930s, the racial hygiene policies adopted in Nazi Germany (1933–45) and given horrific form in the Holocaust have been seen as the epitome of these ideas.

If anti-semitism was not an exclusive German preserve – for example, anti-semitic ideas influenced French politics under the Third Republic (1870–1940) – there was more to racial hygiene in the twentieth century than anti-semitism. The growth of anti-colonial sentiment and nationalist movements in Africa and Asia in the first half of the twentieth century encouraged a reassertion of racial views that affirmed white superiority and control. In South Africa, these anxieties reinforced a segregationist ideology and encouraged mental testing to categorize the black population as intellectually inferior. In Britain, imperialist groups in the 1920s and 1930s sponsored educational tours to promote migration to areas where it was felt 'whiteness' was needed to maintain European hegemony. Racial prejudices that had evolved in a colonial setting were transported back to Europe, helping to structure modern racism. Drawing on the same stereotypes used in the colonies, the inhabitants of southern France, for example, were treated with disdain because of their alleged mongrelization, their laziness, and their smaller brains. Such fears gave expression to racist ideas and saw the adoption of colonial laws to prevent interracial sexual relations and marriage.

The other side of equation was that anti-racial ideologies emerged in the interwar period. Socialists in Germany criticized notions of racial hygiene, while British academics became uncomfortable with the political repercussions of racial analysis. Scientific opposition intensified in the face of Nazism in the 1930s and more leftwing and liberal scientists started to reject racial theories as scientific concepts. In the early 1950s, the international scientific community under the auspices of UNESCO rejected race as a scientific term to identify inherent human difference. Drawing on the new field of cultural anthropology, UNESCO argued that the biological phenomenon of race was a social myth. At a national level, post-war revelations, such as about Vichy France (1940–44), reinforced this process of ideological conversion. However, medicalized racial discourses did not vanish. A dismissal of racial theories did not see a rejection of the belief in mental and physical racial differences. The concept of race continued to have resonance as apparent in French reactions to North African immigrants, and in late twentieth century debate on the health disparities between racial and ethnic communities or on AIDS.

Ideas of race were important in shaping a common culture and belief system that was shared by many European doctors. Colonial medicine had a racist dimension and racial ideas influenced public health policies, but racist theory and practice often diverged. Different forms of racial discrimination existed in different colonial and non-colonial contexts. Although scientific racism, racial stereotyping and European perceptions of a racial hierarchy were deployed to legitimize colonialism, colonial encounters and colonial medicine were shaped not only by racial ideas but also by the problems colonial powers encountered. The next section examines these problems.

Empire and disease

Disease has offered historians an important focus for considering the impact of colonialism and the control strategies colonial powers adopted. Board narratives have been combined with studies of individual diseases, such as malaria, although the focus has often been on the dramatic rather than the everyday. Whereas early studies equated European intervention and colonialism with health gains, scholarship has increasingly emphasized the high mortality associated with colonial expansion and the relative ineffectiveness of Western medicine to tackle tropical diseases. Epidemics became linked to the imperial process and the ways in which colonialism established structures that contributed to morbidity and mortality. Work on Africa, for example, suggests that European conquests before 1930 coincided with a period of ecological and epidemiological disaster. One school of thought argues that changes in population distribution – such as through improved communications, migration or troop movements – encouraged the spread of disease. Another contends that colonization deprived indigenous populations of the ability to control their environment and by destroying the existing ecology created conditions in which disease could flourish. This apocalyptic school has emphasized the devastating impact of colonialism through increased contact and communication, war, agricultural change, and urbanization, as seen in Spanish colonization in fifteenth and sixteenth century South America. Although it is difficult to measure the cost of colonialism, in some ways, imperialism served to perpetuate or extend existing health inequalities; in others, it created new health problems.

The voyages of discovery in the sixteenth century represented a disaster for the peoples encountered. The arrival of the Spanish in the Americas brought diseases like smallpox, plague, measles, chickenpox and influenza from Europe, as well as yellow fever and malaria from Africa, which ravaged not only the Native American Indians but also the Caribbean population. It was not just in the Americas that colonial encounters brought disease. In the eighteenth century, epidemics, such as measles in the Pacific islands and New Zealand, decimated local populations. Although the growth of European imperialism in South Asia or later in Africa did not have the same catastrophic effects on indigenous populations as it had in the Americas, colonialism remained closely associated with epidemics, the introduction of new endemic diseases, such as tuberculosis, and the spread of deficiency diseases, such as beriberi. With an intensification of contacts after 1750, epidemics of cholera, smallpox, influenza and measles increased. As explorers, soldiers and traders penetrated inland, indigenous populations were exposed to new pathogens to which they had little resistance. For example, in northern Australia, the arrival of white settlers had a detrimental effect on the health of the Aboriginal population. Most colonial regions saw a series of epidemics of cholera, smallpox, and then pneumonic plague in the 1890s and 1900s. Contemporary theories attributed these epidemics to non-Europeans representing a 'virgin soil' for disease. Of course, regional geographies and conditions created different patterns of disease, but for Europeans South America, Africa and South Asia all appeared unhealthy places.

Colonial policies contributed to a rise in the level of epidemic and endemic disease. Migration – forced or following work – and the Slave Trade increased exposure and aided the spread of disease. The expansion of trade had a similar effect: for example, smallpox and sleeping sickness followed trade routes. Colonial wars had a direct impact, resulting in the breakdown of social structures and a loss of environmental controls, while rape by colonial soldiers facilitated the spread of venereal diseases. Although these examples are brutal, conquest and colonial policies had an impact on disease patterns in other ways. The expansion of commercial agriculture in South Asia and Africa resulted in ecological changes that altered the local ecology and the pattern of disease. For example, new irrigation canals provided ideal breeding grounds for mosquitoes. Social and political crisis created an environment in which plague could ravage India for two decades after 1896, claiming at least twelve million lives. The country appeared vulnerable given widespread poverty, low immunities to disease, and poor urban conditions, which, when combined with modern networks of transport and trade, facilitated the spread of the disease. Eradication programmes adopted for one disease could allow another to emerge. For example, because yaws and syphilis offer limited cross immunity, moves to eradicate yaws in colonial Kenya in the 1920s and 1930s saw a corresponding increase in syphilis in the 1940s and 1950s. Only by the 1920s did imperialists and their critics start to recognize that colonial policies were contributing to high levels of disease.

It was not just mortality and morbidity patterns among the colonized populations that were affected. It was often European settlers who felt most at risk as they encountered a range of diseases that were unknown or had largely vanished from Europe. Scurvy killed crews on long voyages, at least until the eighteenth century, but settlers also encountered new diseases. Although some, like sleeping sickness, hardly affected settlers, others appeared to threaten colonialism. In

Latin America and the Caribbean, yellow fever was a major problem for settlers and merchants in the eighteenth century. Africa became associated with disease. The imagery of death was employed to describe nineteenth century colonial Africa as the 'white man's grave', especially as colonizers in the pursuit of resources moved into areas often considered unhealthy by local populations. Such imagery became part of popular perceptions of the continent and shaped medical and political responses. But it was not just Africa that took its toll on European colonizers. In South Asia and Latin America, few Europeans settlers were able to escape malaria. Cholera and dysentery exacted a heavy toll; yellow fever seemed more virulent among European settlers than the local population.

Colonial expansion stimulated an examination of the health risks of colonization. A 'hot climate' literature emerged in the seventeenth century as medical writers discussed the effects of high temperatures, humidity and the sun on health. By the first decades of the eighteenth century, a substantial literature existed on tropical disease. Much of this literature initially focused on the Caribbean and East Indies where the British, French and Dutch all had important maritime and trading interests and linked high mortality to environment and climate. Mostly coming from a white, elitist and masculine perspective, writers asserted that Europeans could gain immunity to tropical diseases through a process of acclimatization. The notion of acclimatization offered a scientific rationale that held practical implications for a range of fields from agriculture to medicine and created optimism that it was possible for European settlers to adapt and gain immunity to indigenous diseases. Although ideas of acclimatization remained current in the nineteenth century, notably in botany and agriculture, accounts from external commentators and white settlers in India and Africa painted an increasingly depressing picture of high mortality and a more pessimistic view of European colonization became unmistakable in medical literature and travel writing. Racial ideas were conscripted to explain why colonials faced physiological and mental breakdown in new environments to which, it was argued, their race ill-equipped them. The idea that different races had different immunities to disease proved remarkably resilient: it appealed to European settlers who found it hard to adjust, and was reassuring to those who feared that acclimatization might mean the acquisition of native attributes.

Although Europeans were vulnerable to tropical diseases to which indigenous populations were naturally immune (such as malaria), notions of predisposition were used to explain why equatorial races were susceptible to new diseases. The growing acceptance of bacteriology in explaining disease at the end of the nineteenth century focused attention on the dangers of local disease environments and populations. Although it was argued that indigenous populations were able to adapt to local diseases, they came to be seen as reservoirs of infection, contributing to the myth of the diseased native. The identification of the presence of malaria parasites in the blood provided the foundation for the growing belief that Africans were natural carriers of certain diseases, including leprosy. This belief in the idea that native bodies acted as reservoirs for local pathogens reinforced an enclavist approach, justified draconian intervention by the colonial state, and legitimized ideas of racial segregation as evident in South Africa.

The nature of tropical diseases required a rethinking of European medical knowledge as colonial doctors were confronted with apparently new diseases or familiar ones in new, more virulent forms. Although not all medical practitioners felt this way – some dismissed the idea that climate or geography mattered – an interest in medical topography in the eighteenth and nineteenth centuries strengthened existing ideas that disease was environmentally determined [see 'Public health']. Colonial practitioners drew on these ideas and stressed the role of climate and topology in the production of disease. In India and Africa, Europeans related heat to putrefaction to argue that living at higher altitudes and adopting hygienic routines reduced the risk of diseases like malaria. Even in the 1920s, doctors still endorsed explanations for tropical diseases based around ideas of climate and environment. The idea that succumbing to a hot climate or tropical disease was the result of a biological process provided an explanatory framework that proved reassuring to settlers and influenced colonial medical policies.

Colonial medicine

Although it is important to keep in mind that each colony, each power and each region do not fit into neat categories, medicine, public health and medical practitioners were enlisted in the service of empire. Introducing Western medicine and training indigenous practitioners in Western methods not only asserted the colonial state's credentials to modernity and civilization, but also was perceived as a way of saving indigenous populations from the dangers of local medicine and superstition. Exploration by medical practitioners helped open up new territories and provided information on them as evident in the activities of French medical practitioners in Algeria. Colonial doctors both helped bolster support for colonial rule and shaped administrative policies, with the administration of public health offering insights into how colonial states functioned. Medicine and public health policies also assisted expansion and the retention of colonies: smallpox vaccination and quinine prophylaxis (for malaria) are often represented as crucial in aiding European expansion in Asia and Africa.

Empire may have provided a testing ground (or laboratory) for new technologies, ideas or treatments, but for the most part, colonizers were initially concerned with their own health. The Spanish Crown, for example, concentrated on the health of the military in Spanish America to serve colonial aims. A similar pattern occurred in northern Australia in the second half of the nineteenth century as moves were made to protect minority white settlers. Medical services and sanitary programmes were concentrated in those places where Europeans or their military settled. As a result, urban and costal areas were better supplied than rural locations. Historians have come to refer to this approach as enclavist.

Public health and environmental programmes became essential to efforts to control those diseases that threatened the socioeconomic or military wellbeing of the colony to aid settlement or trade. Sanitary reforms therefore focused on epidemic diseases, such as plague or smallpox, that most affected European soldiers, settlers or colonial interests. In India, for example, the need to send more troops following the mutiny in 1857 came with a high level of disease and focused interest on sanitary reform to reduce mortality among the soldiers sent to secure India from further uprisings. However, there was more to colonial medicine and sanitation than environmental controls, vaccination or quinine. Sanitary policies marked an unprecedented assault on the bodies of the colonized and influenced a policy of racial segregation. In Natal and the Transvaal, for example, fear of epidemics of cholera and smallpox saw efforts to segregate Indians and South Africans to tackle the perceived reservoirs of disease. Responses to epidemics could be draconian. Contravening yellow fever quarantine measures in Senegal could result in anything from the death penalty to life imprisonment or fines. Measures to combat the plague epidemic in India and South Africa in the early twentieth century targeted both individuals and (predominantly poor) areas deemed unsanitary. In India, house and body searches were conducted, buildings were disinfected or demolished, areas were evacuated, and plague suffers were isolated. In South Africa, reactions to the plague were equally harsh: the Cape authorities removed between six and seven thousand Africans to a separate settlement in Uitvlugt. Such responses have been identified as a crucial episode in the creation of a segregated society in South Africa.

These broad generalizations conceal the complexity of medical encounters and policies, overstate their impact, and take little account of the extent that theory and practice operated in different colonies or contexts. The effectiveness of public health measures varied, as did the level of intervention. Where Western medical ideas and policies conflicted with indigenous social mores, their influence was more limited. For example, government policies in India to suppress plague clashed with popular and religious values, provoking opposition and riots, which saw policies modified. Nor were approaches uniform or coherent. Diversity was as important in medicine as it was in other areas of colonial expansion where an often chaotic mix of strategies and practices existed. As Michael Worboys has shown, if in white settler colonies like Australia the main aim was to recreate European medical institutions, in Africa, where a small European military and political administration controlled large, sparsely populated regions, European medicine had a minimal presence and the priority was to maintain military effectiveness.[2] Colonial power and authority were restricted by the distances involved and by resources. The same was true for medical power. Often medical encounters and policies reveal not an omnipresent colonial state apparatus and European hegemony over oppressed colonial subjects, but the limits of power and colonialism. The numbers of colonizers were often small and territories vast, creating obstacles to colonial rule and ensuring that delays occurred in the spread of Western medical practices. Nor was medicine a homogenous entity. European practitioners not only came from different national medical traditions, which shaped their approach, but also worked in different colonial, political, economic, cultural and institutional contexts.

Colonies did different things at different times and colonial powers adopted different policies in different places. For example, medical services in colonial Ceylon (Sri Lanka) where Western-trained indigenous practitioners were used differed from those in British India, despite both colonies being under British control. Regional and local conditions and agencies were important, as was resistance from colonial medical officers, as evident in Nigeria. Local administrators or medical practitioners could hamper central policies, adapt them, or invent new ones. Sanitary measures in the Punjab, for example, were frustrated by professional and administrative disagreements. Local administrators also limited action to prevent unrest or opposition. Nor were sanitary programmes always successful. By the end of the nineteenth century, colonial medical officers tacitly acknowledged that colonial policies had helped perpetuate sanitary problems: in Bombay, for example, efforts to improve water supplies saw areas of the city become saturated with groundwater, creating perfect breeding grounds for water- and insect-borne diseases.

Nor was the colonial state the main or only agent of colonial medicine. Whereas state medical provision was mainly confined to European civilians or soldiers, missionary medicine had a much broader reach. In New Spain, the Catholic Church by the seventeenth century had a major role in hospital provision and in supplying drugs to private practitioners. Christian missionaries emerged as important agents in the provision of Western medicine in China, Japan and India, and later in Africa as the focus of colonial expansion shifted in the late nineteenth century. Formal medical missionary work after 1850 extended missionaries' reach – for missionaries, medicine offered an effective means of challenging the perceived forces of superstition, protected the health of the missionaries themselves, and was a means to secure conversions. The provision of hospitals or dispensaries, such as in China, was often the most visible symbols of this medical missionary work.

Although growing historical interest in the transfer of Western medicine to colonial regions has emphasized resistance, colonial medical encounters were rarely a straightforward process of dominance or resistance. For example, in Japan following the Meiji Restoration (1867–68), the government actively rejected Chinese medicine in favour of Western practices. Elsewhere, neither Western medicine nor traditional healing practices were monolithic. Colonial and indigenous medical theories and practices were often not that fundamentally different, and this allowed an exchange of ideas and practices. In early modern Spanish America, for example, similarities between Spanish, Native American and African medical systems, along with a common faith in the supernatural and in medicinal plants, aided the spread and swapping of ideas. Although differences between indigenous and Western medicine became more marked in the eighteenth and nineteenth centuries, what existed was a process of interaction, not a complete replacement of one system of medicine with another. Just as with other aspects of empire, local traditions and practices were used, particularly where resources were scarce and regions were isolated. Pluralism – or what might be seen as cross-fertilization – was important and the further away Western doctors or nurses were from centres of institutionalized Western medicine the clearer this pluralism.

Some aspects of Western medicine did attract support from local populations. For example, there was some willingness among indigenous populations to try Western drugs, especially as many plant- and mineral-based medicines were similar to local remedies. The creation of hospitals might have given legitimacy to imperial rulers or missionaries, but they were used by local populations and were adapted to local cultures. Encounters worked both ways. Visitors to India in the late seventeenth century commented on the extent to which European medicine was ill-suited to dealing with local diseases, and even in the nineteenth century, colonial settlers were prepared to use traditional practices. For example, Harriet Deacon shows how eighteenth century Dutch-Africans adopted some Khoisan birthing practices, especially for difficult or slow labours, and used black midwives.[3]

This use of indigenous medical knowledge and practitioners persisted in the nineteenth century. In the West and East Indies and Africa, practitioners incorporated some of the medical practices of Native Americans and African slaves. Often indigenous remedies were used as substitutes for more expensive European drugs. Rather than actively stamping out the use of indigenous remedies, European doctors in their choice of medicines were guided by finding remedies for the most prevalent diseases in their locality and by advice from local practitioners about what worked. Elsewhere, such as in Ceylon (Sri Lanka), physicians incorporated local practices as a way of convincing the indigenous population of the efficacy of Western methods. It was only as the technical gap between Western medicine and the healing systems of other cultures widened with improvements in surgery and the development of effective drug therapies and vaccines that Western medical practices were able to strengthen their hold. For much of the nineteenth century, pluralism remained important. Colonial medical encounters were never therefore a simple question of dominance or resistance.

Tropical medicine

Historians have stressed how in the twentieth century imperial medicine moved away from its early environmentalist perspective to focus on those vector-borne parasitic diseases that took the greatest toll on European settlers. Early work on Britain by the historian Michael Worboys critically evaluated the intellectual development of tropical medicine to show how it was linked to the policies, agencies and ideologies of 'constructive imperialism' (see Further Reading). By the 1990s, Worboys's research was influencing other historians who increasingly pointed to a reciprocal relationship between centre and periphery. Although studies revealed how tropical medicine was deployed in different ways depending on local contexts, tropical medicine was shown to aid the medicalization of empire.

The discovery in 1897 by the British physicians Patrick Manson and Ronald Ross that the anopheles mosquito transmitted malaria, and the subsequent research into vector-borne parasitic diseases, has been represented as marking the beginning of tropical medicine. As Britain's leading expert in the field, Manson certainly made this claim. However, tropical medicine did not start with Manson and Ross. Not only were the physicians Amico Bignami and Giuseppe Bastianelli and the zoologist Giovanni Battista Grassi involved in malaria research in Italy at the same time, but also the expansion of bacteriology in the 1880s and 1890s provided the foundation for a shift from an interest in environment to vector-borne parasitic disease and encouraged a focus on specific pathogens. The isolation and cultivation of a number of pathogenic bacteria and research on vaccines appeared to offer practical benefits for combating disease [see 'Science and medicine']. Given the high levels of epidemic and endemic disease, the colonial context created favourable conditions for further work. This approach was evident in the German bacteriologist Robert Koch's studies of cholera in Egypt in the 1880s and in the British trials of antityphoid inoculations in India in the 1890s. As specialists in tropical medicine concentrated on the microorganisms and parasites responsible for tropical diseases, a change occurred from isolating the agents responsible in the laboratory to studying insect vectors, ecology and hygiene in colonial regions.

The parasite-vector mechanism identified for malaria became the model for other researchers. As ideas about tropical disease moved from a focus on germs to the climates in which parasites appeared, topical medicine came to be structured around the life cycles of parasites. Considerable scientific prestige was attached to finding new pathogens and vectors, stimulating the creation of schools of tropical medicine, such as those in Liverpool (1898), Paris (1901) and Brussels (1906), international competition and, over malaria, nationalist posturing. Physicians and bacteriologists worked to understand the aetiology of tropical diseases and catalogue the species of insects associated with them as they endeavoured to understand and eradicate disease. As other parasitic vectors were discovered – for example, the tsetse fly in yellow fever – there was an important practical shift in tropical medicine to emphasize eradicating the parasites – the vector of transmission – and the environment in which they occurred. Tropical medicine was never entirely dependent on European medical theories or practices, however. For example, under the future Nobel Prize winner for physiology Charles Nicolle, the Pasteur Institute of Tunis produced major studies on plague. Colonial practitioners used their experiences to challenge and develop European medical ideas. In many ways, therefore, tropical medicine was developed in a colonial context, with colonial schools offering the main sites through which knowledge about tropical diseases was fashioned.

Other factors were at work that created a favourable context for the application of tropical medicine. These had much to do with the new imperialism of the late nineteenth century. International rivalry among European powers, as apparent in the 'scramble for Africa', the use of empire as a symbolic unifying force, as under the French Third Republic (1870–1940), and attempts to fashion environments in which Europeans could live disease-free to aid the exploitation of colonial resources, persuaded colonial administrators to invest in tropical medicine. This expansion coincided with a series of epidemics which encouraged colonial powers to provide political backing for tropical medicine, as well as substantial investment in research (such as into sleeping sickness). The conquest of malaria, yellow fever and sleeping sickness held political and economic benefits and represented a means through which further European colonialism could be secured. Tropical medicine hence found ready support among those who advocated imperial expansion and was incorporated into colonial health and sanitary programmes.

Tropical medicine came to be regarded as offering a prophylactic means of intervention by killing the parasite or insect-vector or by breaking the cycle of transmission through public health measures. Strategies favoured tackling particular diseases as ideas of eradication gathered momentum – a development that saw tropical medicine become characterized as a colonial tool. Yet often policies were underfunded and were conducted with haste and coercion, as apparent in efforts to tackle sleeping sickness in Northern Zaire or in the Belgian Congo. Attempts were made to manage local ecologies, such as through drainage schemes or deforestation, relocate indigenous populations considered reservoirs of infection, such as in Uganda or northern Australia, or create sanitary cordons for European settlers, a policy energetically pursued in Africa where racial segregation came to be justified on sanitary grounds. Efforts were also made to develop prophylaxis and chemotherapy treatments, an approach favoured by France and Germany. Pesticides were used in an attempt to kill parasites or insects, although these were of limited effectiveness before the introduction of the pesticide DDT in the 1940s. Individual measures were taken: for example, as seen in the move to wearing protective clothing and sleeping under insect nets, routines that became embedded in representations of empire.

However, continuities remained. Voluntary organizations, such as the American Rockefeller Foundation, Christian medical institutions, and missionaries continued to have a crucial role in the development of colonial medical services. In Kenya, for example, the Church of Scotland pioneered the eradication of yaws, adopting methods that were later implemented by the colonial state. Testimonies from a wide cross-section of South African society in the 1940s and 1950s reveal that large numbers were attracted to the Church by their desire to be healed. Medicine when allied to evangelicalism provided a more potent agent of Western medicine than the state or local doctors.

A self-interested emphasis on improving the health of colonial subjects came to characterize colonial medical policy in the 1920s and 1930s as the mortality rates among European settlers improved. The interwar period has often been represented as marking a watershed in imperial rule and colonial medical services as pressure increased for change. Whereas before 1914, colonial medical officials had been mainly responsible for European settlers, in the 1920s colonial powers, such as France in Indochina or Belgium in the Congo, began to develop state medical services for the indigenous population and extended campaigns to eradicate or control single diseases. For example, the British in Uganda resettled inhabitants from areas with tsetse fly to new settlements and, faced with a severe demographic crisis, started to build hospitals and dispensaries for the indigenous population. State medical positions were opened-up to local people with Western medical training and colonial medical colleges were established.

Fears about the role of local populations in spreading disease to white settlers certainly encouraged efforts to extend medical care for indigenous populations. However, colonial powers were seeking to develop colonial economies and medical services in Africa and in the Far East aimed to support these efforts. Elsewhere, growing social unrest and the emergence of nationalist movements focused attention. Colonial powers started to feel a growing obligation to their colonies, which combined with a need to combat anti-colonial sentiment and limit the political and social strength of local healers and rulers. Medicine, particularly public health and government-funded hospitals, became a means of fulfilling this.

Although the market for Western medical services expanded in the twentieth century, as can be seen in India or Kenya, continued ignorance of the needs of indigenous populations, understaffing, financial resources, the limitations of Western medicine, and local opposition, ensured that colonial medical policies were never all encompassing. Disease control policies, such as delousing programmes to control typhus in South Africa, or the isolation of sleeping sickness sufferers in special camps in the Belgian Congo, reflected the ways in which indigenous populations were poorly treated by colonial health authorities and engendered considerable opposition. Fears of hospitalizations discouraged many from seeking Western medical care, and antagonism towards colonial medical policies and faith in indigenous practitioners remained strong.

Despite attempts on the one hand to impose controls to limit indigenous practices, as in Africa, and on the other to resist Western medical incursion, a profusion of therapeutic agencies and practitioners existed. Just as in the nineteenth century, indigenous and Western medical systems in the twentieth century often overlapped. The decision to consult one or the other, or often both, continued to be shaped by choice, local customs and cultures, access and resources, and by the disease needing treatment. Incurable diseases like leprosy saw more openness to indigenous treatments, while local healers were often cheaper. Colonial authorities, especially in Africa, tried to recognize this situation through attempts to regulate local healers while at the same time trying to exclude them from the medical marketplace. But clear regional and geographical differences emerged. Most colonial medical services continued to be concentrated in places where Europeans settled. Although public health services targeted the poor, curative services favoured wealthy urban Europeans. Postcolonial medical reforms continued to replicate these divisions.

Western medicine and the developing world

The process of decolonization, which began in South Asia in the late 1940s and Africa in the late 1950s, not only brought political independence for many former colonies by the mid 1960s, but also a degree of medical independence. However, if greater medical autonomy was achieved, it did not mean that Western medical intervention in Africa or South Asia stopped after 1945. One legacy of colonialism was ongoing medical, economic and political dependency, which was reinforced by internationalism in health and the work of aid agencies that favoured Western solutions. The World Health Organization (WHO) and technical aid programmes by the United States and the Soviet Union had an important role in the provision of medical care and in disease eradication programmes. WHO, for example, sponsored a number of initiatives from child vaccination programmes to the support for public health and primary healthcare provision. Assistance programmes proliferated. Emergency aid schemes (for disaster and famine relief) were established. Yet, WHO's work remained governed by efforts to combat infectious disease as apparent in its immunization programmes. Such policies continued the interests embedded in colonial medicine as WHO and other international agencies were dominated by the top-down biomedical agendas of former colonial powers. For some, such policies were believed to be in compensation for colonial rule. For others, it came from the mistaken belief that poor health was an important cause of economic backwardness in what came to be labelled developing countries.

In the field of medicine, continuities have remained more important than in other areas of postcolonialism. Existing patterns of colonial medical provision and established ideas about indigenous medicine were replicated after 1945. Although in many of the new independent states health policies drew on the idea that healthcare should be extended to the entire population, faith in the superiority of Western medicine, bolstered by immediate post-war developments, encouraged a continued investment in a Western-style, urban and hospital-based approach and in programmes of disease control. African rulers encouraged major efforts to develop medical services to demonstrate their commitment to improving the lives of their citizens, but many imported Western attitudes, medical technology and pharmaceuticals at the expensive of rural services where the majority of the population lived.

Faith in the utility of Western medicine and intervention was often not matched by results. Despite the apparent successes of programmes to eradicate contagious diseases, such as smallpox or yaws, wars, poverty, famine, different medical cultures, the growing influence of global pharmaceutical companies, and limited access to resources, had a marked influence on standards of healthcare in the developing world. For example, restricted access to medical training frequently left postcolonial nations with a shortage of doctors. In some cases, money was often diverted to the creation of expensive Western-style hospitals; in others, the scale of the problem, such as the eradication of malaria, was too great. The failure of some projects reflected an ongoing lack of understanding of local cultures and medical traditions. By the 1960s, the limitations of Western approaches started to become clear. Following an initiative by WHO and UNICEF, attention in the 1970s began to move away from hospital-based and physician-based care towards primary healthcare. As in other areas, rhetoric seldom matched reality. Financial constraints, political sensitivities, and pressure from Western pharmaceutical companies – or Big Pharma – which wanted to protect markets for their drugs, curtailed healthcare in certain areas, such as AIDS programmes, and saw a narrowing of interest to focus on particular health problems.

Conclusions

Whereas tropical medicine was associated with success in the first half of the twentieth century, the emergence of new infectious diseases, such as AIDS, the re-emergence of old diseases, notably malaria, and the growth of lifestyle diseases in Africa and Asia, highlights both the limitations of Western medical intervention and the multifaceted connections that exist between medicine and colonialism. In a colonial context, European knowledge was never a closed system of colonial power, repression, and violence even if medicine served an ideological role in asserting Western ideas and practices. Colonial and tropical medicine had to adjust to shifting political, military, geographical, epidemiological and economic contexts. Often efforts to tackle disease were enclavist in approach, especially outside urban areas, but in many areas, hybrid and plural forms of medical care developed. Colonial policies did have limitations, however. This can be seen in South Africa where socioeconomic conditions and legal controls encouraged the ongoing use of indigenous medicines in the twentieth century. Notwithstanding the global health agenda increasingly pursued by international organizations, medicine in the developing world has remained characterized by a diverse, fragmentary pattern of healthcare systems that were caught between a dependence on private care, self-help and traditional healers and pressure from Big Pharma. Medicine it would seem was never monolithic, unchanging or straightforward in a colonial or postcolonial setting.

Further reading

There are a number of historiographical overviews of medicine and empire, with Shula Marks, 'What is Colonial About Colonial Medicine? And What Has Happened to Imperialism and Health?', *Social History of Medicine* 10 (1997), pp. 205–19, Richard Drayton, 'Science, Medicine, and the British Empire', in Robin W. Winks (ed.), *The Oxford History of the British Empire, vol. 5: Historiography* (Oxford: Oxford University Press, 1999), pp. 264–76, and Waltraud Ernst, 'Beyond East and West', *Social History of Medicine*, 20 (2007), pp. 505–24, providing good starting points. These surveys outline key studies and approaches, but accessible overviews of colonial and tropical medicine can be found in the introduction to David Arnold (ed.), *Warm Climates and Western Medicine: The Emergence of Tropical Medicine 1500–1900* (Amsterdam: Rodopi, 1996) and Michael Worboys, 'Colonial and Imperial Medicine', in Deborah Brunton (ed.), *Medicine Transformed: Health, Disease and Society in Europe 1800–1930* (Manchester: Manchester University Press, 2004), pp. 211–38. The issue of race and medicine is a complex one and is best initially approached through Waltraud Ernst and Bernard Harris (eds), *Race, Science and Medicine 1700–1960* (London: Routledge, 1999) or Warwick Anderson, 'Disease, Race, and Empire', *Bulletin of the History of Medicine*, 70 (1996), pp. 62–67. For medicine as a 'tool of empire', see Daniel Headrick, *Tools of Empire: Technology and European Imperialism in the Nineteenth Century* (New York and Oxford: Oxford University Press, 1981), while the collection edited by Roy Macleod and Milton Lewis (eds), *Disease, Medicine, and Empire: Perspectives on Western Medicine and the Experience of European Expansion* (London: Routledge, 1988) challenges the link between diffusion models of modernization and development. On the relationship between Western medicine and indigenous societies, see David Arnold (ed.), *Imperial Medicine and Indigenous Societies* (Manchester: Manchester University Press, 1988), while Alan Bewell, *Romanticism and Colonial Disease* (Baltimore, MD: Johns Hopkins University Press, 2003) and Ann L. Stoler, *Race and the Education of Desire: Foucault's 'History of Sexuality' and the Colonial Order of Things* (Durham, NC: Duke University Press, 1995) are good examples of the ways in which empire had an impact on Western medical theories. David Arnold, *Science, Technology and Medicine in Colonial India* (Cambridge: Cambridge University Press, 2004) and Mark Harrison, *Public Health in British India: Anglo-Indian Preventive Medicine 1859–1914* (Cambridge: Cambridge University Press, 1994) further illustrate how medical practice in India was accommodated to indigenous environments. There is a large literature on disease patterns: for example, see Noble Cook, *Born to Die: Disease and New World Conquest 1492–1650* (Cambridge: Cambridge University Press, 1998) or Crosby, Alfred, *Ecological Imperialism: The Biological Expansion of Europe 900–1900* (Cambridge: Cambridge University Press, 2004) for the early modern period, and John Farley, *Bilharzia: A History of Imperial Tropical Medicine* (Cambridge: Cambridge University Press, 1991); Maryinez Lyons, *The Colonial Disease: A Social History of Sleeping Sickness in Northern Zaire 1900–40* (Cambridge: Cambridge University Press, 2002) and Philip Curtin, *The Image of Africa: British Ideas and Action 1780–1850* (London: Macmillan, 1965) for the nineteenth and twentieth centuries. Curtin's excellent *Death by Migration: Europe's Encounter with the Tropical World in the Nineteenth Century* (London: Macmillan, 1989) more broadly explores the relationship between colonialism and mortality. On colonial medicine and power, see David Arnold, *Colonizing the Body: State Medicine and Epidemic Disease in Nineteenth-Century India* (Cambridge: Cambridge University Press, 1993) or Megan Vaughan, *Curing their Ills: Colonial Power and African Illness* (Cambridge: Polity Press, 1991). On resistance to colonial medicine, see Luise White, *Speaking with Vampires: Rumour and History in Colonial Africa* (Berkeley, CA: University of California Press, 2000) or Andrew Cunningham and Birdie Andrews (eds), *Western Medicine as Contested Knowledge*

(Manchester: Manchester University Press, 1997). Less has been written about the twentieth century, but Randall M. Packard, 'Postcolonial Medicine', in Roger Cooter and John Pickstone (eds), *Medicine in the Twentieth Century* (London: Routledge, 2000), pp. 97–112, is an excellent overview. This should be supplemented by Sung Lee, 'WHO and the Developing World', in Cunningham and Andrews (eds), *Western Medicine as Contested Knowledge*, ibid, pp. 24–45, and Fraser Brockington, *The Health of the Developing World* (Lewes: Book Guild, 1985), which are both critical of WHO's involvement.

15
Medicine and warfare

Over the past three centuries, medicine has become a significant part of military administration and management. This evolving relationship has encouraged a view that medicine is one of the few beneficiaries of warfare. Developments in surgery have been associated with the invention of gunpowder and the wars of the eighteenth and nineteenth centuries; the Crimean War (1853–56) with nursing reforms, or the South African War (1899–1902) with efforts to organize battlefield medical care. In the First World War (1914–18), new weapons that caused complex wounds saw new surgical techniques introduced and advances made in plastic surgery and orthopaedics as surgeons confronted horrific facial injuries and shattered bones.

However, it is unwise to treat medicine in war as somehow outside the context in which it occurred. Nor is the impact of warfare on medicine straightforward: it could be substantial but episodic. Roger Cooter has led the field in rejecting the idea that war was somehow outside of society to argue that medicine in wartime and peacetime cannot be easily separated (see Further Reading). His work has revealed the ways in which medicine in wartime was not just shaped by technical advances made necessary by wartime conditions, by the need to provide care for sick or maimed soldiers, or by the professional concerns of medical practitioners. As Cooter explains, each war generated particular problems: for example, because of the conditions under which the conflict occurred (trench warfare), the landscape over which it was fought (epidemic conditions in Africa), or because of the type of weaponry used (handheld weapons v. artillery). In assessing the relationship between war and medicine, Cooter draws attention to the necessity of taking into account different ideological and socioeconomic contexts.

The importance of context can be illustrated by examining how political ideologies and resources shaped military medical services. By looking at the English Civil War (1642–49), it becomes possible to see how each side adopted a different approach that owed much to their political beliefs. The Royalist army displayed lukewarm commitment to its casualties and assumed that regimental commanders were responsible. This attitude led commanders to pay lip service to the need for centrally coordinated casualty care. Parliamentary forces adopted a different approach. Concern for common wellbeing combined with control of London's hospitals, large financial resources, and the support of the metropolitan medical and mercantile establishments, saw Parliament accept responsibility for those killed or maimed in its service. This approach was both practical and political. The provision of welfare services for ex-servicemen was equally political, often to prevent revolt. By the end of the nineteenth century, other political factors can be seen at work. Improved literacy and the expansion of the press combined with an extension of the franchise to make governments more conscious of the need to improve military medical care.

Although the socioeconomic, cultural and political context in which war occurred is crucial to understanding the nature of the relationships that existed between medicine and warfare, other forces were at work. Practical or tactical concerns, changing notions of military manpower and attitudes to wastage, or the role of medical or military technology were all important. Taking these basic assumptions into account, this chapter examines the relationship between warfare and medicine, the dangers military personnel faced, the military medical services established, and the impact of warfare on the civilian population and social policy.

The perils of war

The medical problems generated by military campaigns, the diseases and injuries sustained by military personnel, helped determine the nature of military medical services. Public discourses surrounding military action have stressed bloodshed and death tolls, but war did not just see soldiers die in battle. For many, war meant injury, sickness and disability, although exposure to injury and disease often depended on rank, while self-inflicted injuries were not uncommon.

Early modern warfare and colonial expansion exposed soldiers and sailors to a host of injuries and disease. Wounds were inflicted by many sources besides bullets: they came from swords and from blows, such as those from the butt of muskets. Explosions, burns and accidents were an ordinary part of military life. Gunshot wounds presented numerous problems for military surgeons and required new techniques. The systematic mechanization of death Daniel Pick sees in *The War Machine* (1993) as part of the enduring image of conflicts after the 1860s also shaped the injuries sustained. New military technologies – the machine gun, the tank, the long-range bomber, chemical weapons – changed the nature of warfare and the injuries sustained by military personnel and civilians. This relationship between technology, injury and the nature of the military campaigns fought is apparent in the twentieth century and the staggering number of casualties, even excluding the victims of the Holocaust, which resulted from the two world wars. During the First World War, nearly six million Britons and Germans were wounded; over two million permanently disabled. Wounds from small-calibre rifles were outstripped by complex wounds from artillery shells, mines or shrapnel, which could result in disfigurement and disability, including mental disability. Soldiers also faced the threat of gas

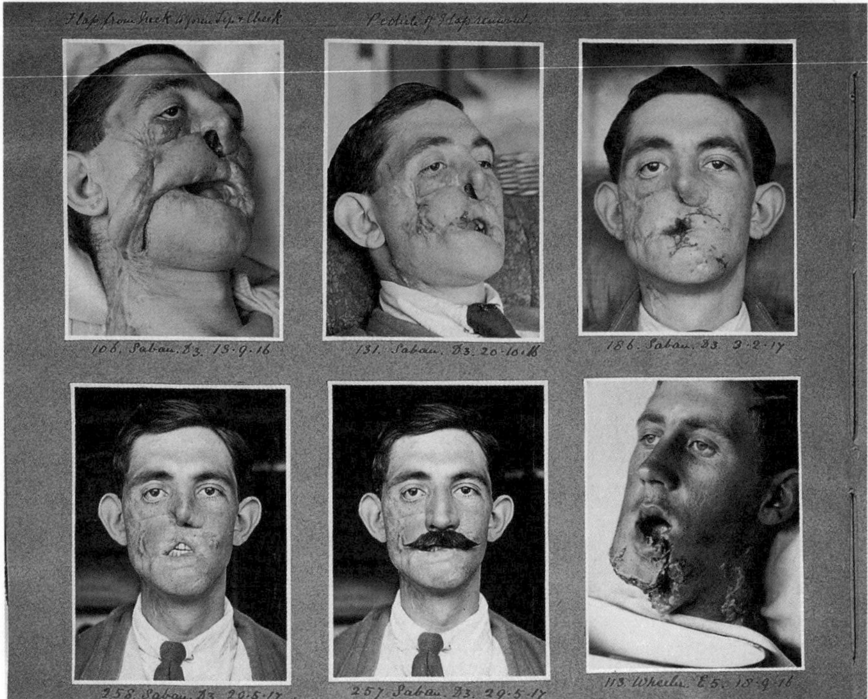

Figure 15.1 Photographs illustrating shrapnel wounds to the face and the treatment received between April 1916 and May 1917. The photographs from the King George Military Hospital in London chart the progress of plastic surgery on one soldier and illustrate the horrific injuries some soldiers sustained during the First World War.

Source: Wellcome Library, London.

gangrene and asphyxia as well as trench foot. As we will see below, complex wounds and the risk of infection posed new medical problems that influenced the nature of military medicine in the First World War.

Modern mechanized warfare produced other types of injury. Although revisionist historians, such as Niall Fergusson, have stressed that soldiers survived modern warfare because they found it an adventure, the psychological impact of war has become widely accepted. The labels shell shock (First World War), battle fatigue (Second World War), Post-Traumatic Stress Disorder (Vietnam), and Gulf War Syndrome used to describe the emotional and psychological trauma of modern warfare reflect the changing medical and military contexts.

The First World War highlights this emotional and mental cost of warfare. If before 1914, the idea that servicemen might suffer mental distress because of combat was barely considered, in part because other labels were used, during the First World War shell shock became a new and disturbing phenomenon. All combatants considered shell shock a threat to morale and fighting strength, but how to measure the extent to which shell shock affected soldiers is problematic as reported levels are notoriously inaccurate and conceal the degree of psychiatric disturbance. Diagnostic confusion meant that some cases were misidentified, whilst the variety of symptoms made shell shock hard to pin down. However, even with these methodological problems, the numbers affected are disproportionate to the contemporary alarm or historical interest generated by shell shock.

Although many soldiers developed a range of strategies to cope with trench warfare – including concentrating on short-term risks, black humour, overestimating personal control, fatalism, superstitious beliefs, or by imposing an imagined order on the chaos – and most coped remarkably well, not all were successful. New recruits were particularly vulnerable, although rank, class and ethnicity shaped the symptoms suffered and reactions. In some cases, shell shock was the result of killing or of watching the maiming or death of a comrade. Others reported the unbearable conflict between ideas of duty and feelings of cowardice. Those who survived battles often found that they had to cope with feelings of intense guilt. Whatever the reason behind the onset of mental disturbance, the label shell shock was stigmatizing.

The realities of shell shock were different from the familiar literary representations found in the writings of the war poets, but why shell shock became a medical and cultural phenomenon during the First World War is subject to considerable debate. Contemporaries, both during and after the war, equated shell shock with moral failure, malingering or weakness, and applied crude class interpretations that cast sufferers as lacking in moral fibre. In Germany, this association of shell shock with weakness was used to explain why the country lost the war. Historians have presented a range of interpretations that have associated shell shock with modernity. In *The Female Malady* (1985), the feminist critic Elaine Showalter argues that shell shock was a crisis of masculinity, but for other historians it was a response to the historical specificity of modern industrialized warfare. Implicit within this explanation is a model of human nature failing to adapt to a changing environment: shell shock hence becomes a protest against the conditions of modern warfare. For Joanna Bourke in *An Intimate History of Killing* (1999) what was unbearable about the First World War was its passivity in the midst of extreme danger, made worse by the monotony of trench life, the nervous exhaustion of conflict, and by the poor conditions under which soldiers lived, which produced tensions and grievances and heightened frustration. However, the highest breakdown rates were not, as Bourke's view implies, among those soldiers who were least active, but among those closely involved in combat. Those most exposed to danger and killing appeared most at risk.

The problems shell-shocked servicemen encountered did not end in 1918. Many physically- and mentally-disabled veterans often faced difficulties readjusting to family and civilian life. Peacetime governments and societies were not always sympathetic. In the 1920s and 1930s, large gaps in the provision of pensions and rehabilitation services existed for disabled veterans, particularly in Britain and Germany. In the latter, the position of psychologically-disabled veterans became a political issue as part of a wider debate over the war, class and welfare provision. Pensions and healthcare were gradually cut and the failure of these veterans to recover was blamed on their moral failure and dependence on welfare. Many psychologically-disabled veterans hence came to feel persecuted.

A concentration on casualties – mental and physical – tells only part of the story. French demographic studies have estimated that in seventeenth century Europe only 10 to 25 per cent of all military deaths occurred in battle. Until the early twentieth century, outbreaks of infectious diseases were the major cause of death during military campaigns. Early modern armies lost roughly between two and four per cent of their fighting force per month from disease, while in the Spanish navy so many sailors were sick that the management of Spain's Mediterranean empire was threatened. Colonial expansion brought with it a host of diseases that ravaged naval vessels and armies until the twentieth century. Geography mattered. Before 1800, European soldiers in tropical areas died from disease at four to five times the rate of those in Europe [see 'Medicine and empire']. Infectious diseases, including cholera, malaria, plague, typhoid, typhus and yellow fever frequently swept through army encampments. The importance of epidemics to military mortality was particularly visible during the Crimean War when disease accounted for nearly two-thirds of deaths in the British, French, Sardinian and Turkish forces. Military encampments were often hastily constructed, overcrowded, and unsanitary and sited in poor locations – ideal settings for the spread of infectious disease. Soldiers' resistance to infection was reduced by fatigue, poor diet, and by stress. Poor management and inadequate supplies compounded these problems. Under these conditions, hygiene and sanitation emerged as important military concerns in the eighteenth century. However, the application of sanitation knowledge was slow to take hold: the outcome of campaigns, especially colonial conquests, affected attitudes toward disease, with military successes often overshadowing high mortality. Although sanitation had improved by 1939, disease remained an important reason for hospital admission for servicemen.

It was not just infectious diseases that caused problems. Until the late eighteenth century, scurvy was a major cause of sickness in the navy. Levels of venereal disease remained a constant source of concern, despite efforts from the seventeenth century onwards to restrict the sexual activity of military personnel. By 1917, sexually transmitted disease had become a major war problem, forcing the French, British and American military to implement measures to prevent infection. Military personnel faced other hazards. Sick and wounded soldiers in eighteenth century French military hospitals and in British prisoner of war camps during the South African War were used for clinical teaching and therapeutic experiments. In the aftermath of the Second World War (1939–45), the 1947 Nuremberg Code sought to prevent such medical experimentation, but conscripts and the enlisted, willingly or otherwise, continued to be used as guinea pigs in medical experiments.

As this section has shown, the changing nature and technology of conflict and the landscape over which military campaigns were waged shaped the types of injuries sustained – both mental and physical – and the nature of the health problems encountered by military authorities. If until 1900, it was deaths from disease rather than from action or wounding that were the major cause of death during military campaigns, for many war meant injury, sickness and disability.

War and medicine

Historians have debated the role of warfare in advancing medicine. Certainly, war seems to have accelerated certain areas of medicine, such as pharmaceutical research during the First and Second World wars, or highlighted others, such as sanitation, as of military importance. However, generalization is difficult. War often had a mixed impact on medicine – hastening some areas, transforming others, while leaving yet others unaffected. Nor was the process a simple one. Military medicine was structured by a multiplicity of actors (medical, military and civic), and by military and medicine technologies. The impact of war on medicine equally depended on the time, place, duration and context of the war, and its aftermath.

In the early modern period, the battlefield became an important school for surgery. The introduction of gunpowder forced a more active response to wound treatment that encouraged the development of innovative surgical techniques as seen in the writings of the sixteenth century French surgeon Ambroise Paré. Army surgeons increasingly adopted a conservative approach to amputation. In the seventeenth century, military surgeons and physicians emphasized the value of specific treatments. Quick and simple cures were favoured and most military physicians and surgeons learnt on the job. The epidemiological cost of war encouraged studies of infectious diseases and an investment in preventive medicine. Work by English military doctors, the physician John Pringle and the surgeon James Lind, in the eighteenth century represented important studies of military hygiene, with Lind's advocacy of citrus fruit leading to a dramatic reduction in scurvy.

The Revolutionary (1792–1802) and Napoleonic (1803–15) wars saw new surgical procedures introduced and established methods were modified or refined. In France, a massive investment in the citizen army required far-reaching reforms to medical education to meet demand for military doctors [see 'Anatomy']. In naval and military engagements, surgeons' skills were repeatedly tested. Plastic surgery for burn victims was introduced along with ambulance care, with later conflicts seeing improvements in battlefield care (see below). Whereas nineteenth century conflicts saw advances in military nursing, sanitation, and changes to the nature of battlefield care, the First World War saw a period of systematic changes to the nature of military medicine. The need to manage compound fractures, deal with wound infection, and provide reconstructive surgery encouraged new surgical treatments, such as continuous irrigation, that led to improved healing. Intravenous saline transfusions and blood transfusions were employed to help treat wounds and shock. Burn treatments were revised as alternative methods (including use of paraffin wax to seal burns) were adopted. Concepts of teamwork, regionalism and hierarchy that became part of interwar discussions of healthcare reform were developed, strengthening professional values.

Further advances were seen during the Second World War. Some followed medical experiments on troops – such as at Britain's Porton Down – or on prisoners of war and civilians. Under the Nazi regime (1933–45), numerous brutal experiments were conducted in concentration camps with the aim of improving military efficiency or determining the effectiveness of certain drugs. Elsewhere, medical advances were driven by wartime conditions and the need to conserve manpower. The unavailability of natural products, like quinine for the treatment of malaria, focused Allied scientific effort on developing new synthetic compounds. Further studies of penicillin saw sufficient quantities produced for seriously ill patients. Other drugs, including streptomycin for tuberculosis, were introduced. Mechanized warfare required mobile medical units. More systematic blood transfusion services were established. Stimulus was given to research into the effect of chemical weapons and to aviation medicine. Under the influence of the British surgeon Archibald McIndoe, improvements were made in reconstructive and plastic surgery.

It is important not to overstress progress. Diverse and contradictory socioeconomic, cultural and medico-political forces influenced the nature of military medicine. The application of new medical technologies or procedures was not always practical. Naval warfare provides a good example of the type of problems encountered. Onboard ship, medical officers had to dispense care in often primitive and cramped conditions, which were ill suited, for example, to the use of anaesthesia, antiseptics or new diagnostic technologies such as X-rays. Surgical intervention was difficult onboard ship and under the impact of shellfire and the resulting fumes and fires. If there were practical limitations, the experiences of one war were not necessarily applicable to future conflicts. The confidence placed in the power of antiseptics to disinfect wounds during the South African War, for example, was misplaced in the trenches of the First World War. Nor did war provide ideal conditions for the development of new medical knowledge: statistics were difficult to gather, military doctors often lacked experience of research, while the need was for quick solutions at the front not lengthy trials. Opposition was equally voiced to new methods. For example, when the compulsory typhoid vaccination of German troops was ordered in 1914, debate erupted in the medical community regarding the safety and effectiveness of vaccination. Nor were soldiers easy to persuade. Antimalarial drugs were resisted, not only because of doubts about their efficacy, but also because of rumours that they caused sexual impotence. Financial and tactical considerations created further obstacles. The introduction of technological innovations in medicine – blood transfusions, new drugs, etc – and the organizational changes they encouraged were not inevitable, but depended on a military culture that saw the benefits.

Developments on the battlefield were not always translated into civilian medicine. Discoveries made in wartime reflected the local or national context of the conflict and did not always have a civilian application. For example, the treatment of trench foot had little immediate relevance to civilian medical practice. In addition, as Roger Cooter has suggested, wartime priorities with obvious civilian uses, such as the treatment of fractures, 'normally reverted to low status in peacetime'.[1] The transfer of knowledge from the battlefield to civilian medicine was complex and slow. For example, the encouragement given to specialisms like plastic surgery or orthopaedics during the First World War remained short-lived, and it was not until the Second World War that further progress was made. The ways in which knowledge and technology were diffused is not therefore a straightforward process.

This is not to ignore the effect of warfare or the military on medicine or attitudes to disease and disability. Innovative surgical techniques, such as those developed in the sixteenth century or in the First World War, offered better methods of wound management. Eighteenth and nineteenth century military hospitals were important centres for experimentation and new styles of medicine and management. New procedures and treatments were trialled in military hospitals, such as the anti-syphilis drug Salvarsan. Military practitioners, journals and societies formed part of the national and international medical mainstream. Doctors entering the armed forces were exposed to advanced or new treatments. Penicillin is the oft-quoted example, but this exposure to the new also extended to sanitation. Military needs also encouraged research and experimentation that could result in civilian applications. Studies of scurvy by the British Admiralty in the eighteenth century and the trials of the pesticide DDT against malarial mosquitoes during the Second World War are just two examples. Culturally, visible symbols of militarization entered nursing and medicine in the nineteenth century. For example, germs became the 'unseen enemy', public health the 'war against disease', while penicillin was the 'magic bullet' that offered 'victory' over infection. Warfare also raised difficult social and medical questions about the strength of the nation as the trauma of the Franco-Prussian War (1870–71) for France or the South African War for Britain reveals. It was a two way street: medical and biological analogies were used to describe warfare (and defeat), while medical advances made during wartime were diffused into civilian medicine through a slow and often complex process.

Medical care for the fighting man

Military medical services have been shaped by a series of interrelated forces: medical and military technology, the context of conflict, tactics, medico-political interests, colonial ambitions and experiences, and by the diseases and injuries encountered. Yet, healthy troops were essential to winning wars: preventing the armed forces from succumbing to epidemic and infectious diseases or scurvy met military needs. Hence, the growing involvement of medicine in the management of warfare focused on reducing wastage, improving efficiency through better battlefield care, and through medical examinations to ensure healthier recruits. After 1800, the need to prevent or reduce medical 'wastage' became increasingly important with the move to mass armies, conscription and modern weapons. Military doctors absorbed these ideas. For example, in the First World War cases with little hope of recovery initially received limited attention from surgeons, but conscription modified this stance and placed greater emphasis on saving the soldiers' lives and bodies. Greater attention was turned to the problem, or threat of malingering, often forcing soldiers to engage in more drastic acts to secure an honourable discharge.

Although healthy soldiers were vital to any war effort, soldiers before the sixteenth century were commonly expected to help themselves or seek assistance from their comrades-in-arms or relatives. The military revolution of the sixteenth century created manpower problems that encouraged improvements in military health services. Changes in military tactics and greater emphasis on standing armies meant that soldiers were no longer to be wasted as high sickness rates were seen to undermine military effectiveness. Healthcare was used to ensure an effective fighting force and to bolster morale. It is no surprise therefore that those countries that first developed standing armies were also the first to organize systems of medical care for their troops. Evidence from seventeenth century France shows the extent to which regiments were investing in medical care. Although most treatment offered at the front followed conventional surgical practice [see 'Surgery'], permanent military hospitals were created. If few states initially rivalled France, other countries with standing armies – Prussia and Russia for example – followed suit.

As armies became larger and more professional in the eighteenth century, and as the number of colonial campaigns increased, medical services were organized to reduce wastage and surgeons and physicians became more actively involved. The battlefield offered surgeons status and professional opportunities, while for others military medicine presented financial advantages as competition in medicine increased [see 'Professionalization']. During the century, coordinated handling of the wounded was established. Greater attention was directed at sanitary measures to combat epidemics. Medical examinations were introduced for recruits. The need to recruit trained practitioners became important, and military doctors were increasingly granted fixed salaries and an equivalent status to officers. Networks of military hospitals were established and special military medical schools were opened to provide qualified medical personnel. Although standards of care were comparable to other areas of medicine, financial shortages limited provision, while at a regimental level medical services often remained minimal.

In the nineteenth century, conflicts between European nations and colonial campaigns drew heavily on manpower resources. The need to reduce casualties and the effects of disease saw medicine assume a greater role in military organization. Growing public and political interest in military welfare necessitated reforms as late nineteenth century governments found that neglecting the health of the armed forces could be politically costly. Medical practitioners and nurses also asserted their professional credentials as military medicine became more specialized and technologically oriented, a transformation that reflected broader trends in military organization and medicine. Evidence of widespread neglect of basic sanitation and a rhetoric that emphasized a connection between war and epidemics saw pressure to improve sanitation from doctors keen to assert their credentials. Although the Crimean War and South African War illustrate the relative failure of sanitary reforms and basic medical care, in the second half of the nineteenth century there was concerted action by most European states to combat infectious disease and improve military medical care and nursing [see 'Nursing']. In Britain, for example, military medicine was reformed in the wake of the Crimean War: the Royal Army Medical Corps was established along with a training hospital at Netley. Imperial exploits exposed troops to high levels of infectious disease, which had to be combated through better sanitation to ensure the effectiveness of occupation and control [see 'Medicine and empire']. Smallpox vaccination was made compulsory for all troops, and in the early twentieth century, the British and Germans started to employ antityphoid inoculations. Controversial measures to prevent the spread of venereal disease in the armed forces were introduced [see 'Women and medicine'], blurring the boundaries between the civilian and military spheres. By 1914, the value of hygiene and sanitation was fully realized by the German and British military.

Since the 1980s, the idea that the First World War marked a watershed in history has been challenged. The war did bring dramatic changes, but also saw continuities. In medicine, it provided a crucial arena for the development of new ways of organizing and dispensing medical care and drew on pre-war plans, cultures of rehabilitation and ideas about the utility of medicine to military campaigns. Medicine and medical expertise became vital for mobilizing manpower and new forms of medical surveillance were introduced which were extended to the civilian population (see below). Fears of venereal disease saw VD hospitals established and more stringent measures introduced, which included the distribution of personal prophylaxis or inspections after visiting prostitutes, to prevent the spread of venereal disease. Trench warfare and heavy artillery encouraged new methods of dealing with the wounded, while escalating casualties and newspaper reports created public pressure for better care for injured and disabled soldiers. Forward treatment at the front was pioneered and clear medical communication lines were created to produce a system of care that was to remain a feature of battlefield medicine throughout the rest of the century. British regimental first aid posts transported the wounded to Casualty Clearing Stations where teams of surgeons worked. Serious cases were then sent to base hospitals to create a line of communication from the battlefield back to 'Blighty'.

In response to high levels of gas gangrene and septicaemia, the French military health service reorganized its surgical facilities and created new temporary facilities out of tents, established a triage system, and recruited additional surgeons. Following conscription, greater effort was directed at the health of the citizen soldier. As evacuation procedures and equipment improved so too did survival and recovery rates.

This growth in military medical services in the First World War represented a bargain with soldiers – healthcare was given in return for fighting – but it is important to remember that the military was only one provider of care. Voluntary organizations also had a crucial role as demonstrated by the influx of middle- and upper-class volunteer nurses into wartime hospitals and the work of the International Red Cross [see 'Nursing']. However, away from the front in northern France, less progress was made. In the Italian campaign, for example, weaknesses in military organization limited medical provision. Gaps also existed in pension and rehabilitation services for soldiers returning from the war as many struggled with the return to civilian life.

By the outbreak of the Second World War, medicine's military potential had been accepted and the role of the military medical officer firmly entrenched. Although medical services were far from perfect, they played a vital role in the conflict. Medical technologies – blood transfusion for example – shaped medical services and when combined with greater mechanization allowed surgical facilities to move nearer to the front. Most combatants established mobile surgical units. These services were assisted by the introduction of new medicines: both the Spanish Civil War (1936–39) and the Second World War saw new drugs, such as antimalarials and penicillin, introduced which reduced recovery times and tackled the problem of wound infection. New medical technologies and greater mobility not only revolutionized treatment and ensured rapid medical assistance, but also dramatically improved survival rates. However, as the experiences in German-occupied Europe, campaigns in Africa, and Japanese responses to disease in Burma reveal, Allied and Axis powers often reacted differently. Whereas Allied investment in medical services continued practices developed during the First World War, medical services were not a high priority for the German Wehrmacht in a culture that stressed masculinity.

There are problems with this account. Some of these developments were short-lived: new military hospitals and schools opened in France during the Revolutionary period were run down under Napoleon. Outside of Germany, where conscription had long been in force, the low status of military medicine, with its dangerous lifestyle, low incomes and poor reputation, lacked appeal for many practitioners. Military life was brutal – physically and morally – and consequently many doctors who entered the army or navy were often poorly qualified or lacking in ability. Other forces were at work. Logistical and financial problems restricted provision. Defeat could quickly turn into sanitary disaster as evident during the Franco-Prussian War. Commanding officers did not always cooperate with doctors, or implement their suggestions. For example, sanitation was frequently neglected, leading to high levels of infectious disease in military encampments. Strategic and military concerns limited medical provision. For example, the difficulties encountered by the German medical corps in treating the wounded during the invasion of southern Yugoslavia, Greece and Crete in 1941 were the result of the impending invasion of Russia and the consequent lack of logistical support. Medical provision and treatments had to be compatible with military interests and tactical concerns, and with financial resources and practical realities.

War and psychiatry

The importance of context and the overriding concern of military medicine to return soldiers to the front are highlighted by the responses to shell shock in the First World War. Although the mental cost of warfare was a feature of military campaigns before 1914, it was during the First World War that the emotional and psychological trauma took a defined military and medical form in the Anglo-Saxon notion of shell shock. Notions of mental trauma have become central to the cultural history of the First World War. As historians in the 1970s started to examine the personal experience of war, shell shock emerged as a metaphor for the nature of modern, industrialized warfare. It was not just culturally that shell shock had an impact. By the end of the war, shell shock was a politically charged question; one that challenged traditional views of the nature and boundaries of mental illness [see 'Asylums'].

Evidence from Italy and Russia demonstrates that psychiatrists were beginning to consider the psychological impact of military life before 1914. The Russo-Japanese War (1904–05) and the First Balkan (or Italo-Turkish) War (1911–12) had seen psychiatric services established. At the beginning of the First World War, German-speaking psychiatrists talked about a *Nervenkrieg* (a war of nerves) and a *Stahlbad* (a curative 'bath of steel'). These expectations were quickly overtaken by the realities of trench warfare. At first doctors on the front were ill equipped to treat the influx of (unexpected) psychological casualties. Services were rapidly established to cope: the aim was to return soldiers to the front and discourage malingering. In Germany, psychiatric services were standardized: military neurological clinics were established and special departments for war neurotics were set up. There were clear advantages for psychiatrists becoming involved. In Italy and Germany, war provided a mechanism for psychiatrists to extend their influence.

Shell shock had a complex and changing identity and raised difficult questions for doctors. Reducing explanations and approaches to simple groupings of doctors is problematic. Although early approaches emphasized physical shock and concussion, most doctors continued to acknowledge the role of physical causes in some cases even if they favoured a more psychological perspective. Most also agreed that heredity and degeneration had some part to play.

Certainly, such organic interpretations of shell shock provided a convenient tool: doctors explored the relationship between shell shock and physical disorders, making links with alcoholism and syphilis, the mainstays of pre-war degenerative psychiatry [see 'Asylums']. As the war progressed, other ideas were advanced that drew on a range of psychological ideas and explanations. Shell shock started to be represented as an escape from the intolerable situation of the trenches, the result of a crisis between the need for self-preservation and the ideals of duty, patriotism and honour. Many in the military were unhappy with this definition. They saw shell shock as a problem of discipline and morale.

Explanations were more complex than a simple binary opposition between organic and psychological models. As Peter Leese explains in *Shell-Shock: Traumatic Neurosis and the British Soldiers of the First World War* (2002), shell shock was a shifting cultural entity, shaped by individual soldiers' distress, medical ideas and cultural responses. Shell shock hence saw a fusion of medical diagnosis and social prejudice. Pre-war ideas about hysteria and degeneration and prevailing notions of class and race structured interpretations. For example, war neurosis in officers was considered different from shell shock in privates. Although little evidence exists that doctors actually stigmatized working-class soldiers rather than officers, mentally disturbed soldiers were readily accused of cowardice, reflecting pre-war industrial and social concerns about productivity, morality and character. The shell-shocked were hence weak and a potential threat to social stability. It was not until the Second World War that these ideas were challenged by a new conception of combat breakdown and group motivation, and not until after the Vietnam War (1965–75) that a medical label found renewed favour.

Just as interpretations of shell shock were mixed and subject to considerable debate, so too were treatments. Historians have retrospectively divided treatments into analytic and disciplinary styles, even if few contemporary commentators thought in these terms. Historians have emphasized the tensions between these two approaches and in particular between classical psychiatry and more psychological methods. Although certain national approaches emerged – for example, German responses to war neurosis drew on existing ideas of hysteria and followed an aggressive approach – research by Leese in *Shell Shock* and Paul Lerner in *Hysterical Men* (2003) revealed that the majority of patients were subject to an eclectic range of treatments that were determined by practical considerations. Treatments evolved from a complex interaction of combat conditions, soldiers' attitudes, military demands, public opinion, political interests (such as over pensions) and conflicting medical opinions. They ranged from suggestion to aversion therapy, isolation, food deprivation, rest, massage, work, and the use of bromides and faradization (electric shock therapy). Few of these methods were new. They were determined by pre-war attitudes, rank, resources and by institutional settings. Drawing from an alternative body of knowledge, some army physicians influenced by Freud's writings, or trained in psychoanalysis, applied cathartic methods to treat soldiers. One school of historical thought suggests that shell shock offered an important introduction to psychotherapy and psychoanalytical approaches that helped reshape interwar psychiatry [see 'Asylums'], but in terms of military psychiatry the lessons learned during the First World War were quickly forgotten.

Military authorities viewed shell shock differently. They wanted quick cures to return the growing number of psychiatric casualties back to the front. As Freud recognized, the psychiatrist's role during the war was 'somewhat like that of a machine gun behind the front line, that of driving back those who fled. Certainly, this was the intent of the war administration'.[2] The result was that cynical therapeutic strategies and the disciplining of patients were encouraged in the interests of military concerns. Many soldiers were persuaded, subtly or otherwise, to return to the front. Even those who endorsed psychotherapeutic approaches were not the benevolent men that novels and later accounts sought to make them out to be. A tension existed between a desire to remove genuinely sick soldiers and those whose presence might encourage low morale, and the need to return soldiers to combat. In many respects, this tension reflected the wider nature of military medicine. Doctors were caught between care and military demands in a system that did not favour the individual.

Civilian health: the example of the First World War

A growing interest in civilian life in wartime and the cultural history of modern warfare has encouraged historians to examine the impact of warfare on civilian health. Easy assumptions that war encouraged epidemics, or that those not on the battlefront escaped relatively unscathed, have not held up to scrutiny. Warfare affected civilian populations in a multitude of ways, with the weak and the vulnerable and those deemed unproductive or marginal to the war effort suffering the most.

Sieges and protracted conflicts could bring a collapse in trade or subsistence crisis for local populations, or leave them homeless, increasing vulnerability to disease. During the English Civil War, advancing parliamentary forces in Scotland laid waste to estates and townships suspected of Royalist sympathies, increasing the civilian death toll. During the Franco-Prussian War and the siege of Paris, typhus, smallpox and typhoid flared up and disease-related deaths tripled during the siege. Armies also aided the spread of disease. The advancing Spanish forces in the New World introduced diseases that devastated the indigenous population, while military campaigns in India and Russia helped spread cholera to Western Europe in the early nineteenth century. Colonial wars and troop movements contributed to the spread of venereal and other diseases in Africa. Demobilization following the First World War has been associated with spreading the 1918–19 influenza pandemic (Spanish Flu) that accounted for more deaths than the conflict itself. It is therefore no surprise that links were made between military and colonial campaigns and epidemics.

In the twentieth century, the move to total warfare increasingly involved civilian populations and blurred the barrier between the civilian and the military sphere. Sixty per cent of deaths during the South African War were among civilians, mainly from epidemics of measles and pneumonia in British concentration camps, but the war also created conditions that encouraged plague to spread in Cape Town and contributed to mortality and morbidity in siege towns. In Russia, roughly seven million died as a direct or indirect result of the Second World War; in London an estimated 30,000 civilians were killed in the Blitz and a further 50,000 injured. More horrifying is the systematic extermination of European Jews (estimated at six million), homosexuals, gypsies and others under the Nazi regime. As demonstrated by the United States' use of nuclear weapons on Hiroshima and Nagasaki (1945), its deployment of Dioxin (Agent Orange) in Vietnam, or its use of depleted uranium shells in the Gulf War (1991), the effects of war on civilians did not always end with peace treaties.

Much of the debate on the impact of war on civilian health has focused on the First World War and Britain. As historians have sought new ways and methods of studying the war and in what ways it affected civilians, they have integrated political, military and demographic history. Initially, scholars emphasized the ways in which the war resulted in at least as many civilian lives lost as deaths in the trenches. Jay Winter, in a series of influential works in the 1970s and 1980s, offered a revisionist view. Using evidence from infant and female mortality returns and increased life expectancy of men over 49 (i.e. those considered too old for conscription), he showed that the paradox of the war was that Britain became a healthier place to live; that those sections of the civilian population who had the poorest health before 1914 gained the most. Winter associated improvement with the unintended consequences of a war economy: the establishment of controls over food supplies (better nutrition), improved welfare provision, and guaranteed work. He went on to argue provocatively that France, Britain and their allies prevailed because they were able to maintain the health of their civilian populations.

Winter's argument attracted considerable support but this did not mean that it went uncontested. Although civilian populations during the First World War were spared the epidemic threats traditionally associated with warfare, other historians have shown how weak and socially disadvantaged groups lost ground. Questions of evidence, and how this evidence should be interpreted, became central to the debate. Critics of Winter rightly argued that general improvements in civilian mortality can tell historians little about the suffering of individuals or families. Nor does the evidence point to a wholesale reduction in mortality or morbidity: levels of health in Germany deteriorated, while mortality in those over sixty years of age rose in Paris and Berlin. Nor was Winter's evidence representative – it mainly referred to skilled and semiskilled workers closely involved in the war economy. Winter himself admitted that gains were not distributed evenly, particularly between nations. Marked differences also existed according to age, sex and involvement in the war effort. For example, deaths among illegitimate children and the elderly increased as they suffered more from relative privations in heating, housing and food. The different experiences of war produced different health experiences: those groups considered marginal to the war effort had the least attention directed to them and suffered most. The debate has resulted in a more mixed assessment of winners and losers.

Looking beyond those civilian deaths caused by direct enemy action through aerial or artillery bombardment, a more balanced analysis would examine the material affects on the lives of the civilian population. Although states did improve healthcare for those sections of the population involved in the war effort (see below), and put in place measures to control infectious diseases, the First World War had a direct and indirect impact on civilian health. Of course, not all countries were affected in the same way. Conditions varied tremendously between countries, regions and towns. In Germany, the demands of total war were extreme. The needs of the civilian population were sacrificed under the 1916 Hindenburg Programme to wartime demands and a large proportion of the population faced severe deprivation, with conditions made worse by the Allied economic blockade and poor management by the government. After 1916, mortality in Germany soared. The German experience was not unique. The population in Belgium equally faced impoverishment and the presence of starving children became a common sight in central and Eastern Europe. The civilian population of Britain and France fared better, but war made existing social problems worse. Assistance for families of soldiers was slow to materialize and in some cases, the delay reduced families to rags. Others suffered deteriorating housing conditions, rising rents and poor working conditions, which saw protests and strikes across Europe.

If the First World War was not accompanied by major epidemics at least until the 1918–19 influenza pandemic, levels of endemic disease did increase. In Italy, the mobilization of male peasants saw women employed on the fields, which exposed a greater number of female workers to malaria to which they had little immunity. Although some diseases, such as gout, virtually disappeared others, such as rickets, syphilis and tuberculosis, increased. There were also hidden health consequences that had long-term effects. Here historians have associated rising levels of cigarette smoking to the increase in cancer rates from the 1930s onwards. Work in munitions factories, with its long hours, poor conditions and exposure to dangerous chemicals, had adverse consequences for those working in them. Governments were aware of the hazards but because of the demands of fighting a modern technological war tended to keep quiet. Holidays became rare and as the war went on the burden of work increased resulting in exhaustion. By 1918, the civilian population of Europe was stretched to breaking point, which in part explains how individuals and states responded to the influenza pandemic that immediately followed the war.

Given this evidence, it is difficult to argue that the First World War saw an improvement in general civilian health. Some civilian groups did better than others – an equation played out at a European level with German civilians suffering most after 1916. Any overall reduction in mortality was due more to long-term trends than to the war itself, which at best saw the pre-war downward trend in mortality slow. This debate over the demographic impact of the First World War is an important reminder that warfare has significant physical, psychological and health consequences for civilian populations. The medical consequences of war should not just be measured in terms of battlefield statistics or the impact of military tactics therefore, but also in terms of its impact on civilian health.

War and civilian healthcare: the twentieth century

Although revisionist historians have downplayed the impact of war on medical policy, studies by Debora Dwork and others have shown in what ways twentieth century conflicts focused concern on the health of the nation and encouraged the extension of medical services.[3] As the historian Mark Harrison makes clear, modern warfare – particularly conflicts after 1850 – eroded the barriers between the 'civilian' and 'military' spheres.[4] In the twentieth century, the shift to total war involved civilian populations in warfare to an unprecedented degree.

The most obvious example of this view associates the creation of the National Health Service in Britain with wartime experiences and the role of the Emergency Medical Service. But the Second World War is not the only example. The shock of the Franco-Prussian War for France and the South African War for Britain intensified debates about social reform and prompted the introduction of a range of medical services as fears were voiced about the health of the nation [see 'Healthcare and the state']. With the outbreak of the First World War, disease became the enemy within as the need to support vast armies saw the welfare of civilians become of military importance. Those nations involved in the conflict established medical and preventive services to protect and promote the health of the nation. Emergency plans were implemented to deal with outbreaks of infectious disease. Public health services in France were extended: measures were put in place to combat the spread of typhoid and vaccination centres were opened to prevent smallpox. Medical surveillance was expanded to combat tuberculosis and venereal disease, which was defined as a major civilian threat. Measures were established to improve health conditions (and hence efficiency) at work. Considerable effort focused on protecting maternal and child health to ensure the health of the future population. These pronatalist policies did not end with the war: efforts continued to be made in Britain, France, Germany and Italy throughout the 1920s and 1930s [see 'Women and medicine'].

Revisionist histories of the post-1945 welfare state have revealed that war, or the common experiences of war, should not be seen as a watershed in social policy [see 'Healthcare and the state']. This debate has encouraged historians to rethink the impact of war on social policy. War could restrict the health services available. During the Franco-Prussian War, for example, Parisian hospitals administered by the state-run Assistance Publique emptied their beds of chronic patients in preparation for battlefield casualties and the priorities of army medical practice dominated Paris. In the First World War, the disruption of the international market for quinine affected Italy's antimalarial campaign and saw a resurgence in the disease. Across Europe, the treatment of wounded soldiers took precedent and fewer civilian patients were admitted to hospitals. The recruitment of doctors and nurses into the armed services also saw a decline in people's ability to access healthcare, especially in rural areas. A similar pattern was repeated in the Second World War. The outbreak of war damaged or retarded civilian health services, as was the case following the German occupation of Poland or the Ukraine. Elsewhere, room was made in civilian hospitals for injured soldiers and preparations for receiving casualties precipitated a crisis in staffing.

Many of the social welfare initiatives taken during wartime in the twentieth century were incomplete or inadequate. They favoured groups deemed essential to the war effort, or for the nation's future health, and were more about damage limitation than a radical departure from previous policy. In the First World War, alarm about the physical conditions of recruits encouraged the extension of existing state medical services. Pronatalist policies were already a feature of social reforms in many European states before 1914. If anything, war disrupted existing infant and maternal welfare initiatives. In terms of the post-1945 period, the Second World War has to be placed in the context of interwar welfare administration. In France, the 1920s and 1930s witnessed unprecedented moves to extend welfare provision and 'democratize' access to hospital care. In Britain, the 1930s saw not only a growth of municipal healthcare, but also an increasing number of reports that emphasized the need for a state health service [see 'Healthcare and the state']. Rather than marking a watershed in welfare, war can therefore be seen as accelerating existing trends in social policy rather than forging new ones.

Conclusions

Was warfare good for medicine? How you answer this question depends on the socioeconomic, cultural and political context in which war occurred, on the timeframe adopted, and on the status of the combatants. Rather than a simple model of 'progress through bloodshed', the connections between warfare and medical advance, and between warfare and social policy, were not straightforward. Medicine in wartime responded to particular demands that resulted in changes to how military medicine was delivered and how servicemen were cared for, but these were not always translated back into civilian medicine.

Further reading

Although there are few overviews of early modern and modern military medicine, Roger Cooter, 'War and Modern Medicine' in W.F. Bynum and Roy Porter (eds), *Companion Encyclopaedia of the History of Medicine*, vol. 2 (London: Routledge, 1997), pp. 1536–73, and Mark Harrison, 'Medicine and the Management of Modern Warfare', *History of Science* 34 (1996), pp. 379–410, offer excellent introductions. The edited collection by Roger Cooter, Mark Harrison and Steve Sturdy (eds), *Medicine and Modern Warfare* (Amsterdam: Rodopi, 1999) examines medicine and modern warfare in a European perspective. For an introduction to the literature on war and health, see Roger Cooter, 'Of War and Epidemics: Unnatural Couplings, Problematic Conceptions', *Social History of Medicine* 16 (2003), pp. 283–302. Less attention has been focused on early modern medicine and warfare, although Laurence Brockliss and Colin Jones' exhaustive *The Medical World of Early Modern France* (Oxford: Clarendon Press, 1997) shows how military medicine contributed to medicalization, while Eric Gruber von Arni, *Justice to the Maimed Soldiers: Nursing, Medical Care and Welfare for Sick and Wounded Soldiers and their Families during the English Civil Wars and Interregnum 1642–1660* (Aldershot: Ashgate, 2001) focuses on soldiers. Anne Summers, *Angels and Citizens: British Women as Military Nurses 1854–1914* (London: Routledge, 1988) provides a seminal account of the role of warfare in nursing reform. The literature on the First World War is extensive. On the impact on the war on medicine, see for example, Roger Cooter, *Surgery and Society in Peace and War: Orthopaedics and the Organization of Modern Medicine 1880–1948* (Basingstoke: Palgrave Macmillian, 1993) or Jeffrey Reznick, *Healing the Nation: Soldiers and the Culture of Caregiving in Britain during the First World War* (Manchester: Manchester University Press, 2005). On the treatment of disabled soldiers after the war, see Deborah Cohen, *The War Come Home: Disabled Veterans in Britain and Germany 1914–39* (Berkeley, CA: University of California Press, 2001) and Patrick Kelly, *Creating a National Home: Building the Veterans' Welfare State 1860–1900* (Cambridge, MA: Harvard University Press, 1997). In terms of civilian health, Jay Winter, *The Great War and the British People*, 2003 edn (Basingstoke: Palgrave Macmillan, 2003) provides a provocative assessment of the impact of the First World War, while Linda Bryder, 'The First World War: Healthy or Hungry?', *History Workshop Journal* 24 (1987), pp. 141–55, puts forward a counter-argument. There is a large literature on shell shock, with Ben Shephard's *A War Of Nerves: Soldiers and Psychiatrists 1914–1994* (Cambridge, MA: Harvard University Press, 2002) providing the best existing overview on the subject, with Joanna Bourke's *Dismembering the Male: Men's Bodies, Britain and the Great War* (London: Reaktion Books, 1999) a seminal study of war and the politics of the body. The literature on the Second World War is more limited, although Mark Harrison, *Medicine and Victory: British Military Medicine in the Second World War* (Oxford: Oxford University Press, 2008) gives a detailed overview of Britain. On the war and the NHS, see D.M. Fox, *Health Policies, Health Politics: The British and American Experience 1911–1965* (Princeton, NJ: Princeton University Press, 1992) or Charles Webster, *The Health Service since the War, I: Problems of Health Care* (London: HMSO, 1988) for an exhaustive introduction. For those seeking an introduction to military history, Jeremy Black, *Introduction to Global Military History: 1775 to the Present Day* (London: Routledge, 2005) offers a global perspective.

16

The rise of the asylum

We like to imagine asylums in the past in certain ways, as apparent in literary representations of the Victorian asylum found in Wilkie Collins, *The Woman in White* (1860) or Sarah Waters, *Fingersmith* (2002). Assumptions have been made about what went on in these institutions, and the desperate and sometimes dangerous treatments that were used. Scholarship on the history of psychiatry initially appeared to confirm many of our enduring images of the asylum as dark and repressive institutions. These studies were dominated by famous institutions, such as Bedlam or the Quaker York Retreat, and by the work of psychiatrists, such as Philippe Pinel, Emil Kraepelin, Jean-Martin Charcot or Sigmund Freud. Although these accounts emphasized modernization, this did not mean that they were prone to glorification: if anything, they condemned past treatments to emphasize the extent to which psychiatry had progressed since the 1790s. A number of psychiatric revolutions were identified: moral management in the eighteenth century was equated with the rise of the asylum, a psychoanalytical revolution was associated with Freud, and a psychopharmacological revolution with the introduction of psychotropic drugs and deinstitutionalization in the second half of the twentieth century.

Encouraged by the antipsychiatry movement of the 1960s and a new style of social history more concerned with class and agency, a new generation of historians in the 1970s and 1980s came to reject this overarching narrative as they rethought the process of institutionalization and how societies and doctors responded to mental illness. Although no single revisionist school emerged, historians openly or implicitly drew on sociology and some of the assumptions of the antipsychiatry movement to re-examine the process of institutionalization, the role of the medical profession, and the ways in which insanity was defined. New sources and a closer examination of the history of individual asylums were used to cast doubt on the chronology of confinement and the reasons behind institutionalization to reveal the complexities of asylum life. Old myths, such as the uniform horrors of Bedlam or Pinel's casting-off the chains of patients at Bicêtre, were debunked. The idea that asylums represented what the sociologist Erving Goffman called 'total' (or closed) institutions, or were convenient places to detain inconvenient people, gave way to the notion that boundaries inside and outside the asylum were fluid. What became clear is that asylums had to be placed in context if they were to be understood, not only in terms of periodization, but also in terms of their socioeconomic, cultural, political and professional milieu.

However, as we shall see in this chapter, although earlier interpretations of the history of psychiatry have been challenged, the asylum remains central to our understanding of responses to mental illness in the past. Focusing on the key historiographical questions, this chapter first examines Foucault's notion of the 'great confinement' and the reasons why asylums came to dominate the treatment of mental illness. In the following sections, the chapter addresses both the changes in treatments that occurred in the nineteenth and twentieth centuries and the major challenges to the asylum. Throughout, questions are asked about the influence of doctors and the importance of socioeconomic contexts.

The 'great confinement'

Care of the insane in early modern Europe was mainly organized around the care provided by family members, housekeepers, friends and neighbours, or by communities. Only a small number of institutions dealt with the insane, and these were mainly for paupers. Some of the earliest were established in fifteenth century Spain and were closely related to religious institutions. Of these early asylums, the most notorious was St Mary of Bethlehem (Bethlem or Bedlam) in London, which began to admit 'lunatiks' almost by accident in the fifteenth century. Local parishes also made limited provision for the insane: if they were deemed harmless, outdoor relief was provided in the form of medicines, nursing care, clothing or food, while the more difficult or violent were placed in poorhouses or other parish institutions. Overall, the numbers admitted to early modern institutions remained small.

In *Madness and Civilization* (1965), the French philosopher and historian Michel Foucault put forward the notion of the 'great confinement' (*grand renfermement*) to explain how the mid seventeenth to eighteenth century was a crucial turning point in the treatment of the insane. As in much of his work, Foucault argued that change should not be associated with progress [see 'Historiography']. Instead, he outlined a more sinister grand narrative of institutional growth and the intellectual classification of insanity, which he associated with the literal shutting-up of the insane in the rapidly growing number of state institutions that emerged from the mid seventeenth century onwards. Foucault argued that the rise of Absolutism, which he identified with the accession of Louis XIV to the French throne in 1643, ushered in new responses to unreason as the insane were incarcerated along with other deviant groups in a range of state institutions from Paris's Hôspital Général to the *Zuchthäuser* in German-speaking territories. Foucault claimed that in a society increasingly concerned with deviant behaviour, asylums were an economic means of isolating and dealing with the deviant – those who could not or would not work – to contain and discipline rather than to care or cure. Drawing on evidence from France, Foucault demonstrated how municipal authorities were required to provide institutional facilities for the poor insane and how measures were introduced that permitted families to have their insane relatives confined in an asylum and deprived of their legal rights. This confinement was more than just the physical segregation of the insane: it represented the imposition of new rules of normality through the science of psychiatry.

Historians have vigorously debated the merits of Foucault's argument. As explained in Chapter 1, Foucault's work has been attacked for its empirical weaknesses, for confusing intellectual ideas, institutional reforms and social reforms, and for concentrating on a few leading men and exaggerating the impact of medical ideas. Although the number of madhouses and asylums did rise during the eighteenth century, few of these institutions conform to Foucault's model, even in France. Rather than being driven by Absolutist states, many were charitable or private enterprises, with industrializing Britain seeing the largest increase in institutions for the mentally ill. Charitable institutions, such as St Luke's Hospital in London, drew on similar impetuses that fuelled the voluntary hospital movement [see 'Hospitals']. More widespread was the growth of private madhouses as part of what the British historian Parry-Jones has labelled the 'trade in lunacy'. Between 1774 and 1815, approximately seventy-two provincial and metropolitan private madhouses were established in Britain.[1] Most were initially built on the small-scale domestic arrangements that had characterized care in the early modern period and few resembled the large-scale institutions Foucault associates with the eighteenth century. Nor were they primarily aimed at the poor. Although it was those institutions that admitted paupers that generated most contemporary concern – often because of the scandals associated with them – private madhouses admitted patients from the middling orders and from the poor, with some established for a rich clientele.

Although the process of a European 'great confinement' from the mid seventeenth to the eighteenth century does not hold up to scrutiny, it was during the nineteenth century that the number of state asylums rose dramatically. In Russia, for example, reforms were initiated under Tsar Nicholas I who set out to construct a network of regional asylums. In the Nordic countries, the main period of asylum building occurred after 1850. By the mid nineteenth century, most European governments required municipal authorities to care for the insane and passed legislation to regulate the mechanisms through which they were committed. During the second half of the nineteenth century, the number and size of these publicly-funded asylums rose along with the number of mentally ill patients in state institutions. The exact timing varied between countries. In England, the number of certified lunatics in public asylums doubled between 1844 and 1860s, while in Germany the main move to asylum care occurred between 1880 and 1910. Notwithstanding the involvement of national governments in regulation, many of these asylums were local institutions designed to serve a defined geographical area.

Historians have advanced a number of explanations to account for this process of institutionalization. Some have located the reasons for institutionalization in the wider socioeconomic changes associated with industrialization in the eighteenth and nineteenth centuries. Others have pointed to the importance of medical or professional factors. In practice, socioeconomic and medical factors are often hard to separate, and the remainder of this section will explore the various arguments and counter-arguments that have been put forward to explain the rise of the asylum as the accepted place for the care of the insane.

Contemporaries associated the growing willingness of families to seek institutional support for their insane relatives with a range of social factors. Historians have similarly pointed to the importance of the sweeping socioeconomic changes that were affecting eighteenth and nineteenth century Europe. For many, the connection between the rise of the asylum and a move to a capitalist economy in the late eighteenth and nineteenth centuries has proved appealing. One way of looking at this process is to argue that capitalism left in its wake mounting numbers of human casualties that required institutional responses. In *Museums of Madness* (1979), Andrew Scull offered a sophisticated reading of these forces in the context of England as the first industrial nation. Scull was interested in the social, legal and professional responses to mental illness and the approach he adopted reflected contemporary arguments in social history and the social sciences. Highly critical of *Madness and Civilization,* Scull's carefully researched and provocative argument connected the rising numbers of asylums to the growth of industrial capitalism and the structural and social changes he associated with the reorganization of English society along market principles. For Scull, the massive social upheavals attributed to this process broke down traditional social hierarchies and responsibilities, weakening social and familial ties. Scull claimed that as a consequence poor families could no longer either cope with their insane relatives or afford to care for them at home. The result was that they dumped their unproductive or dangerous relatives – those 'inconvenient' people who were unable to function in the new market economy – in the asylum.

Scull's view of the destabilizing effects of industrialization is appealing, especially as many contemporaries responded to industrialization with considerable anxiety. Although varying patterns of industrialization might account for the different timing of institutionalization – such as in Sweden – there was a general European trend as industrialization, population growth and urbanization resulted in deep-seated social changes that necessitated institutional solutions. Admissions to the Santa Maria della Pietà mental hospital in Rome support this argument. They show how many of those admitted were those on the margins of society and were without traditional family support networks or economic means.

Since Scull published *Museums of Madness* in 1979, a more sceptical response to institutionalization has emerged as historians have become more cautious about connecting asylum reform to a particular chronology of capitalism following research that revealed that the process of industrialization had a longer history than previously assumed. Subsequent scholarship has questioned interpretations that position the rise of institutional psychiatry as simply a response to the emergent capitalist economy. Ireland provides a good example of how there could be a substantial increase in the number of asylums with only limited industrialization, urbanization or population growth. In his work on eighteenth century England, Roy Porter suggests that the expansion in asylum provision was not simply about capitalism, but was a response to the growth of a 'myriad of renegotiations of social responsibility in an economy in which services were increasingly provided by cash payments'.[2] Part of the explanation for the growing number of madhouses therefore lies in commercialization, demand and rising affluence. To what extent this growth was due to a breakdown in social hierarchies is harder to determine, but work on individual asylums in Paris, England, Scotland and elsewhere, and on the reasons for admission to nineteenth century asylums, has provided only limited evidence to support claims that economic factors were solely responsible for admission. Given the stigma associated with mental illness, many first sought to cope with their insane relatives within the family. As admission records demonstrate, it was only when their behaviour became too troublesome, bizarre or violent that families or communities sought committal.

Why families and communities turned to the asylum to care for those people they found too difficult or dangerous to look after remains unclear. For the historian Jonathan Andrews, reforms to the nature of the asylum made it more attractive for families.[3] From the mid eighteenth century, those running asylums argued for the curative benefits of institutional care. The growing use of moral management and moral therapy, or what might be seen as a psychological approach (see below), in the late eighteenth and early nineteenth centuries embodied this curative idea. For Scull, these ideas promoted what he called the 'domestication of madness' in well-managed asylums under medical control. They found favour with middle-class reformers who joined with doctors to promote a particular style of asylum care. Legislation reflected these values, creating legal systems of certification and confinement that placed the asylum at the centre of treatment for mental illness.

Given the faith placed in the asylum and in management to cure insanity, attempts were made by asylum mangers, doctors and government inspectors in the nineteenth century to ensure a disciplined regime that was considered essential to moral management. More and better-trained staff were appointed, and if coercion and violence – from staff and from other inmates – occurred, they were increasingly represented as abuses. Although a wide range of evidence supports late nineteenth century claims that conditions in public asylums were poor and overcrowded, effort was made to make them appear more domestic and less prison-like. If in some institutions improvements were little more than a question of cheering-up the wards with cheap wallpaper and a few prints, those running public asylums attempted to do what they could with limited funds. Most asylums acquired a library and organized concerts, dances and plays. Cricket pitches and other amenities, as well as workrooms, were added. These served a therapeutic purpose – work and recreation were perceived to have physical and psychological benefits – but such facilities also made asylums more acceptable to families. This is not to underplay the monotonous, bureaucratized or drab conditions that existed in many asylums, or to ignore the extent to which some patients experienced sexual abuse, violence or coercion. Evidence from inquiries and from patients reveals the extent to which this domestication could conceal abuses, but the gradual rejection of physical forms of restraint, the adoption of new approaches, such as work therapy, and a resourceful use of the asylum environment helped convince families that asylums were a viable last resort for the care of difficult or dangerous people.

A further set of arguments connects the rise of the asylum with social control. The notion of social control has been widely used in sociology to refer to the social processes by which the behaviour of individuals or groups is regulated. For sociologists, the issue is not the existence of social control, but determining the mechanisms at work. A common distinction is made between coercive forms of control and the softer ideological methods that operated by shaping values and attitudes. Medical definitions of mental illness could be used, therefore, to classify individuals as socially, morally or politically deviant or dangerous, with the asylum there to contain them. This approach suggests that the appearance of growing numbers of the insane, criminals and paupers in the eighteenth and nineteenth centuries was met by incarcerating them in purpose-built institutions to segregate them in environments that inculcated bourgeois values. The committal process in nineteenth century Ireland, which criminalized the mentally ill, or the policies adopted in Nazi Germany (1933–45), are good examples of this process.

Eighteenth and nineteenth century medical ideas about insanity did have an important moral dimension. This can be located within a moralizing discourse that was part of a larger cultural movement towards the internalization of bourgeois discipline. If this was vividly embodied in the definition of moral insanity advanced by the English physician James Cowles Pritchard, certain types of behaviour from drunkenness to masturbation came to be associated with mental illness in the nineteenth century as doctors extended the definition of insanity over conditions that had previously been labelled sinful. As demonstrated in Chapter 4, women were often the victims of these definitions. Numerous examples exist of patients being admitted to asylums because they transgressed social or legal norms. In the *Politics of Madness* (2006), Melling and Forsythe present a comprehensive analysis of asylum committals in the English county of Devon that shows how many asylum inmates had broken the boundaries of acceptable or respectable behaviour, whatever their class.

Contemporaries were concerned about how the asylum was used. Fears of wrongful confinement were given voice in literature from Daniel Defoe in *Augasta triumphans* (1728) to Wilkie Collins in *The Woman in White*, in newspaper reports, and in well-publicized legal cases. In Germany, a lunatics' rights movement (*Irrenrechtsreformbewegung*) emerged in the 1890s that provided a focus for protest against the perceived abuses associated with confinement, while in France complaints about committal were regularly reported to the Ministers of the Interior and Justice. There were broader cultural anxieties about the possibility and stigma of being mislabelled as insane and locked away with no prospect of escape or legal rights.

Although the social control argument is an influential one, little evidence exists that asylums were systematically used to control or discipline the socially, morally or politically deviant. A gap exists between how insanity was defined and how committal functioned. Many cases of wrongful confinement were motivated by familial greed or convenience rather than being conspiracies on the part of doctors or the state. As research on Paris and Switzerland demonstrates, most asylum inmates were often admitted during periods of crisis (public or familial), or when other alternatives had failed. Asylum inmates were invariably those too difficult or dangerous for families to look after, or were individuals who lacked familial or communal networks for support, a pattern that reflects admissions to other institutions [see 'Hospitals'].

A further set of socioeconomic explanations for the rise of the asylum can be advanced. Asylums fitted well with late eighteenth and nineteenth century evangelical and reform movements that aimed to improve the condition of the poor. They reflected a bureaucratic faith in institutional solutions that characterized nineteenth century responses to a range of social problems, but they were also a cost-effective solution to the problem of insanity. Asylums were represented as money saving ventures, while confidence in their ability to cure allowed cost-saving compromises to be made about their nature, size and quality.

Other historians have looked to medical and professional explanations to understand the growing role of the asylum. If which came first the asylum or new approaches is akin to the chicken or the egg argument, two broad strands can be detected. The first associates the rise of the asylum with changing explanations about insanity. Revisionists like Roy Porter in *Mind Forg'd Manacles* (1987) have argued that the Enlightenment (eighteenth century) was crucial in reshaping ideas about the nature of mental illness that made treatment viable and institutionalization desirable. The notion of human malleability advanced by the English philosopher John Locke argued that insanity was the result of uncontrollable imagination and false principles, and in doing so rejected earlier assumptions that linked insanity to permanent irrationality and bestial insensibility. Such ideas combined with a growing interest in anatomy and nerves influenced by mechanical philosophy [see 'Anatomy']. Both supported new approaches that connected mind and body and proposed that mental illness was curable. That insanity was attracting increased attention in the eighteenth century should not be seen as surprising. The Enlightenment was marked by a faith in the importance of reason, by optimism about the ability to improve humanity, and by a growing sensibility to the plight of the distressed.

Encouraged by these ideas, a growing number of eighteenth century doctors

– or alienists – started to make nervous disorders their speciality and drew on their practical experiences. In the process, they rejected carceral regimes in favour of reformist therapies that emphasized management and the use of methods that engaged with the intellect and emotions. These ideas were embodied in 'moral treatment' (*traitement moral* in France) or moral therapy. This approach has been associated with the English physician William Battie at St Luke's, with the Quaker York Retreat, and with the mythic activities of Philippe Pinel in the asylums he ran in Paris – Salpêtrière (for women) and Bicêtre (for men) – where he was reported to have cast-off the chains of the inmates. All asserted what might be labelled psychological methods. In effect, this meant the power of the alienist over inmates and the rejection of the primacy of physical restraint in an approach that placed the alienist, as Scull argues in *Museums of Madness*, in the role of moral entrepreneurs. Although it is a mistake to make a straightforward connection between moral management and kindness – room remained for fear and discipline – new strategies concentrated on patients' minds rather than on merely their bodies through a combination of gentleness, subjugation and distraction. These ideas spread outwards from Britain and France to other European states.

Although Foucault and other scholars have argued that these new methods represented restraint by other means, general historical opinion holds with the view that moral management represented a turning point in treatment, even if it is difficult to reduce this approach to a precise formula. With insanity increasingly seen as a disorder of the mind, the aim was to return patients to sanity by resocializing them through a combination of work and recreation, privileges and discipline. This was shown to only be possible through the well-ordered asylum where the entire environment from the building and furnishings to the strict hierarchies in place (seen in how inmates were segregated according to sex and condition) and how the day was organized, were designed to re-educate and cure the patient. Alienists eagerly promoted these ideas and argued that because insanity was ultimately rooted in the brain, asylums should be under their control. This model was embodied in the new legislative measures introduced in Britain, France, Belgium and elsewhere in the first half of the nineteenth century that supported medical certification and institutionalization of the insane in public asylums. Until the 1850s, the effectiveness of this approach appeared to be confirmed by the number of patients discharged as cured. Changing medical ideas about insanity hence drove institutionalization.

A second strand in medical explanations associates the asylum with the growing authority of alienists over definitions of insanity and its treatment. For Scull, asylums offered a vehicle of what he termed 'professional imperialism', a mechanism by which alienists asserted their dominance over insanity as agents of the bourgeois social order. We have already seen how alienists claimed the asylum and mental illness as their sphere and how they asserted their role in defining and treating insanity. This claim was supported by legislation. For example, in France in 1838 and in Britain in 1845 legislation gave doctors a clear role in confinement and in the management of insanity. The well-managed asylum was central to the process. It provided both a site for observation and experimentation, and for defining and treating mental illness. Patronage, academic networks and personal factors, as demonstrated by the careers of John Conolly in Britain and Jean-Étienne Dominique Esquirol in France, were also important in extending alienists' authority. Just as in other fields, specialist journals, professional bodies and qualifications were established in the nineteenth century that helped define psychiatry as a specialism [see 'Professionalization']. The science of asylum management became the cornerstone of this emerging psychiatric profession and legitimized professional power.

Assumptions about professional imperialism can be challenged to demonstrate how the extent of medical influence has been exaggerated. In France and Britain, doctors often had little to do with the treatment of the insane until the late eighteenth century. The same was true for Russia in the nineteenth century: here administrative reforms and a programme of asylum building was driven by Tsar Nicholas I. Moral management was initially non-medical in nature and was only gradually medicalized. Medical power over committal was equally limited. Studies of individual asylums and admission records reveal how families and friends were important actors in determining the location and nature of care. They negotiated admission (and discharge) and asylum doctors often merely confirmed the diagnosis already made by families, neighbours or by non-medical authorities. Alienists were peripheral in other ways. In Britain, Poor Law authorities were important in first identifying insane paupers and second in determining who was sent to public asylums. In Paris, the police and the *Infermerie spéciale* served a similar role.

Medical power was limited in other ways. Those working in public asylums often had little control over the institution, and their decisions were liable to be overturned by lay asylum managers. Politicians and lawyers challenged medical definitions of insanity in other ways. In France, the magistracy openly questioned medical expertise in legal cases and a similar situation existed in Britain. The debate generated by accusations of wrongful confinement in Britain and Germany raised questions about the power and competency of alienists. In Germany, a popular movement (*Irrenrechtsreformbewegung*) endeavoured to regain some lay control over the definition and treatment of mental illness. In these movements, concern was directed at what appeared to be the arbitrary and contested power of medical experts.

It is hard to separate medical ideas from their socioeconomic contexts. Socioeconomic explanations and arguments that favour medical or professional factors have their advantages, but as this section has shown, it is also possible to advance a series of counter-arguments. Although Foucault's model of a great confinement does not hold up to scrutiny, the mid nineteenth century did witness the heyday of the asylum movement. Support was not just expressed by alienists as part of what might be seen as professional imperialism. Public asylums had the support of reformers, municipal authorities and governments, and broadly from the public. Although at one level this is evident in the asylum reform movement that characterized Britain and France in the early nineteenth century, it is also visible in the rising number of admissions to public asylums. Asylums may have been the last resort for the families or friends of those committed, but the reasons for their growth reflected the medical and socioeconomic forces that shaped them.

Asylum care: 1850–1914

In the second half of the nineteenth century, the early optimism about the curative benefits of the asylum had evaporated and asylums started to be seen as problematic institutions, or in Scull's memorable words 'warehouses for the insane'. Scull's idea that early enthusiasm for asylum care gave way under the pressure of overcrowding to favour large custodial institutions continues to hold sway in much of the historical literature. On the surface the view that asylums after 1860 became large impersonal and custodial institutions in which overcrowding, material misery, absence of therapeutic activities and widespread abuse were believed to be commonplace is borne out by the growing size of asylum populations. Table 16.1 reveals the extent to which asylums in England and Wales grew between 1850 and 1920.

The pattern was repeated elsewhere in Europe: in Germany, the proportion of the population in an asylum rose from 1 in 5,300 in 1852 to 1 in 500 by 1911, while in Italy the asylum population trebled between 1874 and 1907. In Russia, despite the dramatic growth in the number of asylums after 1850, many were overcrowded and understaffed, conditions that frustrated efforts at treatment. Contemporaries spoke of asylums becoming silted-up with incurable patients. As

Table 16.1 County asylums in England and Wales, 1850–1920

Year	*Number of institutions*	*Total number of patients*	*Average per asylum*
1850	24	7,140	297
1860	41	15,845	386
1870	50	27,109	542
1880	61	40,088	657
1890	66	52,937	802
1900	77	74,004	961
1910	91	97,580	1,072
1920	94	93,648	966

Source: Annual Reports of the Lunacy Commissioners to 1910; Annual Reports of the Board of Control for 1920.

asylums grew in size, patients lost their individuality, and treatment and care became wholesale. New drugs, such as chloral hydrate, were introduced to make patients more manageable and were greeted with enthusiasm as alienists grappled with overcrowding and growing numbers of chronic and intractable patients. Although a reliance on what contemporaries labelled chemical restraint did not preclude other treatments, such as hydrotherapy or electrical treatments to stimulate nerves, overcrowding ensured that routine and discipline became central to creating well-ordered asylums. It was in these large public institutions that the drift to custodialism can be detected.

One obvious explanation for this growing asylum population is the rise in the general population in the period. However, the numbers in asylums grew at a faster rate than the general population. Contemporaries worried that deteriorating urban conditions and the nature of urban life promoted a range of social problems from drinking and promiscuity to mental illness, while in France the defeat of the Franco-Prussian War (1870–71) and the events of the Paris Commune (1871) suggested growing physical and moral decadence. These fears contributed to hereditarian and degenerationist ideas (see below). Other reasons were advanced for why asylum populations had grown which reflected changing attitudes to social welfare. Contemporaries noted a growing willingness of families and individuals to seek aid from the state, and commented on how patients previously cared for at home were now being admitted to state-funded institutions. They also emphasized better diagnostic methods and pointed to an increasingly eagerness among doctors to certify people insane. The asylums and alienists can be represented, therefore, as victims of their own success: contemporary accounts certainly point to alienists' willingness to diagnose a growing range of symptoms as mental illness, while new guidelines for committal expanded the boundaries of what constituted insanity.

Yet professional imperialism was not the only reason for growth. Economy favoured large asylums, especially when provision was paid for locally. Internal factors also played a part. Evidence from Surrey and Lancashire country asylums demonstrates how only a third of those admitted were discharged within twelve months. Although turnover was higher when one takes into account that between 10 and 18 per cent of inmates died within a year of admission, a large body of patients remained. They formed a growing population of long-stay patients, many of whom were old or infirm. These patients lay behind overcrowding as public asylums struggled to expand.

Alienists advanced other explanations that reflected professional insecurities and mounting doubts about their ability to cure the majority of asylum inmates. Many turned to ideas of degeneration and heredity to explain why asylums had become overcrowded. In the mid nineteenth century, physical and physiological explanations had begun to displace earlier associations of insanity with moral disorders as attempts were made to move psychiatry closer to mainstream medicine. The importation of ideas from anthropology, evolutionary theory and social Darwinism encouraged alienists to think in these terms. As Chapter 12 demonstrates, in the last decades of the nineteenth century ideas about heredity and degeneration acquired a new significance as part of wider discourses about the state of European nations, empires and race that reflected the socio-political pessimism of the period. This interest in heredity, degeneration and insanity was given form in the works of Joseph Moreau (de Tours) and Benedict Augustine Morel in France, and by Henry Maudsley in England. They were instrumental in outlining theories of mental degeneracy as a psuedosomatic explanation for mental illness. Because of the vagueness of these ideas, and because by providing a physical explanation for mental illness they brought psychiatry closer to medicine, theories of mental degeneracy gained widespread acceptance as alienists became increasingly disenchanted with the curative power of the asylum. As the work of Cesare Lombroso in Italy or Richard von Krafft-Ebing in Germany demonstrates, alienists started to argue that some forms of madness were passed from generation to generation and that for certain patients little could be done. These ideas helped cast a new role for the asylum as a means of protecting society from the pollution represented by insanity.

In his *The History of Psychiatry* (1997), Edward Shorter argues that an interest in heredity was not entirely negative. Whereas Shorter claims that nineteenth century alienists pioneered an understanding of genetics and neuroscience, most historians agree that degenerationist concerns in psychiatry emerged from a sense of failure and from profession concerns. They diverted attention from the therapeutic shortcomings of late nineteenth century asylums and brought psychiatry into a closer relationship with medicine and with contemporary debates on nation, race and empire. In contributing to debates on degeneration, alienists provided explanations for a range of social problems from criminality and pauperism to venereal disease and alcoholism that served to assert the worth of psychiatry.

However, it is wrong to characterize late nineteenth century psychiatry as hidebound by ideas of degeneration. Connections between physiology, pathology, brain functions and mental illness equally were sought as attempts were made to medicalize insanity and associate it with empirical laboratory examinations. This reflected approaches in other branches of medicine [see 'Science and medicine']. Work on phrenology earlier in the century had already established links between cerebral regions and mental faculties, but where these findings were spurious, phrenology encouraged a broader interest in the organic nature of mental illness. This trend initially found expression in Germany. Although German-speaking states had opened asylums, a closer connection existed here between university psychiatric clinics and research, which encouraged an environment that favoured empirical and organic interpretations. Given the strength of clinical and pathological anatomy in medicine and mid-century work in physiology, early work on the organic nature of mental illness had an anatomical focus [see 'Anatomy']. It aimed to localize and associate psychiatric conditions with specific areas of the brain through neuropathology. This approach is evident in the work of the Berlin neurologist Wilhelm Griesinger who argued that all mental diseases were in effect brain diseases. His neurological approach to mental illness was adopted by his successors who sought to wed psychiatry to neurology, neuropathology and the materialism of the laboratory. Although well-versed in ideas of heredity, the influential work of Emil Kraepelin at the Heidelberg clinic was informed by this interest in neurological diseases. Kraepelin produced the classic clinical portrait of manic-depressive insanity and dementia praecox (later labelled schizophrenia by Paul Eugen Bleuler). In equating psychoses with a morbid deterioration of the brain, Kraepelin emphasized organic brain symptoms and his work proved highly influential in asylum medicine.

This interest in the organic nature of mental illness and the desire to find objective symptoms based on clinical observations influenced the Viennese neurologist Sigmund Freud. This biological dimension has often been overlooked in accounts that have associated psychoanalysis with a transformation in Western society encouraged by secularization and a growing sense of crisis in *fin de siècle* Europe. Although a founding myth has been constructed around Freud, psychoanalysis was part of a larger contemporary psychotherapeutic and psychogenic movement. Given that functional nervous disorders like hysteria and the new category of neurasthenia were not easily explained by neuropathology, neurophysicians like Jean-Martin Charcot in France looked for other explanations that did not have the same negative associations as mental degeneracy. Having become disheartened with existing remedies in the face of overcrowding, alienists were turning to new approaches and the idea that if psychotic patients belonged in the asylum, a new group of neurotic patients were amenable to treatment and in particular to hypnotic and suggestive therapies, an approach lead by Charcot at Salpêtrière and Bernheim at Nancy. Trained in neurology, Freud was influenced by Charcot's work, but in trying to understand the less severe mental illnesses that were the focus of his practice in Vienna, Freud rejected neuropathological explanations. In response, he advanced an alternative psychodynamic theory of the mind, which he named psychoanalysis.

As with Charcot, Freud used hysteria as the basis for his ideas, but interpreted the physical signs of hysteria as reflecting emotional and psychological symptoms. In doing so, Freud put forward a theory of the self that was internally conflicted and complex – ego, superego and id – to argue that unconscious impulses influenced behaviour. Freud gradually developed his techniques of analysis, first with hypnotherapy and later through free association and the analysis of dreams. In his later work, Freud focused on the role sexuality played in motivation and in the development of the human psyche, which culminated in 1903 in what he called the Oedipus complex. Freud came to consider neuroses and sexual perversions as two forms of expression of the breakdown of normal sexual development.

Psychoanalysis had numerous benefits: it offered a range of treatments suited to office-based practice, but more importantly made sense of a range of mental phenomena that could not otherwise be explained. Others adopted and adapted

Freud's ideas. For example, the Swiss psychiatrist Carl Jung proposed a less sexualized vision of the unconscious, while Pierre Janet in France advanced theories of personality development. The result was a range of psychodynamic approaches that helped alienists extend their field of expertise (see below). Often the differences between these approaches have been emphasized – for example, Jungian psychology or the object relations school of Melanie Klein – but they shared a common psychological dimension and a strong interest in sexuality, instincts, familial relations, emotion and dreams.

Historians have mixed views about Freudian analysis and the reception of his methods. Many have been critical, arguing that psychoanalysis was characterized by intense controversy, or have shown how Freud's approach was ill-suited to asylum practice. Freud's ideas did encounter professional hostility and psychoanalysis was a troubled discipline, marked by divisions. Freud's controversial ideas met with initial resistance in Vienna, where Freud felt shunned, but elsewhere Freudianism was at first viewed as a fashionable fad. His methodological approach was criticized by asylum psychiatrists, especially as they were of little use in the treatment of chronic psychotic cases. Many were sceptical of hypnotism, arguing that it manipulated the patient, while Freud's interest in sex was considered distasteful. However, if psychoanalytical techniques made little headway in asylums where the intensive methods were not practicable, numerous psychiatrists did experiment with free association and with the analysis of dreams, while Freud's ideas had a profound impact on office-based psychiatry, particularly in the United States. Freudian ideas equally had a marked impact on art and literature, and influenced other fields of medical inquiry, such as endocrinology and gynaecology, and the sexual reform movement. The public were also more accommodating than alienists. Although journalists and other writers shared the medico-psychological community's distaste of Freud's sexual theories, they disseminated a selective view that asserted the value of his theory of the unconscious.

By the 1920s, professional attitudes to psychoanalysis had started to alter. As alienists were reinventing themselves as psychiatrists and expanding their realm, they started to employ psychotherapeutic methods. Hostility remained, but as we shall see in the next section, psychiatrists in the 1920s and 1930s were beginning to carve out new roles for themselves that had less to do with the asylum. In these new arenas – infants and delinquent children, industry, alcoholism, marital affairs – psychotherapeutic and psychological methods had a particular utility.

Social psychiatry and mental hygiene: 1918–39

The First World War (1914–18) altered attitudes to mental illness. The experiences of the trenches and the emergence of shell shock contributed to the medicalization of the mind [see 'War and medicine']. During the war, military psychiatrists developed new diagnostic technologies, such as the intelligence test, and established institutional alliances between psychiatric clinics, military authorities, and local and national administrations. In Italy, for example, the war created a need for mass mental care and provided Italian psychiatrists with opportunities to reinforce their social role. The war gave a greater number of doctors firsthand experience of treating the mentally disturbed and cast doubt on assumptions about degeneration that had characterized psychiatry before 1914. Experiences with shell-shocked soldiers associated some forms of mental collapse with temporary incapacity and therefore with recoverability. In addition, the treatment of shell-shocked soldiers on the frontline without admission to an asylum, not only suggested that early treatment was possible, and indeed desirable under certain circumstances, but also raised questions about the role of the asylum. Although these ideas had found some expression before 1914 in Germany and the United States, where several psychiatric clinics were opened, and in France where enthusiasm was shown in voluntary admission, in the years after 1919 these ideas gained greater currency in Europe as support was expressed for social psychiatry and mental hygiene. The 1920s and 1930s saw a proliferation of sites outside of the asylum for the treatment of mild or borderline cases along with growing popular and professional interest in the boundaries of mental health.

It is hard to separate enthusiasm for social psychiatry and non-institutional treatment from a growing strand of criticism about the asylum that existed in the last decades of the nineteenth century. Overcrowding and the rising cost of institutionalization encouraging an interest in new responses to mental illness. Critics drew on ideas of degeneration and heredity to demonstrate that asylum care was not working to argue that intervention should occur earlier in the process of mental breakdown. As interest in psychiatry moved from the major psychoses to milder or borderline cases, which included neuroses and other functional disorders, psychiatrists began to suggest that there were certain groups who did not need institutionalization. Good examples of this new categorization are neurasthenia and hysteria, with the former associated with nerve weakness or exhaustion and mainly applied to middle-class patients (and in particular women). In the years after the First World War, new concepts about the nature of mental incapacity were added that drew on experimental physiology and psychology. This new understanding of mental illness is apparent in Adolf Meyer's concept of maladjustment, which suggested that mental disorders were an outcome of inadequate responses to the challenges of everyday life. In this rethinking of the nature and boundaries of mental illness, experiences with shell-shocked soldiers provided evidence for new psychiatric models. Such experiences also demonstrated the value of psychoanalytical and psychodynamic approaches as treatments for borderline or temporary cases of mental collapse that did not require institutionalization. Other approaches were developed, such as active therapy in Germany, which aimed to make patients more responsible for their behaviour. Together, these new ideas and approaches opened up opportunities for treating and supporting patients outside of the asylum, interests reinforced by a desire to diminish the financial burden of care and reduce asylum overcrowding in favour of cheaper, non-institutional responses.

It is possible to be cynical and suggest that for a branch of medicine that had a low status these claims were a bid to raise the standing of psychiatry by making it relevant to the management of health and society. Psychiatrists were certainly endeavouring to associate themselves with a preventive model that was gaining increasing support throughout the 1920s and 1930s [see 'Public health']. Through social psychiatry, they equated mental with physical health and hygiene and attempted to move psychiatry closer to other branches of medicine.

It is easy to associate mental hygiene with eugenics and campaigns for the segregation and sterilization of those groups identified as mentally defective. The connections historians have made between mental hygiene, race and eugenics in Nazi Germany (1933–45) and the resulting sterilization and euthanasia programmes provides a brutal example of how social psychiatry could be used. Although moves to sterilize certain categories of patient was not unique – for example, similar policies were adopted in Scandinavia – the euthanasia programme (or Aktion T4) is a chilling example of Nazi racial hygiene policies [see 'Healthcare and the state']. For example, in Austria under the Nazis over 60 per cent of all patients in state psychiatric hospitals were killed. However, there was more to social psychiatry and mental hygiene than eugenic campaigns or Nazi euthanasia programmes. Psychiatrists did draw on eugenicists' discourses to both highlight those areas in which mental illness might occur, and to argue that if mental illness was caught early, serious breakdown could be prevented and a mentally-healthy society promoted. New services were offered through outpatient clinics to provide early treatment to those with mild nervous or psychological disorders. In Britain, a growing number of asylums opened outpatient clinics, such as in Cardiff in 1919, while some twenty Dutch towns had established some form of outpatient care by the 1930s. Education, child welfare and industry presented further arenas for the application of new psychological methods, and psychological and psychiatric services were extended into these areas as part of a mental hygiene movement. This enthusiasm for social psychiatry is apparent in the growth of child guidance clinics. It was felt that intervention during childhood helped prevent mental problems in adulthood as it was argued that many later disorders were a cumulative result of mental habits acquired in childhood. Child guidance clinics combined attempts to medicalize child welfare with a desire to promote a mental health agenda that benefitted the child, the family and society. In Britain, demand for these services had outstripped supply by the 1930s.

The 1920s and 1930s were therefore a time when the boundaries of mental illness were being reworked. Psychiatry was trying to move closer to medicine and through social psychiatry was able to expand into a range of areas. New ideas about the nature of mental illness were being advanced and new centres for treatment outside the asylum were being established. These clinics became the hub of mental hygiene movements, which in merging various forms of surveillance contributed to what Nikolas Rose in the *Psychological Complex* (1985) has referred to as the psychologization of the mundane. However, as we shall see in the following section, social psychiatry and mental hygiene only in part characterize the changes that were occurring in interwar psychiatry.

Physical therapies: 1918–45

In the previous section, we have seen how social psychiatry was used to expand the boundaries of psychiatry, but the 1920s and 1930s were also marked by a new organicism that drew on neuropathological ideas developed in the last decades of the nineteenth century. Whereas in the nineteenth century, Britain and France had pioneered new approaches to mental illness, the focus in the 1920s and 1930s shifted to Austria, Germany, Hungary and Poland and to treatments developed by neurologists. The introduction in the 1920s of malarial therapy to prevent patients with tertiary syphilis (or general paralysis of the insane) deteriorating further and the development of prolonged-sleep therapies for psychotic disorders offered powerful new therapies. The apparent success of malarial therapy and the possibilities it raised for intervention encouraged the search for other forms of physical treatment. Psychiatrists increasingly turned their attention to schizophrenia, a disease not amenable to existing treatments and one considered responsible for asylum overcrowding. The result was a heady period of experimentation. Insulin coma therapy (1933) was devised by the Austrian neurophysiologist Manfred Joshua Sakel and was followed by Cardiazol treatment (1934), which was developed by the Hungarian neurologist Ladislaus Meduna, and then by electroconvulsive therapy (ECT), which was first used by Ugo Cerletti and Lucio Bini in Rome. Apart from insulin, all produced a series of controlled fits in the belief that there was a negative correlation between schizophrenia and epilepsy.

However, it is psychosurgery or lobotomy – proposed by the Portuguese neurologist Egas Moniz and first performed in 1935 – that has come to characterize approaches to mental illness in the 1930s and 1940s. The procedure, which involved damage to the frontal lobes of the brain through surgery, was reported to tranquilize patients and alter their behaviour and personality. It appeared to be particularly useful in the treatment of schizophrenia. Early operative procedures underwent modifications as neurosurgeons endeavoured to reduce the dangers of the procedure.

Although the theory behind shock therapies proved erroneous, when these new treatments were reported asylum psychiatrists quickly adopted them. Enthusiasm for psychosurgery, for example, soon led to its extension to a range of psychiatric disorders. Psychiatrists believed that these methods promised a new curative approach. They were hence introduced with little investigation or attention to the possible side effects. Although lobotomy was discredited in the 1950s, ECT became a mainstay in the treatment of severe depression.

These therapies have retrospectively come to be associated with brutal and damaging treatments. Evidence shows that their application was invariably terrifying, while they were often used on patients (and especially female patients) against their will. However, rather than simply arguing that these treatments were brutal aberrations, they should be seen in context. First, it is unwise to see the initial enthusiasm that surrounded shock therapies as unique. Various psychiatric treatments, particularly drugs, followed a similar trajectory of initial enthusiasm, therapeutic optimism and then reactions against them. Second, although shock therapies can be placed within this broader trend, the therapeutic pessimism that existed in psychiatry in the early twentieth century in part explains their rapid adoption. With mainstream medicine able to cite a series of successful therapies and new chemotherapeutic agents, psychiatrists sought to embrace a medical approach and wanted similar successes. For example, although lobotomies had become an historical embarrassment by the 1960s, psychosurgery built on research into the chemistry of the brain and cerebral localization. Similar connections with mainstream medicine can be detected for other physical treatments introduced in the 1930s. Third, many of the new treatments were directed at traditionally intractable diseases, such as schizophrenia or in the case of malarial therapy tertiary syphilis, which were held responsible for asylum overcrowding, and where it was felt there was little hope of recovery. Fourth, these new treatments appeared to work. Although initially limited to female schizophrenics, Cardiazol promised high cure rates, while ECT provided relief for severe depression that reduced treatment times. The final point to remember is that although these treatments were debated at the time, they were also popular and were endorsed by leading clinicians.

In the 1920s and 1930s, there was a growing enthusiasm for physical and shock therapies. Rather than being aberrations, these new treatments were a response to professional concerns, ideas about the organic nature of mental illness, overcrowding in asylums, and therapeutic pessimism. They offered asylum psychiatrists effective treatments for chronic and previously intractable cases that appeared to work. Although this is not to minimize their often traumatic or damaging nature, or their side effects, the introduction of shock therapies helped reverse the therapeutic nihilism of the early twentieth century. They also confirmed an organic interpretation of mental illness that was to prove central to psychiatry after 1945.

The psychopharmacological revolution

The introduction of antipsychotics and psychopharmacology in the 1950s and 1960s has frequently been hailed as a breakthrough in the treatment of mental illness. Yet a longer history can be seen. Psychiatrists had been seeking a pharmaceutical panacea for mental illness since the mid nineteenth century. Enthusiasm for chemical restraint in the late nineteenth century and the continuing use of large quantities of drugs in asylums had seen experimentation with sedatives and stimulants. Asylum staff came to favour the use of barbiturates like Veronal and Medinal to sedate patients, while depressed patients were prescribed stimulants, mainly in the form of brandy and whisky until Benzedrine, a drug that produced a sense of euphoria, started to be prescribed in the 1930s. With the introduction of shock therapies in the 1930s, further investigations were made following the successes of insulin and Cardiazol as chemotherapies. However, these experiments were overshadowed by the development of a new group of drugs that, like shock therapies, took the psychiatric profession by storm. Of these, chlorpromazine was the first to be introduced.

Chlorpromazine was initially developed as a possible treatment for morning sickness, but following the use of the drug by two Parisian psychiatrists in calming manic patients, chlorpromazine was rapidly adopted, as it appeared to offer a cure in some cases of schizophrenia and a general reduction of symptoms in all cases. Chlorpromazine was hailed as a revolutionary breakthrough that launched an era of psychopharmacology. Pharmaceutical companies rushed to produce a range of drugs with similar effects to cash in on chlorpromazine's success. The first of the tricyclic and neuroleptic drugs followed in 1957. Various tranquilizers were introduced, the most common of which was Valium (1963). These transformed the treatment of depression and were quickly adopted by psychiatrists disillusioned with the empirical methods of the physical treatment available. One result was that psychiatric hospitals became extensions of pharmaceutical laboratories, and psychiatrists the customers and researchers of the pharmaceutical companies. This fortified psychiatry's dependence on drugs. Further tricyclic, neuroleptic and psychoactive drugs were developed in the 1970s. An investment in the search for new drugs was matched by laboratory and clinical studies into the physical dimension of major mental illnesses, studies that strengthened the biological basis of mental illness. These focused on neurochemistry and neuroendocrinology and brought clinical rewards. Work on the chemical pharmacology of serotonin, for example, led to the development of powerful psychoactive drugs and selective serotonin re-uptake inhibitors, such as Prozac, while research into dopamine produced new antidepressants and antipsychotic agents.

Many commentators felt that with psychopharmacological advances psychiatry had escaped from the hazardous and irreversible treatments that had characterized asylums. However, like the shock therapies of the 1930s, the side effects of these new drugs were frequently ignored because the benefits appeared too great, while critics showed that the introduction of new drugs into psychiatric hospitals was as much about control as it was about cure. Although these new drugs did little to treat underlying pathologies, they were used with increasing frequency inside psychiatric hospitals and by general practitioners. Numbers in psychiatric institutions fell in response in what Scull has described as a process of 'decarceration'. In England, for example, the number of residents in psychiatric institutions declined from 83,320 in 1976 to 49,417 in 2009–10. Although not all countries followed Britain's lead in closing old asylums, the number of psychiatric beds in Europe was scaled-down in favour of non-institutional treatments in a process of deinstitutionalization. New outpatient clinics, halfway houses, old-age homes, and community services were created and psychiatric social work was extended. New patterns of mental healthcare services resulted that concentrated on clinics, day hospitals and the care provided through general practitioners. In the 1980s and 1990s, psychiatric patients increasingly lived and worked outside of psychiatric hospitals, and the number of long-term admissions had dropped significantly in many European countries.

To simply associate changes to the structure of mental healthcare and deinstitutionalization with the introduction of new and apparently effective drugs ignores other factors. Changes in social policy, rising welfare costs and the global economic downturn of the 1970s combined with the growth of psychiatric social work, revelations about conditions in asylums, and ongoing professional desires to align psychiatry with medicine, to encourage non-institutional responses. The antipsychiatry movement of the 1960s and 1970s gave voice to increasing disquiet about the nature of psychiatry, questioning its scientific status and the notion of mental illness. The psychiatrist Thomas Szasz, for example, argued that mental illness was a 'myth' manufactured by doctors to control individuals whom society considered deviant. Influenced by these ideas, the antipsychiatry movement pressed for demedicalized and deinstitutionalized care in the community, while the post-war investment in social psychiatry offered viable alternatives to institutional care. However, the development of chemotherapies for a range of nonpsychotic mental states did open up new possibilities for psychiatry. Many of these did not require institutionalization and although the reasons for the fall in the number of beds in psychiatric hospitals cannot be attributed to any one cause, the emphasis on somatic treatments and biological psychiatry dramatically altered responses to mental illness. If the nineteenth century was the asylum era, the late twentieth century became the antidepressant era.

Conclusions

This chapter has examined the rise of the asylum in the late eighteenth and nineteenth centuries as the main response to mental illness and the arguments and counter-arguments for their growth. It has illustrated how the growth of asylums follows a different chronology to Foucault's great confinement, and how neither socioeconomic nor medical or professional arguments alone are sufficient in explaining the rise of the asylum. If there was more to the asylum than the broader social changes associated with industrialization, there are also problems with thinking about growth in terms of social control or professional imperialism. The result is a more complex history of the asylum, but as later sections have revealed, the dominance of the asylum was already beginning to be questioned in the last decades of the nineteenth century. In part, this reflected growing pessimism and ideas about heredity and degeneration, but also new organic interpretations of mental illness. Two strands emerged – social psychiatry and psychotherapeutic methods on the one hand, and renewed interest in physical treatments on the other. In the twentieth century, both were to influence psychiatry and encourage the development of non-institutional solutions that questioned the role of the asylum in treating all forms of mental illness. Hence, rather than the First World War and shell shock representing a decisive turning point, the changes in psychiatry in the 1920s and 1930s can be located in a longer chronology, while there are connections between the shock therapies in the 1920s and 1930s and the development of antipsychotics and psychopharmacology after 1945. Whereas this chapter has pointed to greater continuities, it has also shown how the history of the asylum cannot be reduced to simple pessimistic or optimistic explanations, but how both need to be seen in their socioeconomic, cultural, political and professional contexts.

Further reading

There are a number of synoptic studies of the history of psychiatry. Edward Shorter, *A History of Psychiatry: From the Era of the Asylum to the Age of Prozac* (New York: John Wiley & Sons, 1998) and Michael Stone, *Healing the Mind: A History of Psychiatry from Antiquity to the Present* (New York: W.W. Norton, 1998) provide different approaches. Few interested in the history of psychiatry can afford not to start with Michel Foucault, *Madness and Civilization: A History of Insanity in the Age of Reason* (New York: Pantheon Books, 1965). Readers interested in Foucault's work and its impact should consult Colin Jones and Roy Porter (eds), *Reassessing Foucault: Power, Medicine and the Body* (London: Routledge, 1994). The collections edited by Arthur Still and Irving Velody (eds), *Rewriting the History of Madness* (London: Routledge, 1992) and by Mark Micale and Roy Porter (eds), *Discovering the History of Psychiatry* (New York and Oxford: Oxford University Press, 1994) also contain perceptive critiques of Foucault along with historiographical surveys. The journal *History of Psychiatry* provides numerous case studies of psychiatrists, mental disorders and asylums in different national contexts, as well as periodic assessments of the literature. The three volumes of *The Anatomy of Madness* (London: Tavistock, 1985–88) edited by Roy Porter and W.F. Bynum and the essays in Roy Porter and David Wright (eds), *The Confinement of the Insane: International Perspectives 1800–1965* (Cambridge: Cambridge University Press, 2003) provide an international perspective, while Jonathan Andrews et al, *The History of Bethlem* (London: Routledge, 1997) provides a mixed examination of the most (in)famous asylum that also explores many of the changes examined in this chapter. On the York Retreat and moral management, readers should turn to Anne Digby's excellent *Madness, Morality and Medicine: A Study of the York Retreat 1796–1914* (Cambridge: Cambridge University Press, 1985), and on Pinel see Dora B. Weiner's '"*Le geste de Pinel*": The History of a Psychiatric Myth', in Mark Micale and Roy Porter (eds), *Discovering the History of Psychiatry*, pp. 232–47. For the psychiatric profession, Andrew Scull, Charlotte MacKenzie and Nicholas Hervey, *Masters of Bedlam: The Transformation of the Mad-Doctoring Trade* (Princeton, NJ: Princeton University Press, 1999) contains case studies of individual British alienists and their ideas. Given the focus of the revisionist historiography, there is a large literature on Britain, but the obvious starting points are Andrew Scull, *Museums of Madness: The Social Organization of Insanity in Nineteenth-Century England* (London: Allen Lane, 1979) and Roy Porter, *Mind-Forg'd*

Manacles: A History of Madness in England from the Restoration to the Regency (London: Penguin, 1990), while Peter Bartlett and David Wright (eds), *Outside the Walls of the Asylum: The History of Care in the Community 1750–2000* (London: Athlone Press, 1999) explore non-institutional responses. Andrew Scull, *The Most Solitary of Afflictions: Madness and Society in Britain 1700–1900* (New Haven, CT: Yale University Press, 2005) offers a revised edition of *Museums of Madness* and is one of the best accounts of psychiatry in the eighteenth and nineteenth centuries, with the collection edited by Joseph Melling and Bill Forsythe (eds), *Insanity, Institutions and Society 1800–1914* (London: Routledge, 1999) containing chapters responding to Scull's ideas. Detailed examinations of French psychiatry are provided by Jan Goldstein, *Console and Classify: The French Psychiatric Profession in the Nineteenth Century* (Cambridge: Cambridge University Press, 2002) and Ian Dowbiggin, *Inheriting Madness: Professionalization and Psychiatric Knowledge in Nineteenth-Century France* (Berkeley, CA: University of California Press, 1991). On women and insanity, Elaine Showalter, *The Female Malady: Women, Madness and English Culture 1830–1980* (London: Virago, 1987) is the obvious starting point with a critique provided by Joan Busfield, *Men, Women and Madness: Understanding Gender and Mental Disorder* (Basingstoke: Palgrave Macmillan, 1996). The Further Reading in Chapter 12 outlines the literature on degeneration, although Ian Dowbiggin, 'Degeneration and Hereditarianism', in the first volume of *The Anatomy of Madness* (London: Tavistock, 1987) and the chapter on Henry Maudsley in *Masters of Bedlam* are good on the detail related to Britain and France, with mental deficiency examined in David Wright and Anne Digby (eds), *From Idiocy to Mental Deficiency: Historical Perspectives on People with Learning Disabilities* (London: Routledge, 1996). Much has been written on Freud and readers should look at Sonu Shamdasani, 'Psychoanalytic Body', in Roger Cooter and John Pickstone (eds), *Companion to Medicine in the Twentieth Century* (London: Routledge, 2003), pp. 307–22, and Peter Gay, *Freud: A Life for Our Time* (London: Papermac, 1989). Those interested in shell shock should consult the Further Reading in Chapter 15. Less has been written on the history of psychiatry in the twentieth century. The special volume of the *Medical History* journal (vol 48(4), 2004) edited by Michael Neve examines the growth of social psychiatry in Britain, the Netherlands and Germany. While Shorter's *History of Psychiatry* presents an overview of the shock therapies, his approach should be balanced against Andrew Scull, 'Somatic Treatments and the Historiography of Psychiatry', *History of Psychiatry* 5 (1994), pp. 1–12, and the subsequent responses by Merskey et al in the same volume which offer insights into shock therapies from different perspectives. More has been written on psychosurgery, with Jack Pressman, *The Last Resort: Psychosurgery and the Limits of Medicine* (Cambridge: Cambridge University Press, 2002) and German E. Berrios, 'Psychosurgery in Britain and Elsewhere', in German E. Berrios and Hugh Freeman (eds), *150 Years of British Psychiatry 1841–1991* (London: Gaskell, 1991), pp. 180–96 providing thought-provoking studies. David Healy, *The Antidepressant Era* (Cambridge, MA: Harvard University Press, 1999), E.M. Tansey, '"They used to call it psychiatry": Aspects of the development and impact of psychopharmacology', in Marijke Gijswijt-Hofstra and Roy Porter (eds), *Cultures of Psychiatry and Mental Health Care in Postwar Britain and the Netherlands* (Amsterdam: Rodopi, 1998), pp. 79–101, and David Healy, *Creation of Psychopharmacology* (Cambridge, MA: Harvard University Press, 2002) provide good introductions to the development of antipsychotics and psychopharmacology, while Andrew Scull deals with de-institutionalization in *Decarceration* (Chapel Hill, NC: Rutgers University Press, 1984) and Peter Sedgwick, *Psychopolitics* (London: Pluto Press, 1982) with the antipsychiatry movement. For those readers interested in definitions of mental illness, German E. Berrios and Roy Porter (eds), *A History of Clinical Psychiatry* (London: Athlone Press, 1999) mixes clinical with historical accounts.

Afterword

Any conclusions about the last five hundred years of medicine in Europe can appear superficial and overgeneralized and can be accused of ignoring diversity and national or regional contexts in favour of reading broad trends as representative. One such generalization would be that medicine has 'progressed' over the last five centuries with the post-1945 period being associated with the most radical transformation in the nature of medicine and delivery of healthcare. It is hard to escape from the fact that medicine in 2010 is very different from medicine in 1500. Innovations in medical care and medical science can be identified from changes in anatomical thinking and the ways in which the body was understood in the seventeenth century to successful transplant surgery, the development of chemotherapies, and an increasingly genetic model of disease in the twentieth century. Changes have occurred in how healthcare is delivered, in how medical practice is policed, in the relationships between healers and their patients, and in the burden of infectious disease (at least in Western Europe).

However, ideas of change, innovation and development do not necessarily have to support a view of inevitable modernization or that medicine neatly progressed from an early modern humoral understanding of disease in which surgery was a bloody art or hospitals were gateways to death to a superior science-based technocratic medicine in the twenty first century. If the extent to which everyday life has been medicalized has been exaggerated, several long-term developments converged during the nineteenth and twentieth centuries, but how to measure 'progress' – when? where? who for? – innovation and change, and what 'progress' meant for contemporaries are important questions for which there are no simple answers. As this volume has shown, changes in the nature and landscape of medicine and medical care were seldom as sudden, extensive or inevitable as might first be presumed. If there have been important changes – if not major discontinuities – in the way, for example, that disease has been understood, in the treatments used by healers, in surgery or in nursing, it is possible to find analogous practices/circumstances in contemporary medicine and medicine in the past. For example, although health came to be viewed as a normal state in the twentieth century, it was no less desired in the past, while we are just as likely to purchase over-the-counter medicines as our contemporaries did in the nineteenth century when confronted with minor or everyday complaints. Continuities can be detected. Medical practices and practitioners have never been without their critics as medicine and health have always been intimate parts of everyday life. Over the last five hundred years, connections between social and biological disorders have remained an integral part of political, cultural and social representations of disease – be it plague or AIDS – and the meanings given to diseases have often gone beyond their biological manifestations. Continuities can equally be found in how medicine has continued to be shaped by subtle shifts in power relations and by commercial concerns.

Whereas some of the problems facing medicine in the twenty first century might on the surface appear familiar to those encountered by contemporaries in the past, to over-emphasize the comparisons and continuities runs the risk of underplaying the intricate connections that have existed between, for example, diseases, ideas, practices, individuals, practitioners, institutions, societies, cultures and politics in the past. Medicine was always more than a set of intellectual and practical or material resources that healers could use, and over the last five hundred years medicine has come to mean many things, none of which should be viewed as pre- or un-scientific. The development of medical ideas about the body, the distribution of medical services, the creation and consolidation of professions and institutions, the incidence of disease, and representations of health, gender or race, are not independent of the cultural, socioeconomic, political or national contexts in which they existed or were produced and used. By thinking about these contexts, and the shifting power-relations in medicine, such as between practitioners and patients or individuals and the state, it is possible to gain insights into the complex and rich world that has characterized medicine in Europe since 1500.

If the social history of medicine covers an eclectic collection of approaches and sub-disciplines, it continues to offer exciting ways to examine this rich history of medicine that does not over-privilege ideas of progress, great men and women, technology or institutions. As this volume has demonstrated, considerable room remains for the discipline to develop. The twentieth century is a fertile field for investigation, particularly of the cultural history of medicine, while oral histories continue to be needed to uncover (or recover) people's experiences and narratives of health, illness and medicine. Ideas of periodization also need to be re-interrogated to write longer histories of the twentieth century. More generally, particular countries – for example, Spain, Greece, Finland, Russia – warrant scrutiny, as do local and regional experiences. New questions can be asked about the nature of early modern and modern medicine. For example, whereas historians have concentrated on the canonical settings of medicine – the hospital or university for example – and the urban, considerable scope remains for examining the rural dimensions of health and medicine. Equally, histories of the relationship between religion and medicine in the nineteenth and twentieth centuries are required that do not over-privilege a narrative of secularization, along with studies of warfare and medicine that look beyond the First World War (1914–18). Although scholars have used the model of the medical marketplace to help understand the choices patients have made, the patient's perspective, both in relation to the canonical settings of medicine and within the more informal and private sphere, and how families fit in with negotiating or providing care requires further study. What was meant by the healthy body, the disabled body, the sick body, the racial body, the gendered body, etc, and how these different constructions of the body influenced experiences of health and medicine in the past would also offer fertile fields for investigation. As historians are driven (subtly or otherwise) by theoretical reflections and increasingly by their engagement with histories of meaning and identity, further questions will be added as they continue to explore the socially and culturally contextualized history of medicine.

Notes

Preface

1 Ilana Löwy, 'The Social History of Medicine: Beyond the Local', *Social History of Medicine* 20 (2007), p. 465.

1 Understanding the social history of medicine: historiography

1 George Rosen, 'People, Disease and Emotion', *Bulletin of the History of Medicine* 4 (1967), pp. 5–23.
2 Charles Webster, 'Abstract of Presidential Address', *Society for the Social History of Medicine Bulletin* 19 (1976), p. 1.
3 Mary Douglas, *Purity and Danger: An Analysis of Concepts of Pollution and Taboo*, 2010 edn (London: Routledge).
4 Paul Weindling, 'Medicine and Modernization', *History of Science* 24 (1986), 277.
5 Nicholas Jewson, 'Medical Knowledge and the Patronage System in Eighteenth-Century England', *Sociology* 8 (1974), pp. 369–85.
6 Andrew Wear, 'Introduction', in Andrew Wear (ed.), *Medicine in Society: Historical Essays* (Cambridge: Cambridge University Press, 1992), p. 2.
7 Roy Porter, 'The Patient's View: Doing Medical History from Below', *Theory and Society* 14 (1985), p. 175.
8 Ibid, p. 174.
9 Ludmilla Jordanova, 'The Social Construction of Medical Knowledge', *Social History of Medicine* 8 (1995), p. 367.
10 Ibid, p. 367.
11 Charles Rosenberg, 'Disease and Social Order, Definitions and Expectations', *Milbank Quarterly* 64 (1986), pp. 34–55.
12 David Harley, 'Rhetoric and the Social Construction of Sickness and Healing', *Social History of Medicine* 12 (1999), p. 432.
13 Ibid, n. 11.
14 Ludmilla Jordanova, 'Has the Social History of Medicine Come of Age?', *Historical Journal* 36 (1993), pp. 437–49.
15 Roger Cooter, 'After the Cultural Turn', in Frank Huisman and John Harley Warner, (eds), *Locating Medical History. The Stories and their Meanings* (Baltimore, MD: John Hopkins University Press, 2004), p. 22.
16 Harley, 'Rhetoric and the Social Construction', n 12, p. 432.

2 Disease, illness and society

1 B.R. Mitchell, *International Historical Statistics: Europe 1750–1993* (London: Palgrave Macmillan, 1998).

3 Medicine and religion

1 Jonathan Barry, 'Piety and the Patient: Medicine and Religion in Eighteenth-century Bristol', in Roy Porter (ed.), *Patients and Practitioners: Lay Perceptions of Medicine in Pre-Industrial Society* (Cambridge: Cambridge University Press, 1985), pp. 151, 162, 172.
2 Rhodri Hayward, 'Demonology, Neurology, and Medicine in Edwardian Britain', *Bulletin of the History of Medicine* 78 (2004), pp. 37–58.

4 Women, health and medicine

1 Nancy Theriot, 'Negotiating Illness: Doctors, Patients, and Families in the Nineteenth Century', *Journal of the History of Behavioural Sciences* 37 (2001), p. 355.

5 Medical self-help and the market for medicine

1 Ute Frevert, 'Professional Medicine and the Working Classes in Imperial Germany', *Journal of Contemporary History* 20 (1980), p. 650.
2 Colin Jones, 'The Great Chain of Buying: Medical Advertisement, the Bourgeois Public Sphere, and the Origins of the French Revolution', *American Historical Review* 101 (1996), p. 25.
3 See Neil McKendrick, *The Birth of Consumer Society* (Bloomington, IN: Indiana University Press, 1982).
4 Matthew Ramsey, 'Academic Medicine and Medical Industrialism: The Regulation of Secret Remedies in Nineteenth-Century France', in Mordechai Feingold, and Ann La Berge (eds), *French Medical Culture in the Nineteenth Century* (Amsterdam: Rodopi, 1994), p. 25.
5 James Woycke, 'Patient Medicines in Imperial Germany', *Canadian Bulletin of the History of Medicine* 9 (1992), p. 52.

6 Anatomy and medicine

1 Cited in Philip Wilson, 'An Enlightenment Science: Surgery and the Royal Society', in Roy Porter (ed.), *Medicine in the Enlightenment* (Amsterdam: Rodopi, 1995), p. 378.

7 Surgery

1 Thomas Schlich, 'Emergency of Modern Surgery', in Deborah Brunton (ed.), *Medicine Transformed: Health, Disease and Society in Europe, 1800–1930* (Manchester: Manchester University Press, 2004), p. 61.
2 This section draws on Christopher Lawrence, 'Divine, Democratic and Heroic', in Christopher Lawrence (ed.), *Medical Theory, Surgical Practice. Studies in the History of Surgery* (London: Routledge, 1992), pp. 1–47.
3 Christopher Lawrence and Richard Dixey, 'Practicing on Principle: Joseph Lister and the Germ Theories of Disease', in Lawrence, *Medical Theory, Surgical Practice*, ibid, pp. 153–215.

9 Practitioners and professionalization

1 Margaret Pelling and Charles Webster, 'Medical Practitioners', in Charles Webster (ed.), *Healing, Medicine and Mortality in the Sixteenth Century* (Cambridge: Cambridge University Press, 1979), pp. 165, 182–88.
2 Ibid, pp. 182–88.
3 Laurence Brockliss and Colin Jones, *The Medical World of Early Modern France* (Oxford: Clarendon Press, 1997), pp. 527, 630–31.
4 George Weisz, 'The Emergence of Medical Specialization in the Nineteenth Century', *Bulletin of the History of Medicine* 77 (2003), pp. 536–75.
5 Lindsay Granshaw, '"Fame and Fortune by Means of Bricks and Mortar": The Medical Profession and Specialist Hospitals in Britain 1800–1948', in Lindsay Granshaw and Roy Porter (eds), *The Hospital in History* (London: Routledge, 1989), pp. 199–220.
6 Oscar Wilde, *Collins Complete Words* (London: Collins, 1999), p. 1074.

10 Science and the practice of medicine

1 For such an account, readers should turn to one of the overviews referred to in the Further Reading.
2 John Harley Warner, 'Introduction to Special Issue on Rethinking the Reception of Germ Theories of Disease', *Journal of the History of Medicine and Allied Sciences* 52 (1997), pp. 7–16.

11 Nursing

1 Monica Baly, 'Florence Nightingale and the Establishment of the First School at St Thomas's', in Vern Bullough et al (eds), *Florence Nightingale and Her Era: A Collection of New Scholarship* (1990), pp. 8–13.

12 Public health

1 Christopher Hamlin, 'Muddling in Bumbledom: On the Enormity of Large Sanitary Improvements in Four British Towns, 1855–1885', *Victorian Studies* 32 (1988), pp. 55–83.
2 *Twenty-Sixth Report on the Sanitary Condition of Merthyr Tydfil* (1901), p. 8.
3 Dorothy Porter, 'From Social Structure to Social Behaviour in Britain after the Second World War', *Contemporary British History* 16 (2002), pp. 58–80.

14 Medicine and empire

1 Warwick Anderson, 'How's the Empire?', *Journal of the History of Medicine and Allied Sciences* 63 (2003), p. 464.
2 Michael Worboys, 'Colonial and Imperial Medicine', in Deborah Brunton (ed.), *Medicine Transformed: Health, Disease and Society in Europe, 1800–1930* (2004), pp. 211–38.
3 Harriet Deacon, 'Midwives and Medical Men in the Cape Colony before 1860', *Journal of African History* 39 (1998), p. 289.

15 Medicine and warfare

1 Roger Cooter, 'War and Modern Medicine', in W.F. Bynum and Roy Porter (eds), *Companion Encyclopaedia of the History of Medicine* vol. 2 (London: Routledge, 1997), p. 1550.
2 Hans Binneveld, *From Shellshock to Combat Stress: A Comparative History of Military Psychiatry* (Amsterdam: Amsterdam University Press, 1997), p. 135.
3 Deborah Dwork, *War is Good for Babies and Other Young Children: A History of the Infant and Child Welfare Movement in England 1898–1918* (London: Tavistock, 1987).
4 Mark Harrison, 'Medicine and the Management of Modern Warfare', *History of Science* 34 (1996), p. 381.

16 The rise of the asylum

1 William Parry-Jones, *The Trade in Lunacy* (London: Routledge and Kegan Paul, 1972), p. 30.
2 Roy Porter, 'Madness and its institutions', in Andrew Wear (ed.), *Medicine in Society: Historical Essays* (Cambridge: Cambridge University Press, 1992), p. 287.
3 Jonathan Andrews, 'The Rise of the Asylum in Britain', in Deborah Brunton (ed.), *Medicine Transformed: Health, Disease and Society in Europe, 1800–1930* (Manchester: Manchester University Press, 2004), pp. 314–16.

Further Reading A-Z

Abbott, Andrew, *The System of Professions: Essay on the Division of Expert Labour* (Chicago, IL: University of Chicago Press, 1988).

Ackerknecht, Erwin H., *Medicine at the Paris Hospital, 1794–1848* (Baltimore, MD: Johns Hopkins University Press, 1967).

Adams, M.B., (ed.), *The Wellborn Science: Eugenics in Germany, France, Brazil and Russia* (New York and Oxford: Oxford University Press, 1990).

Alexander, John, *Bubonic Plague in Early Modern Russia* (Oxford: Oxford University Press, 2003).

Anderson, Warwick, 'Disease, Race, and Empire', *Bulletin of the History of Medicine*, 70 (1996), pp. 62–67.

Andrews, Jonathan et al, *The History of Bethlem* (London: Routledge, 1997).

Arnold, David (ed.), *Imperial Medicine and Indigenous Societies* (Manchester: Manchester University Press, 1988).

Arnold, David, *Colonizing the Body: State Medicine and Epidemic Disease in Nineteenth-Century India* (Cambridge: Cambridge University Press, 1993).

Arnold, David (ed.), *Warm Climates and Western Medicine: The Emergence of Tropical Medicine 1500–1900* (Amsterdam: Rodopi, 1996).

Arnold, David, *Science, Technology and Medicine in Colonial India* (Cambridge: Cambridge University Press, 2004).

Arrizabalaga, Jon, Henderson, John and French, Roger, *The Great Pox: The French Disease in Renaissance Europe* (New Haven and London: Yale University Press, 1997).

Baldwin, Peter, *The Politics of Social Solidarity: Class Bases of the European Welfare State 1875–1975* (Cambridge: Cambridge University Press, 1992).

Baldwin, Peter, *Contagion and the State in Europe, 1830–1930* (Cambridge: Cambridge University Press, 2005).

Baldwin, Peter, *Disease and Democracy: The Industrialized World Faces Aids* (Berkeley and London: University of California Press, 2005).

Baly, Monica, *Florence Nightingale and Nursing Legacy*, 1997 edn (Oxford: Blackwell, 1997).

Barnes, David, *The Making of a Social Disease: Tuberculosis in Nineteenth-Century France* (Berkeley and London: University of California Press, 1995).

Barnes, David, *The Great Stink of Paris and the Nineteenth-Century Struggle against Filth and Germs* (Baltimore, MD: Johns Hopkins University Press, 2006).

Barry, Jonathan, 'Piety and the Patient: Medicine and Religion in Eighteenth Century Bristol', in Porter, Roy (ed.), *Patients and Practitioners: Lay Perceptions of Medicine in Pre-Industrial Society* (Cambridge: Cambridge University Press, 1985), pp. 145–75.

Barry, Jonathan and Davies, Owen (eds), *Witchcraft Historiography* (Basingstoke: Palgrave Macmillan, 2007).

Bartlett, Peter and Wright, David (eds), *Outside the Walls of the Asylum: The History of Care in the Community 1750–2000* (London: Athlone Press, 1999).

Bashford, Alison, *Purity and Pollution: Gender, Embodiment and Victorian Medicine* (Basingstoke: Palgrave Macmillan, 1998).

Beier, Lucinda, *Sufferers and Healers: The Experience of Illness in Seventeenth-Century England* (London: Routledge, 1987).

Berg, Manfred and Cocks, Geoffrey (eds), *Medicine and Modernity: Public Health and Medical Care in Nineteenth- and Twentieth-Century Germany* (Cambridge: Cambridge University Press, 2002).

Berger, Stefan, Feldner, Heiko and Passmore, Kevin (eds), *Writing History: Theory and Practice* (London: Hodder Arnold, 2003).

Berridge, Virginia, *Health and Society in Britain since 1939* (Cambridge: Cambridge University Press, 1999).

Berridge, Virginia and Strong, Philip (eds), *AIDS and Contemporary History* (Cambridge: Cambridge University Press, 2002).

Berrios, German E., 'Psychosurgery in Britain and Elsewhere', in Berrios, German E. and Freeman, Hugh (eds), *150 Years of British Psychiatry 1841–1991* (London: Gaskell, 1991).

Berrios, German E. and Porter, Roy (eds), *A History of Clinical Psychiatry* (London: Athlone Press, 1999).

Bewell, Alan, *Romanticism and Colonial Disease* (Baltimore, MD: Johns Hopkins University Press, 2003).

Bivins, Roberta, *Alternative Medicine: A History* (Oxford: Oxford University Press, 2007).

Black, Jeremy, *Introduction to Global Military History: 1775 to the Present Day* (London: Routledge, 2005).

Blume, Stuart, *Insight and Industry: On the Dynamics of Technological Change in Medicine* (Cambridge, MA: MIT Press, 1992).

Bonner, Thomas N., *To the Ends of the Earth: Women's Search for Education in Medicine* (Cambridge, MA: Harvard University Press, 1992).

Bonner, Thomas N., *Becoming a Physician: Medical Education in Britain, France, Germany, and the United States, 1750–1945* (New York and Oxford: Oxford University Press, 1995).

Bourke, Joanna, *Dismembering the Male: Men's Bodies, Britain and the Great War* (London: Reaktion Books, 1999).

Bourke, Joanna, *An Intimate History of Killing: Face-to-Face Killing in Twentieth-Century Warfare* (London: Granta Books, 1999).

Bowler, Peter J. and Morus, Iwan R., *Making Modern Science* (Chicago, IL: University of Chicago Press, 2005).

Brieger, Gert, 'The Historiography of Medicine', in Bynum, W.F. and Porter, Roy (eds), *Companion Encyclopaedia of the History of Medicine*, vol. 1 (London: Routledge, 1997), pp. 24–44.

Broberg, Gunnar and Roll-Hansen, Nils (eds), *Eugenics and the Welfare State: Sterilization Policy in Denmark, Sweden, Norway and Finland* (East Lansing, MI: Michigan State University Press, 2005).

Brockington, Fraser, *The Health of the Developing World* (Lewes: Book Guild, 1985).

Brockliss, Laurence and Jones, Colin, *The Medical World of Early Modern France* (Oxford: Clarendon Press, 1997).

Bruce, Steve (ed.), *Religion and Modernization* (Oxford: Clarendon Press, 1992).

Brundage, Anthony, *The English Poor Laws 1700–1930* (Basingstoke: Palgrave Macmillan, 2001).

Bryder, Linda, 'The First World War: Healthy or Hungry?', *History Workshop Journal* 24 (1987), pp. 141–55.

Bryder, Linda, *Below the Magic Mountain: A Social History of Tuberculosis in Twentieth-Century Britain* (Oxford: Clarendon Press, 1988).

Budd, Robert, *The Uses of Life: A History of Biotechnology* (Cambridge: Cambridge University Press, 1993).

Bullough, Vern et al (eds), *Florence Nightingale and Her Era: A Collection of New Scholarship* (New York and London: Garland, 1990).

Burleigh, Michael, *Death and Deliverance* (London: Pan, 2002).

Burnham, J.C., 'How the Concept of Profession Evolved in the Work of Historians of Medicine', *Bulletin of the History of Medicine* 70 (1996), pp. 1–24.

Busfield, Joan, *Men, Women and Madness: Understanding Gender and Mental Disorder* (Basingstoke: Palgrave Macmillan, 1996).

Bynum, W.F., *Science and the Practice of Medicine in the Nineteenth Century* (Cambridge: Cambridge University Press, 1994).

Bynum et al, W.F., *The Western Medical Tradition, 1800 to 2000* (Cambridge: Cambridge University Press, 2006).

Bynum, W.F. and Porter, Roy (eds), *Medical Fringe and Medical Orthodoxy, 1750–1850* (London: Routledge, 1987).

Carmichael, Ann, *Plague and the Poor in Renaissance Florence* (Cambridge: Cambridge University Press, 1986).

Cherry, Steve, *Medical Services and the Hospitals 1860–1939* (Cambridge: Cambridge University Press, 1996).

Christiansen, N.E. and Petersen, K., 'The Nordic Welfare States', *Scandinavian Journal of History* 26 (2001), pp. 153–56.

Cipolla, Carlo, *Fighting the Plague in Seventeenth-Century Italy* (Madison. WI: University of Wisconsin Press, 1981).

Cocks, Geoffrey and Jarausch, Konrad (eds), *German Professions, 1800–1950* (New York and Oxford: Oxford University Press, 1982).

Cohen, Deborah, *The War Come Home: Disabled Veterans in Britain and Germany 1914–39* (Berkeley, CA: University of California Press, 2001).

Collins, Harry and Pinch, Trevor, *Dr Golem: How to Think About Medicine* (Chicago, IL: University of Chicago Press, 2005).

Cook, Harold, *The Decline of the Old Medical Regime in Stuart London* (Ithaca, NY: Cornell University Press, 1986).

Cook, Noble, *Born to Die: Disease and New World Conquest 1492–1650* (Cambridge: Cambridge University Press, 1998).

Cooter, Roger, *Studies in the History of Alternative Medicine* (Basingstoke: Palgrave Macmillan, 1988).

Cooter, Roger, *Surgery and Society in Peace and War: Orthopaedics and the Organization of Modern Medicine, 1880–1948* (London: Macmillan, 1993).

Cooter, Roger, 'War and Modern Medicine' in Bynum, W.F. and Porter, Roy (eds), *Companion Encyclopaedia of the History of Medicine* vol. 2 (London: Routledge, 1997), pp. 1536–73.

Cooter, Roger, 'Of War and Epidemics: Unnatural Couplings, Problematic Conceptions', *Social History of Medicine* 16 (2003), pp. 283–302.

Cooter, Roger, 'After Death/After-"life": The Social History of Medicine in Post-Modernity', *Social History of Medicine* 20 (2007), pp. 441–64.

Cooter, Roger, Harrison, Mark and Sturdy, Steve (eds), *Medicine and Modern Warfare* (Amsterdam: Rodopi, 1999).

Cooter, Roger and Luckin, Bill (eds), *Accidents in History: Injuries, Fatalities and Social Relations* (Amsterdam: Rodopi, 1997).

Cooter, Roger and Pickstone, John (eds), *Medicine in the Twentieth Century* (London: Routledge, 2000).

Condrau, Flurin, 'The Patient's View Meets the Clinical Gaze', *Social History of Medicine* 20 (2007), pp. 525–40.

Conrad, Lawrence et al, *The Western Medical Tradition 800BC to AD1800* (Cambridge: Cambridge University Press, 1995).

Crosby, Alfred, *Ecological Imperialism: The Biological Expansion of Europe 900–1900* (Cambridge: Cambridge University Press, 2004).

Crowther, M. Anne and Dupree, Marguerite, *Medical Lives in the Age of Surgical Revolution* (Cambridge: Cambridge University Press, 2007).

Cunningham, Andrew, *The Anatomical Renaissance: The Resurrection of Anatomical Practices of the Ancients* (Aldershot: Scolar, 1997).

Cunningham, Andrew and Andrews, Birdie (eds), *Western Medicine as Contested Knowledge* (Manchester: Manchester University Press, 1997).

Curtin, Philip, *The Image of Africa: British Ideas and Action 1780–1850* (London: Macmillan, 1965).

Curtin, Philip, *Death by Migration: Europe's Encounter with the Tropical World in the Nineteenth Century* (London: Macmillan, 1989).

D'Antonio, Patricia, 'Revisiting and Rethinking the Rewriting of Nursing History', *Bulletin of the History of Medicine* 73 (1999), pp. 268–90.

Daston, Lorraine and Galison, Peter, *Objectivity* (New York: Zone, 2007).

Davidson, Roger and Hall, Lesley (eds), *Sex, Sin and Suffering: Venereal Disease and European Society since 1870* (London: Routledge, 2001).

Debus, A.G., *Man and Nature in the Renaissance* (Cambridge: Cambridge University Press, 1978).

Digby, Anne, *Madness, Morality and Medicine: A Study of the York Retreat 1796–1914* (Cambridge: Cambridge University Press, 1985).

Digby, Anne, *Making a Medical Living: Doctors and their Patients in the English Market for Medicine, 1720–1911* (Cambridge: Cambridge University Press, 1994).

Digby, Anne, *The Evolution of British General Practice 1850–1948* (Oxford: Oxford University Press, 1999).

Dingwall, Robert, Rafferty, Anne Marie and Webster, Charles, *An Introduction to the Social History of Nursing* (London: Routledge, 1988).

Dingwall, Robert et al, *An Introduction to the Social History of Nursing* (London, Routledge, 2002).

Dixon, Anna and Mossialos, Elias, *Health Care Systems in Eight Countries* (European Observatory on Health Care Systems, 2002).

Dobson, Mary, *Contours of Death and Disease in Early Modern England* (Cambridge: Cambridge University Press, 2003).

Doel, Ronald and Söderqvist, Thomas (eds), *The Historiography of Contemporary Science, Technology, and Medicine: Writing Recent Science* (London: Routledge, 2007).

Dowbiggin, Ian, 'Degeneration and Hereditarianism', in Bynum, W.F., Porter, Roy and Shepherd, Michael (eds), *The Anatomy of Madness* (London: Tavistock, 1987).

Dowbiggin, Ian, *Inheriting Madness: Professionalization and Psychiatric Knowledge in Nineteenth-Century France* (Berkeley, CA: University of California Press, 1991).

Drayton, Richard, 'Science, Medicine, and the British Empire', in Winks, Robin W. (ed.), *The Oxford History of the British Empire, vol. 5: Historiography* (Oxford: Oxford University Press, 1999), pp. 264–76.

Duden, Barbara, *The Woman Beneath the Skin: A Doctor's Patients in Eighteenth Century Germany* (Cambridge, MA: Harvard University Press, 1991).

Duffin, Jacalyn, *History of Medicine: A Scandalously Short Introduction* (Toronto: University of Toronto Press, 1999).

Durbach, Nadja, *Bodily Matters: The Anti-Vaccination Movement in England, 1853–1907* (Durham, NC: Duke University Press, 2005).

Dwork, Deborah, *War is Good for Babies and Other Young Children: A History of the Infant and Child Welfare Movement in England 1898–1918* (London: Tavistock, 1987).

Ellis, Jack, *The Physician-Legislators of France: Medicine and Politics in the Early Third Republic* (Cambridge: Cambridge University Press, 1990).

Ernst, Waltraud (ed.), *Plural Medicine, Tradition and Modernity, 1800–2000* (London: Routledge, 2002).

Ernst, Waltraud, 'Beyond East and West', *Social History of Medicine*, 20 (2007), pp. 505–24.

Ernst, Waltraud and Harris, Bernard (eds), *Race, Science and Medicine 1700–1960* (London: Routledge, 1999).

Evans, Richard, *Death in Hamburg: Society and Politics in the Cholera Years, 1830–1910* (London: Penguin, 1991).

Farley, John, *Bilharzia: A History of Imperial Tropical Medicine* (Cambridge: Cambridge University Press, 1991).

Field, M.G., 'Soviet Medicine', in Cooter, Roger and Pickstone, John (eds), *Medicine in the Twentieth Century* (London: Routledge, 2000), pp. 51–66.

Fisher, Kate, *Birth Control, Sex and Marriage in Britain, 1918–1960* (Oxford: Oxford University Press, 2006).

Fissell, Mary, *Patients, Power and the Poor in Eighteenth Century Bristol* (Cambridge: Cambridge University Press, 1991).

Fissell, Mary, 'Gender and Generation: Representing Reproduction in Early Modern England', *Gender and History* 7 (1995), pp. 433–56.

Fissell, Mary, *Vernacular Bodies: The Politics of Reproduction in Early Modern England* (Oxford: Oxford University Press, 2004).

Fissell, Mary, 'Introduction: Women, Health and Healing in Early Modern Europe', *Bulletin of the History of Medicine* 82 (2008), pp. 1–17.

Flexner, Abraham, *Medical Education* (New York: Macmillan, 1925).

Foucault, Michel, *Madness and Civilization: A History of Insanity in the Age of Reason* (New York: Pantheon Books, 1965).

Foucault, Michel, *The Birth of the Clinic* (London: Tavistock, 1973).

Foucault, Michel, *The History of Sexuality*, vols 1–3 (London: Penguin, 1997–8).

Fox, D.M., *Health Policies, Health Politics: The British and American Experience 1911–1965* (Princeton, NJ: Princeton University Press, 1992).

Fraser, Derek, *The Evolution of the British Welfare State* (Basingstoke: Palgrave Macmillan, 1973).

French, Roger, *Medicine Before Science: The Business of Medicine from the Middle Ages to the Enlightenment* (Cambridge: Cambridge University Press, 2003).

French, Roger and Wear, Andrew (eds), *The Medical Revolution of the Seventeenth Century* (Cambridge: Cambridge University Press, 1989).

Gaudilliere, Jean-Paul and Löwy, Ilana (eds), *The Invisible Industrialist: Manufacturers and the Construction of Scientific Knowledge* (Basingstoke: Palgrave Macmillan, 1999).

Gay, Peter, *Freud: A Life for Our Time* (London: Papermac, 1989).

Geison, Gerald, '"Divided We Stand" Physiologists and Clinicians in the American Context', in Vogel, Morris and Rosenberg, Charles (eds), *The Therapeutic Revolution:*

Essays in the Social History of American Medicine (Philadelphia, PA: University of Pennsylvania Press, 1979), pp. 67–90.

Geison, Gerald, *Michael Foster and the Cambridge School of Physiology* (Princeton, NJ: Princeton University Press, 1987).

Gelfand, Toby, *Professionalizing Modern Medicine: Paris Surgeons and Medical Science and Institutions in the Eighteenth Century* (Westport, CT: Greenwood Press, 1980).

Gelis, Jacques, *History of Childbirth: Fertility, Pregnancy and Birth in Early Modern Europe* (London: Polity, 1991).

Gentilcore, David, *Healers and Healing in Early Modern Italy* (Manchester: Manchester University Press, 1998).

Gilbert, Pamela, *Cholera and Nation* (Albany, NY: State University of New York Press, 2008).

Gilfoyle, Timothy, 'Prostitutes in History', *American Historical Review* 104 (1999), pp. 117–41.

Gilman, Sander, *Disease and Representation: Images of Illness from Madness to AIDS* (Ithaca, NY: Cornell University Press, 1988).

Goldstein, Jan, *Console and Classify: The French Psychiatric Profession in the Nineteenth Century* (Cambridge: Cambridge University Press, 2002).

Gorsky, Martin, Mohan, John and Willis, Tim, *Mutualism and Health Care: British Hospital Contributory Schemes in the Twentieth Century* (Manchester: Manchester University Press, 2006).

Granshaw, Lindsay, '"Fame and Fortune by Means of Bricks and Mortar": The Medical Profession and Specialist Hospitals in Britain 1800–1948', in Granshaw, Lindsay and Porter, Roy (eds), *The Hospital in History* (London: Routledge, 1989), pp. 199–200.

Granshaw, Lindsay, '"Upon this Principle I have based a practice": The development and reception of antisepsis in Britain, 1867–90', in Pickstone, John (ed.), *Medical Innovations in Historical Perspective* (Basingstoke: Palgrave Macmillan, 1992), pp. 16–46.

Granshaw, Lindsay and Porter, Roy (eds), *The Hospital in History* (London: Routledge, 1989).

Green, Monica, 'Gendering the History of Women's Healthcare', *Gender and History* 20 (2008), pp. 487–518.

Grell, Ole Peter and Cunningham, Andrew (eds), *Medicine and the Reformation* (London: Routledge, 1993).

Grell, Ole Peter and Cunningham, Andrew (eds), *Health Care Provision and Poor Relief in Northern Europe 1500–1700* (London: Routledge, 1996).

Grmek, Mirko, Maulitz, Russell and Duffin, Jacalyn, *History of AIDS: Emergence and Origin of a Modern Pandemic* (Princeton, NJ: Princeton University Press, 1992).

Gross Solomon, Susan and Hutchinson, John F. (eds), *Health and Society in Revolutionary Russia* (Bloomington, IN: Indiana University Press, 1990).

Hamlin, Christopher, *Cholera: The Bibliography* (Oxford: Oxford University Press, 2009).

Hamlin, Christopher, *Public Health and Social Justice in the Age of Chadwick: Britain 1800–54* (Cambridge: Cambridge University Press, 2009).

Hannaway, Caroline, 'Medicine and Religion in Pre-Revolutionary France', *Social History of Medicine* 2 (1989), pp. 315–19.

Hannaway, Caroline and La Berge, Ann (eds), *Constructing Paris Medicine* (Amsterdam: Rodopi, 1998).

Hardy, Anne, *The Epidemic Streets: Infectious Diseases and the Rise of Preventive Medicine, 1856–1900* (Oxford: Clarendon Press, 1993).

Hardy, Anne, *Health and Medicine in Britain since 1860* (Basingstoke: Palgrave Macmillan, 2001).

Harris, Ruth, 'Possession on the Borders: The "Mal de Morzine" in Nineteenth-Century France', *Journal of Modern History* 69 (1997), pp. 451–71.

Harrison, Mark, *Public Health in British India: Anglo-Indian Preventive Medicine 1859–1914* (Cambridge: Cambridge University Press, 1994).

Harrison, Mark, 'Medicine and the Management of Modern Warfare', *History of Science* 34 (1996), pp. 379–410.

Harrison, Mark, *Disease and the Modern World: 1500 to the Present Day* (London: Polity Press, 2004).

Harrison, Mark, *Medicine and Victory: British Military Medicine in the Second World War* (Oxford: Oxford University Press, 2008).

Hayward, Rhodri, '"Much Exaggerated": The End of the History of Medicine', *Journal of Contemporary History* 40 (2005), pp. 167–78.

Headrick, Daniel, *Tools of Empire: Technology and European Imperialism in the Nineteenth Century* (New York and Oxford: Oxford University Press, 1981).

Healy, David, *The Antidepressant Era* (Cambridge, MA: Harvard University Press, 1999).

Healy, David, *Creation of Psychopharmacology* (Cambridge, MA: Harvard University Press, 2002).

Healy, Margaret, *Fictions of Disease in Early-modern England: Bodies, Plagues and Politics* (Basingstoke: Palgrave Macmillan, 2001).

Henderson, John, *The Renaissance Hospital: Healing the Body and Healing the Soul* (New Haven, CT: Yale University Press, 2006).

Henderson, John, Horden, Peregrine and Pastore, Alessandro (eds), *The Impact of Hospitals 300–2000* (Bern: Peter Lang, 2007).

Henry, John, *The Scientific Revolution and the Origins of Modern Science* (Basingstoke: Palgrave Macmillan, 2008).

Hong, Young-sun, 'Neither Singular Nor Alternative: Narratives of Modernity and Welfare in Germany, 1870–1945', *Social History* 30 (2005), pp. 133–153.

Howell, Joel, *Technology in the Hospital: Transforming Patient Care in the Early Twentieth Century* (Baltimore, MD: Johns Hopkins University Press, 1995).

Huisman, Frank, 'Shaping the Medical Market: On the Construction of Quackery and Folk Medicine in the Dutch Historiography', *Medical History* 43 (1999), pp. 359–75.

Huisman, Frank, and Warner, John Harley (eds), *Locating Medical History. The Stories and their Meanings* (Baltimore, MD: Johns Hopkins University Press, 2004).

Hurren, Elizabeth, *Dying for Victorian Medicine* (Basingstoke: Palgrave Macmillan, 2011).

Immergut, Ellen, *Health Politics: Interests and Institutions in Western Europe* (Cambridge: Cambridge University Press, 1992).

Jenner, Mark and Wallis, Patrick (eds), *Medicine and the Market in England and Its Colonies, c.1450–c.1850* (Basingstoke: Palgrave Macmillan, 2007).

Jones, Colin, 'Sisters of Charity and the Ailing Poor', *Social History of Medicine* 2 (1989), pp. 339–48.

Jones, Colin, *The Charitable Imperative: Hospitals and Nursing in Ancien Régime and Revolutionary France* (London: Routledge, 1989).

Jones, Colin and Porter, Roy (eds), *Reassessing Foucault: Power, Medicine and the Body* (London: Routledge, 1994).

Jones, Helen, *Health and Society in Twentieth-Century Britain* (London: Longman, 1994).

Jordanova, Ludmilla, 'The Social Construction of Medical Knowledge', *Social History of Medicine* 8 (1995), pp. 361–81.

Kelly, Patrick, *Creating a National Home: Building the Veterans' Welfare State 1860–1900* (Cambridge, MA: Harvard University Press, 1997).

Kinzelbach, Annemarie, 'Hospitals, Medicine and Society', *Renaissance Studies* 15 (2001), pp. 217–28.

Kinzelbach, Annemarie, 'Infection, Contagion and Public Health in Late Medieval and Early Modern German Imperial Towns', *Journal of the History of Medicine and Allied Sciences* 61 (2006), pp. 369–89.

Kiple, Kenneth (ed.), *The Cambridge World History of Human Disease* (Cambridge: Cambridge University Press, 1993).

Klestinec, Cynthia, 'A History of Anatomy Theatres in Sixteenth-Century Padua', *Journal of the History of Medicine* 59 (2004), pp. 375–412.

Kohler, Robert, *From Medical Chemistry to Biochemistry: The Making of a Biomedical Discipline* (Cambridge: Cambridge University Press, 1982).

Kohn, George (ed.), *Encyclopaedia of Plague and Pestilence from Ancient Times to the Present* (New York: Facts on File Inc, 2001).

Koven, Seth and Michel, Sonya, 'Womanly Duties', *American Historical Review* 95 (1990), pp. 1076–108.

La Berge, Ann, *Mission and Method* (Cambridge: Cambridge University Press, 1992).

Laqueur, Thomas, *Making Sex: Body and Gender from the Greeks to Freud* (Cambridge, MA: Harvard University Press, 1991).

Latour, Bruno, *The Pasteurization of France* tr. Sheridan, A. and Law, J. (Cambridge, MA: Harvard University Press, 1988).

Lawrence, Chris, Hardy, Anne and Tansey, Tilly in Bynum, W.F. et al, *The Western Medical Tradition, 1800 to 2000* (Cambridge: Cambridge University Press, 2006).

Lawrence, Christopher, 'Incommunicable Knowledge: Science, Technology and the Clinical Art in Britain, 1850–1914', *Journal of Contemporary* 20 (1985), pp. 503–20.

Lawrence, Christopher, 'Divine, Democratic and Heroic', in Lawrence, Christopher (ed.), *Medical Theory, Surgical Practice. Studies in the History of Surgery* (London: Routledge, 1992), pp. 1–47.

Lawrence, Christopher, *Medicine in the Making of Modern Britain 1700–1920* (London: Routledge, 1994).

Lawrence, Christopher and Dixey, Richard, 'Practicing on Principle: Joseph Lister and the Germ Theories of Disease', in Lawrence, Christopher (ed.), *Medical Theory, Surgical Practice* (London: Routledge, 1992), pp. 153–215.

Lawrence, Christopher and Treasure, Tom, 'Surgeons', in Cooter, Roger and Pickstone, John (eds), *Medicine in the Twentieth Century* (London: Routledge, 2000), pp. 653–670.

Lawrence, Susan, 'Medical education', in Bynum, W.F. and Porter, Roy (eds), *Companion Encyclopaedia of the History of Medicine*, vol. 2 (London: Routledge, 1997), pp. 1151–79.

Lawrence, Susan, *Charitable Knowledge: Hospital Pupils and Practitioners in Eighteenth-Century London* (Cambridge: Cambridge University Press, 2002).

Lee, Sung, 'WHO and the Developing World', in Cunningham, Andrew and Andrews, Bridie (eds), *Western Medicine as Contested Knowledge* (Manchester: Manchester University Press, 1997), pp. 24–45.

Leese, Peter, *Shell-Shock: Traumatic Neurosis and the British Soldiers of the First World War* (Basingstoke: Palgrave Macmillan, 2002).

Lee Downs, Laura, *Writing Gender History* (London: Hodder Arnold, 2004).

Lerner, Paul, *Hysterical Men: War, Psychiatry, and the Politics of Trauma in Germany, 1890–1930* (Ithaca, NY: Cornell University Press, 2003).

Lesch, John, *Science and Medicine in France: The Emergence of Experimental Physiology, 1790–1855* (Cambridge, MA: Harvard University Press, 1984).

Lightman, Bernard, *Victorian Popularizers of Science: Designing Nature for New Audiences* (Chicago, IL: University of Chicago Press, 2007).

Lindemann, Mary, *Medicine and Society in Early Modern Europe,* 2010 edn (Cambridge: Cambridge University Press, 2010).

Loudon, Irvine, *Death in Childbirth: An International Study of Maternal Care and Maternal Mortality, 1800–1950* (Oxford: Clarendon Press, 1980).

Loudon, Irvine, *Medical Care and the General Practitioner, 1750–1850* (Oxford: Oxford University Press, 1986).

Loudon, Irvine (ed.), *Western Medicine: An Illustrated History* (Oxford: Oxford University Press, 1997).

Lyons, Maryinez, *The Colonial Disease: A Social History of Sleeping Sickness in Northern Zaire 1900–40* (Cambridge: Cambridge University Press, 2002).

MacCulloch, Diarmaid, *Reformation: Europe's House Divided 1490–1700* (London: Penguin, 2005).

Macleod, Roy and Lewis, Milton (eds), *Disease, Medicine, and Empire: Perspectives on Western Medicine and the Experience of European Expansion* (London: Routledge, 1988).

Maehle, A.H. and Geyer-Kordesch, J. (eds), *Historical and Philosophical Perspectives on Biomedical Ethics* (Aldershot: Ashgate, 2002).

Marks, Lara, *Sexual Chemistry* (New Haven and London: Yale University Press, 2001).

Marland, Hilary, *Medicine and Society in Wakefield and Huddersfield, 1780–1870* (Cambridge: Cambridge University Press, 1987).

Marks, Harry, *The Progress of Experiment* (Cambridge: Cambridge University Press, 1997).

Marks, Shula, 'What is Colonial About Colonial Medicine? And What Has Happened to Imperialism and Health?', *Social History of Medicine* 10 (1997), pp. 205–19.

Maulitz, Russell, *Morbid Appearances: The Anatomy of Pathology in the Nineteenth Century* (Cambridge: Cambridge University Press, 1988).

McClelland, Charles, *The German Experience of Professionalization* (Cambridge: Cambridge University Press, 2002).

McGann, Susan and Mortimer, Barbara (eds), *New Directions in the History of Nursing: International Perspectives* (London: Routledge, 2005).

McKeown, Thomas, *The Rise of Modern Populations* (London: Hodder and Stoughton, 1976).

McLaren, Angus, *A History of Contraception* (Oxford: Blackwell, 1990).

McLarren Caldwell, Janis, *Literature and Medicine in Nineteenth-Century Britain* (Cambridge: Cambridge University Press, 2004).

Melling, Joseph and Forsythe, Bill (eds), *Insanity, Institutions and Society 1800–1914* (London: Routledge, 1999).

Melling, Joseph and Forsythe, Bill, *The Politics of Madness: The State, Insanity and Society in England, 19845–1914* (London: Routledge, 2006).

Mercer, Alex, *Disease, Mortality and Population in Transition* (London and New York: Continuum, 1990).

Merians, Linda (ed.), *The Secret Malady: Venereal Disease in Eighteenth-Century Britain and France* (Lexington, KY: University Press of Kentucky, 1996).

Micale, Mark and Porter, Roy (eds), *Discovering the History of Psychiatry* (New York and Oxford: Oxford University Press, 1994).

Morone, James and Goggin, Janice, 'Health Policies in Europe', *Journal of Health Politics, Policy and Law* 20 (1995), pp. 557–69.

Nutton, Vivian, 'Humanist Surgery', in Wear, Andrew, French, Roger and Lonie, Iain (eds), *The Medical Renaissance of the Sixteenth Century* (Cambridge: Cambridge University Press, 1985), pp. 75–99.

Nutton, Vivian, 'Wittenberg Anatomy', in Grell, Ole Peter and Cunningham, Andrew (eds), *Medicine and the Reformation* (London: Routledge, 1993), pp. 11–32.

Nye, Robert, 'The Rise and Fall of the Eugenics Empire: Recent Perspectives on the Impact of Biomedical Thought in Modern Society', *Historical Journal* 36 (1993), pp. 687–700.

Nye, Robert, *Sexuality* (Oxford: Oxford University Press, 1999).

Nye, Robert, 'The Evolution of the *Concept of Medicalization* in the Late Twentieth Century', *Journal of History of the Behavioral Sciences* 39 (2003), pp. 115–29.

Oakley, Ann, *The Captured Womb: History of the Medical Care of Pregnant Women* (Oxford: Blackwell, 1986).

Packard, Randall M., 'Postcolonial Medicine', in Cooter, Roger and Pickstone, John (eds), *Medicine in the Twentieth Century* (London: Routledge, 2000), pp. 97–112.

Pedersen, Susan, *Family, Dependence, and the Origins of the Welfare State: Britain and France 1914–1945* (Cambridge: Cambridge University Press, 1995).

Pelling, Margaret, *Cholera, Fever and English Medicine 1825–1865* (Oxford: Clarendon Press, 1978).

Pelling, Margaret, *Medical Conflicts in Early Modern London: Patronage, Physicians, and. Irregular Practitioners, 1550–1640* (Oxford: Oxford University Press, 2003).

Phillips, Howard and Killingray, David (eds), *The Spanish Influenza Pandemic of 1918* (London: Routledge, 2003).

Pick, Daniel, *Faces of Degeneration: A European Disorder c.1848–1918,* 1993 edn (Cambridge: Cambridge University Press, 1993).

Pick, Daniel, *The War Machine: The Rationalization of Slaughter in the Modern Age* (New Haven, CT: Yale University Press, 1993).

Pickstone, John, *Medicine and Industrial Society: A History of Hospital Development in Manchester and its Region, 1752–1946* (Manchester: Manchester University Press, 1985).

Pickstone, John, *Ways of Knowing* (Manchester: Manchester University Press, 2000).

Pierson, Christopher, *Beyond the Welfare State?* (Cambridge: Polity Press, 2007).

Porter, Dorothy (ed.), *The History of Public Health and the Modern State* (Amsterdam: Rodopi, 1994).

Porter, Dorothy, 'The Mission of the Social History of Medicine', *Social History of Medicine* 8 (1995), pp. 345–59.

Porter, Dorothy, *Health, Civilization and the State: History of Public Health from Ancient to Modern Times* (London: Routledge, 1999).

Porter, Roy, *Patients and Practitioners: Lay Perceptions of Medicine in Pre-Industrial Society* (Cambridge: Cambridge University Press, 1985).

Porter, Roy, 'The Patient's View: Doing Medical History from Below', *Theory and Society* 14 (1985), pp. 167–74.

Porter, Roy, *Health for Sale: Quackery in England 1660–1850* (Manchester: Manchester University Press, 1989).

Porter, Roy, *Mind-Forg'd Manacles: A History of Madness in England from the Restoration to the Regency* (London: Penguin, 1990).

Porter, Roy (ed.), *The Cambridge Illustrated History of Medicine* (Cambridge: Cambridge University Press, 1996)

Porter, Roy, *The Greatest Benefit to Mankind: A Medical History of Humanity from Antiquity to the Present* (London: HarperCollins, 1997).

Porter, Roy, *Quacks: Fakers and Charlatans in Medicine* (Stroud: Tempus, 2003).

Porter, Roy and Bynum, W.F., *The Anatomy of Madness,* vol 1–3 (London: Tavistock, 1985–88).

Porter, Roy and Bynum, W.F., *Companion Encyclopaedia of the History of Medicine*, volume 1 and 2 (London: Routledge, 1993).

Porter, Roy and Porter, Dorothy, *In Sickness and in Health: The British Experience 1650–1850* (London: Fourth Estate, 1988).

Porter, Roy and Wright, David (eds), *The Confinement of the Insane: International Perspectives 1800–1965* (Cambridge: Cambridge University Press, 2003).

Pressman, Jack, *The Last Resort: Psychosurgery and the Limits of Medicine* (Cambridge: Cambridge University Press, 2002).

Pullan, Brian, 'The Counter-Reformation, Medical Care and Poor Relief', in Grell, Ole Peter, Cunningham, Andrew and Arrizabalaga, Jon (eds), *Health Care and Poor Relief in Counter-Reformation Europe* (London: Routledge, 1999), pp. 18–39.

Pullan, Brian, *Rich and Poor in Renaissance Venice: The Social Institutions of a Catholic State to 1620* (ACLS History E-Book Project, 2008).

Rafferty, Anne Marie, *The Politics of Nursing Knowledge* (London: Routledge, 1996).

Ramsey, Matthew, *Professional and Popular Medicine in France 1770–1830* (Cambridge: Cambridge University Press, 1988).

Ranger, Terence and Slack, Paul (eds), *Epidemics and Ideas: Essays on the Historical Perception of Pestilence* (Cambridge: Cambridge University Press, 1995).

Reiser, Stanley J., *Medicine and the Reign of Technology* (Cambridge: Cambridge University Press, 1982).

Reznick, Jeffrey, *Healing the Nation: Soldiers and the Culture of Caregiving in Britain during the First World War* (Manchester: Manchester University Press, 2005).

Richardson, Ruth, *Death, Dissection and the Destitute* (London: Penguin, 1989).

Riley, James, *Sick, not Dead: The Health of British Workingmen during the Mortality Decline* (Baltimore, MD: Johns Hopkins University Press, 1997).

Riley, James, *Rising Life Expectancy: A Global History* (Cambridge: Cambridge University Press, 2001).

Risse, Guenter, *Hospital Life in Enlightenment Scotland: Care and Teaching at the Royal Infirmary of Edinburgh* (Cambridge: Cambridge University Press, 1986).

Risse, Guenter, *Mending Bodies Saving Souls: A History of Hospitals* (New York and Oxford: Oxford University Press, 1999).

Rivett, Geoffrey, *From Cradle to Grave: Fifty years of the NHS* (London: King's Fund, 1998).

Rose, Nikolas, *Psychological Complex: Psychology, Politics and Society in England, 1869–1939* (London: Routledge and Kegan Paul, 1985).

Rose, Nikolas, *The Politics of Life Itself* (Princeton, NJ: Princeton University Press, 2007).

Rosen, George, *From Medical Police to Social Medicine* (New York: Science History Publications, 1974).

Rosenberg, Charles and Golden, Janet (eds), *Framing Disease: Studies in Cultural History* (Chapel Hill, NC: Rutgers University Press, 1992).

Rupke, Nicolaas (ed.), *Vivisection in Historical Perspective* (London: Routledge, 1987).

Russell, Colin, *Science and Social Change, 1770–1900* (Basingstoke: Palgrave Macmillan, 1983).

Savage, J. and Heijnen, S. (eds), *Nursing in Europe* (World Health Organization, 1997).

Schiebinger, Londa (ed.), *Feminism and the Body* (Oxford: Oxford University Press, 2000).

Schultheiss, Katrin, *Bodies and Souls: Politics and the Professionalization of Nursing in France, 1880–1922* (Cambridge, MA: Harvard University Press, 2001).

Scull, Andrew, *Museums of Madness: The Social Organization of Insanity in Nineteenth-Century England* (London: Allen Lane, 1979).

Scull, Andrew, *Decarceration* (Chapel Hill, NC: Rutgers University Press, 1984).

Scull, Andrew, 'Somatic Treatments and the Historiography of Psychiatry', *History of Psychiatry* 5 (1994), pp. 1–12.

Scull, Andrew, *The Most Solitary of Afflictions: Madness and Society in Britain 1700–1900* (New Haven, CT: Yale University Press, 2005).

Scull, Andrew, MacKenzie, Charlotte and Hervey, Nicholas, *Masters of Bedlam: The Transformation of the Mad-Doctoring Trade* (Princeton: Princeton University Press, 1999).

Sedgwick, Peter, *Psychopolitics* (London: Pluto Press, 1982).

Shamdasani, Sonu, 'Psychoanalytic Body', in Cooter, Roger and Pickstone, John (eds), *Companion to Medicine in the Twentieth Century* (London: Routledge, 2003), pp. 307–22.

Shapin, Steven and Schaffer, Simon, *Leviathan and the Air-Pump: Hobbes, Boyle, and the Experimental Life* (Princeton, NJ: Princeton University Press, 1985).

Shapin, Steven, *A Social History of Truth: Civility and Science in Seventeenth-Century England* (Chicago, IL: University of Chicago Press, 1996).

Shapin, Steven, *The Scientific Revolution* (Chicago, IL: University of Chicago Press, 1996).

Shephard, Ben, *A War Of Nerves: Soldiers and Psychiatrists 1914–1994* (Cambridge, MA: Harvard University Press, 2002).

Shorter, Edward, *A History of Psychiatry: From the Era of the Asylum to the Age of Prozac* (New York: John Wiley & Sons, 1998).

Shortt, S.E.D., 'Physicians, Science, and Status: Issues in the Professionalization of Anglo-American Medicine in the Nineteenth Century', *Medical History* 27 (1983), pp. 51–68.

Showalter, Elaine, *The Female Malady: Women, Madness and English Culture 1830–1980* (London: Virago, 1987).

Siraisi, Nancy, *Medieval and Early Renaissance Medicine* (Chicago, IL: University of Chicago Press, 1990).

Siraisi, Nancy, 'Vesalius and the Reading of Galen's Teleology', *Renaissance Quarterly* 1 (1997), pp. 1–37.

Sismondo, Sergio, *An Introduction to Science and Technology Studies* (Oxford: Blackwell, 2004).

Slack, Paul, *Poverty and Policy in Tudor and Stuart England* (London: Longman, 1990).

Slack, Paul, *The Impact of the Plague in Tudor and Stuart England* (Oxford: Clarendon Press, 1990).

Smith, Timothy, *Creating the Welfare State in France, 1880–1940* (Montreal: McGill-Queen's University Press, 2003).

Snow, Stephanie, *Operations Without Pain: The Practice and Science of Anaesthesia in Victorian Britain* (Basingstoke: Palgrave Macmillan, 2006).

Sontag, Susan, *Illness as Metaphor and AIDS and its Metaphors* (London: Penguin Classics, 2009).

Stanley, Peter, *For Fear of Pain: British Surgery, 1790–1850* (Amsterdam: Rodopi, 2003).

Stevenson, Christine, *Medicine and Magnificence: British Hospital and Asylum Architecture, 1660–1815* (New Haven, CT: Yale University Press, 2000).

Still, Arthur and Velody, Irving (eds), *Rewriting the History of Madness* (London: Routledge, 1992).

Stoler, Ann L., *Race and the Education of Desire: Foucault's 'History of Sexuality' and the Colonial Order of Things* (Durham, NC: Duke University Press, 1995).

Stone, Michael, *Healing the Mind: A History of Psychiatry from Antiquity to the Present* (New York: W.W. Norton, 1998).

Summers, Anne, *Angels and Citizens: British Women as Military Nurses 1854–1914* (London: Routledge, 1988).

Swann, John, *Academic Scientists and the Pharmaceutical Industry* (Baltimore, MD: Johns Hopkins University Press, 1988).

Szreter, Simon, 'The Importance of Social Intervention in Britain's Mortality Decline, c.1850–1914: A Reinterpretation of the Role of Public Health', *Social History of Medicine* 1 (1988), pp. 1–37.

Tansey, E.M., '"They used to call it psychiatry": Aspects of the development and impact of psychopharmacology', in Gijswijt-Hofstra, Marijke and Porter, Roy (eds), *Cultures of Psychiatry and Mental Health Care in Postwar Britain and the Netherlands* (Amsterdam: Rodopi, 1998), pp. 79–101.

Taylor, Becky, Stewart, John and Powell, Martin, 'Central and Local Government and the Provision of Municipal Medicine, 1919–39', *English Historical Review* 122 (2007), pp. 397–426.

Theriot, Nancy, 'Negotiating Illness: Doctors, Patients, and Families in the Nineteenth Century', *Journal of the History of Behavioural Sciences* 37 (2001), pp. 349–68.

Thompson, John and Goldin, Grace, *The Hospital* (New Haven, CT: Yale University Press, 1975).

Timmerman, Carsten, 'Rationalization "Folk Medicine" in Interwar Germany: Faith, Business and Science at "Dr Madaus & Co."', *Social History of Medicine* 14 (2001), pp. 459–82.

Tuchman, Arleen M., *Science, Medicine and the State in Germany: The Case of Baden, 1815–1871* (Oxford: Oxford University Press, 1993).

Vaughan, Megan, *Curing their Ills: Colonial Power and African Illness* (Cambridge: Polity Press, 1991).

von Arni, Eric Gruber, *Justice to the Maimed Soldiers: Nursing, Medical Care and Welfare for Sick and Wounded Soldiers and their Families during the English Civil Wars and Interregnum 1642–1660* (Aldershot: Ashgate, 2001).

Vrettos, Athena, *Somatic Fictions: Imagining Illness in Victorian Culture* (Stanford, CA: Stanford University Press, 1995).

Waddington, Keir, *Charity and the London Hospitals, 1850–1898* (Woodbridge: Boydell, 2000).

Wallis, Patrick and Jenner, Mark (eds), *Medicine and the Market in England and its Colonies, c.1450–c.1850* (Basingstoke: Palgrave Macmillan, 2007).

Wangensteen, Owen and Wangensteen, Sarah, *The Rise of Surgery from Empiric Craft to Scientific Discipline* (Folkestone: Dawson, 1978).

Warner, John Harley, 'The History of Science and the Sciences of Medicine', *Osiris* 10 (1995), pp. 164–93.

Wear, Andrew, *Knowledge and Practice in English Medicine, 1550–1680* (Cambridge: Cambridge University Press, 2000).

Weatherall, Miles, *In Search of a Cure: A History of Pharmaceutical Discovery* (Oxford: Oxford University Press, 1990).

Webster, Charles, *The Great Instauration: Science, Medicine and Reform, 1626–60* (London: Duckworth, 1975).

Webster, Charles, 'Medical Practitioners' in Webster, Charles (ed.), *Healing, Medicine and Mortality in the Sixteenth Century* (Cambridge: Cambridge University Press, 1979), pp. 165–236.

Webster, Charles, *The Health Services since the War. Volume I: Problems of Health Care. The National Health Service before 1957* (London: HMSO, 1988).

Webster, Charles, *The National Health Service: A Political History* (Oxford: Oxford University Press, 2002).

Weindling, Paul (ed.), *The Social History of Occupational Health* (London: Routledge, 1985).

Weindling, Paul, 'The Modernization of Charity in Nineteenth Century France and Germany', in Barry, Jonathan and Jones, Colin (eds), *Medicine and Charity before the Welfare State* (London: Routledge, 1991), pp. 190–206.

Weindling, Paul, *Health, Race and German Politics between National Unification and Nazism 1879–1945* (Cambridge: Cambridge University Press, 1993).

Weindling, Paul (ed.), *International Health Organizations and Movements, 1918–1939* (Cambridge: Cambridge University Press, 1995).

Weiner, Dora B., *The Citizen-Patient in Revolutionary and Imperial Paris* (Baltimore, MD: Johns Hopkins University Press, 1993).

Weiner, Dora B., '"*Le geste de Pinel*": The History of a Psychiatric Myth', in Micale, Mark S. and Porter, Roy (eds), *Discovering the History of Psychiatry* (New York and Oxford: Oxford University Press, 1994), pp. 232–47.

Weisz, George, 'The Emergence of Medical Specialization in the Nineteenth Century', *Bulletin of the History of Medicine* 77 (2003), pp. 536–75.

White, Luise, *Speaking with Vampires: Rumour and History in Colonial Africa* (Berkeley, CA: University of California Press, 2000).

Wiesner-Hanks, Merry, *Gender in History* (Malden, MA: Blackwell, 2001).

Wilsford, David, 'States Facing Interests', *Journal of Health Politics, Policy and Law* 20 (1995), pp. 571–613.

Wilson, Adrian, *The Making of Man-Midwifery: Childbirth in England, 1660–1770* (Cambridge, MA: Harvard University Press, 1995).

Winter, Jay, *The Great War and the British People,* 2003 edn (Basingstoke: Palgrave Macmillan, 2003).

Witz, Ann, *Professions and Patriarchy: The Gendered Politics of Occupational Closure* (London: Routledge, 1995).

Wohl, Anthony S., *Endangered Lives: Public Health in Victorian Britain* (London: Methuen, 1983).

Worboys, Michael, *Spreading Germs: Disease Theories and Medical Practice in Britain, 1865–1900* (Cambridge: Cambridge University Press, 2000).

Worboys, Michael, 'Colonial and Imperial Medicine', in Brunton, Deborah (ed.), *Medicine Transformed: Health, Disease and Society in Europe 1800–1930* (Manchester: Manchester University Press, 2004), pp. 211–38.

Woycke, James, 'Patient Medicines in Imperial Germany', *Canadian Bulletin of the History of Medicine* 9 (1992), pp. 41–56.

Wright, David and Digby, Anne (eds), *From Idiocy to Mental Deficiency: Historical Perspectives on People with Learning Disabilities* (London: Routledge, 1996).

Index